Texas Woman's University
School of Occupational Therapy
P.O. Box 425648
Denton, TX 76204-5648

OCCUPATIONAL THERAPY WITH ELDERS

WITH ELDERS

Strategies for the **COTA**

Shadows and Sunlight

I remember being young and wild,
Although my body forgets and betrays me.
I peer out of this aging body
With a mind that still knows
Who, when, where and how.
When did fifty
Or even sixty seem like young?
Birthdays only serve as a yardstick for the outside.
How can you measure what I feel on the inside?

My heart tears seeing friends disappear
Into places I only fear.
My memories of yesteryear seem crystal clear.
I close my eyes and feel myself running in the breeze.
The crowds along the college track applauding my triumph,
When the sound of my therapist
Cheering my toddling in a walker wakes me.
I laugh out loud
And people shake their heads as if I am half crazed.
So many losses totaling into this single moment.

The respect I had as a working man
Still fills my chest with pride.
My dearest Rosalie leaving me on Earth so quickly.
Our dreams of travel and leisurely walks are gone.
Saying goodbye to my neighborhood of 43 years,
To move into a room with a stranger.
Overhearing the hushed voices of my son and daughter
As they discuss the exorbitant costs of my care outside my door.
Then the frustrated voices in deciding who will take Dad home.

How did the tables get turned so fast?
Ironically my children become my caretakers now.
How can I express to those I love,
Do not grieve for my losses so deeply.
As I still intend to live
As best I can,
As much as you will allow me.
Keep open the windows of possibilities.
Do not shut the door of life just yet.

YOLANDA **G**RIFFITHS (Used by permission)

OCCUPATIONAL THERAPY WITH ELDERS

Strategies for the COTA

HELENE **L**OHMAN, MA, OTR/L
Assistant Professor
Department of Occupational Therapy
School of Pharmacy and Allied Health Professions
Creighton University
Omaha, Nebraska

RENÉ **L. P**ADILLA, MS, OTR/L
Assistant Professor
Department of Occupational Therapy
School of Pharmacy and Allied Health Professions
Creighton University
Omaha, Nebraska

SUE **B**YERS-**C**ONNON, BA, COTA/L, ROH
Instructor
Occupational Therapy Assistant Program
Mt. Hood Community College
Gresham, Oregon

WITH ILLUSTRATIONS BY RENÉ L. PADILLA, MS, OTR/L
WITH PHOTOS BY KEVIN CALLAHAN, OTAS

with 42 contributors
with 131 illustrations

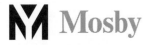 Mosby

An Affiliate of Elsevier Science

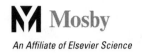
Mosby
An Affiliate of Elsevier Science

Printed in the United States of America

Mosby, Inc.
11830 Westline Industrial Drive
St. Louis, MO 63146

Library of Congress Cataloging-in-Publication Data

Occupational therapy with elders : strategies for the COTA / [edited
  by] Helene Lohman, René L. Padilla, Sue Byers-Connon ; with
  illustrations by René L. Padilla, with photos by Kevin Callahan ;
  with 42 contributors, with 131 illustrations.
       p.   cm.
    Includes bibliographical references and index.
    ISBN 0–8151–3724–9
    1. Occupational therapy for the aged.   2. Occupational therapy
assistants.   I. Lohman, Helene.   II. Padilla, René L.   III. Byers-
Connon, Sue.
    [DNLM: 1. Occupational Therapy—in old age.   2. Aging.
3. Rehabilitation—in old age.   WB 555 0157 1997]
RC953.8.0220246   1997
615.8'515'0846—dc21
DNLM/DLC   97–18554

03 04 05 / 9 8 7 6 5

Contributors

MARLENE J. AITKEN, BA, MS, PhD
Associate Professor
Occupational Therapy Department
School of Pharmacy and Allied
Health Professions
Creighton University
Omaha, Nebraska

PATTY L. BARNETT, COTA/L, ROH
Assistant Coordinator of Clinical
Education
Division of Occupational Therapy
School of Health Related Professions
University of Alabama at Birmingham
Birmingham, Alabama

SHIRLEY A. BLANCHARD, MS, OTR/L
Assistant Professor
Occupational Therapy Department
School of Pharmacy and Allied
Health Professions
Creighton University
Omaha, Nebraska

ADA BOONE, BS, COTA
Staff COTA
Department of Occupational Therapy
Rehab Works, Inc.;
Instructor
Occupational Therapy Department
Division of Allied Health
Sacramento City College
Sacramento, California

REBECCA PLAS BOTHWELL, OTR
Staff Occupational Therapist
The Rehabilitation Institute
Kansas City, Missouri

KATE H. BROWN, PhD
Associate Professor
Occupational Therapy Department
School of Pharmacy and Allied
Health Professions; Faculty Associate
Center for Health Policy and Ethics
Creighton University
Omaha, Nebraska

KRIS R. BROWN, BS, OTR/L
Staff Therapist
NovaCare
Dakota Dune, South Dakota

PAMELA BROWN, OTR/L
Rehabilitation Program Manager
Advanced Rehabilitation Systems
Boston, Massachusetts

LESLIE BRUNSTETER-WILLIAMS, BSOT
Staff Occupational Therapist
Acute Care, In-Patient, and
Out-Patient Services
Rehabilitation Services Department
Trinity Lutheran Hospital
Kansas City, Missouri

SUE BYERS-CONNON, BA, COTA/L, ROH
Instructor
Occupational Therapy Assistant
Program
Mt. Hood Community College
Gresham, Oregon

CLAUDELLE A. H. CARRUTHERS, OTR, PT,
PhD
Assistant Professor
Researcher
Occupational Therapy and Physical
Therapy Departments
The College of St. Catherine
St. Paul, Minnesota

BRENDA M. COPPARD, MS, OTR/L
Assistant Professor
Occupational Therapy Department
School of Pharmacy and Allied
Health Professions
Creighton University
Omaha, Nebraska

JANA K. CRAGG, MA, OTR
Program Director
Occupational Therapy Assistant
Program
Allied Health Department
St. Philip's College
San Antonio, Texas

TERRYN DAVIS, COTA
Certified Occupational Therapy
Assistant
Occupational Therapy Department
San Jose State University
San Jose, California

L. MARGARET DRAKE, PhD, OTR/L, ATR,
FAOTA
Associate Professor
Occupational Therapy Department
School of Pharmacy and Allied
Health Professions
Creighton University
Omaha, Nebraska

BARBARA FLYNN, PharmD
Assistant Professor
Department of Pharmaceutical and
Administrative Sciences
School of Pharmacy and Allied
Health Professions
Creighton University
Omaha, Nebraska

KAI GALYEN, OTR/L
Occupational Therapy Department
Benedictine Nursing Center
Mount Angel, Oregon

CORALIE H. GLANTZ, OTR/L, FAOTA
Glantz/Richman Rehabilitation
Associates, Inc.
Riverwoods, Illinois

YOLANDA GRIFFITHS, MHR, OTR/L
Academic Fieldwork Coordinator
Assistant Professor
Occupational Therapy Department
School of Pharmacy and Allied
Health Professions
Creighton University
Omaha, Nebraska

MAJ. KAROLINE D. HARVEY, OTR
Assistant Chief
Occupational Therapy
Brooke Army Medical Center
Fort Sam Houston, Texas

JEAN T. HAYS, COTA
Instructor
Occupational Therapy Assistant
Program
St. Philip's College
San Antonio, Texas

CARLY R. HELLEN, OTR/L
Director of Alzheimer's Care
The Wealshire
Lincolnshire, Illinois

TYROME HIGGINS, BBA, COTA, ROH
C Company 426th FSB
U.S. Army
Fort Campbell, Kentucky

SHERRY HOFF, MPH, OTR
Assistant Professor
School of Occupational Therapy
Pacific University
Forest Grove, Oregon

JODI LANE, COTA/L
Occupational Therapy Assistant
Providence St. Vincent Home Care
Rehabilitation Department
Portland, Oregon;
Part-Time Instructor
Occupational Therapy Assistant
Program
Mt. Hood Community College
Gresham, Oregon

PENNI JEAN LAVOOT, MS, COTA
Occupational Therapy Assistant
Certified Driver Rehabilitation
Specialist
Occupational Therapy Department
Rancho Los Amigos Medical Center
Downey, California

HELENE LOHMAN, MA, OTR/L
Assistant Professor
Occupational Therapy Department
School of Pharmacy and Allied
Health Professions
Creighton University
Omaha, Nebraska

DEBORAH MORAWSKI, OTR
Supervisor
Occupational Therapy Department
Community Hospital of Los Gatos
Los Gatos, California

MEG NIEMAN, MS, OTR/L
Assistant Professor, Occupational
Therapy
Math, Science, and Allied Health
Department
Manchester Community Technical
College
Manchester, Connecticut

SANDRA HATTORI OKADA, MSG, OTR
Gerontologist
Occupational Therapist
Clinical Gerontology Services
Department
Occupational Therapy Drivers
Training Program
Ranchos Los Amigos Medical Center
Downey, California

RENÉ L. PADILLA, MS, OTR/L
Assistant Professor
Occupational Therapy Department
School of Pharmacy and Allied
Health Professions
Creighton University
Omaha, Nebraska

CLAIRE PEEL, PhD, PT
Associate Professor
Division of Physical Therapy
The University of Alabama at
Birmingham
Birmingham, Alabama

ANGELA M. PERALTA, COTA
Adjunct Intructor
Occupational Therapy Assistant
Program
Touro College
New York, New York

CLAUDIA GAYE PEYTON, MS, OTR/L
Chair
Occupational Therapy Department
School of Pharmacy and Allied
Health Professions
Creighton University
Omaha, Nebraska

SHERRELL POWELL, MA, OTR
Professor and Director
Occupational Therapy Assistant
Program
Natural and Applied Science
Department
LaGuardia Community College
City University of New York
Long Island, New York

NANCY RICHMAN, OTR/L, FAOTA
Glantz/Richman Rehabilitation
Associates, Inc.
Riverwoods, Illinois

BARBARA JO RODRIGUES, OTR
Lead Occupational Therapist
Occupational Therapy Department
Mental Health Unit
Dominican Santa Cruz Hospital
Santa Cruz, California

CAROL J. SCHWOPE, MA, COTA/L
Staff Therapist and Student
Coordinator
Rehabilitation Services
Health South at St. Mary's Hospital
Huntington, West Virginia

ELLEN SPERGEL, MS, OTR
Professor and Chair
Occupational Therapy Assistant
Program
Occupational Therapy Department
Rockland Community College
Suffern, New York

SHARON STOFFEL, MA, OTR, FAOTA
Assistant Professor
Occupational Therapy
College of St. Catherine
St. Paul, Minnesota

LORI TAYLOR, COTA/L
Occupational Therapy Assistant
RehabVisions
Omaha, Nebraska

JEAN VANN, OTR/L
Occupational Therapist, semi-retired
Hospice Team
Legacy Visiting Nurse Association
Portland, Oregon

To the elders, including my parents and grandparents, who have been role models in my life. To my students who inspire me to write.

Helene

To my family, Kathy, Sam and Joel.

René

To the elders I have known, for the valuable lessons they have taught me. To my mother for teaching me the value of life, the joy of living, and the acceptance of death.

Sue

Acknowledgments

It is true that writing a book is not a simple process or one that one person can undertake alone. We wish to acknowledge many people for their contribution to this project:

- The contributing authors, for their dedication, hard work, and belief in this project;
- Coralie H. Glantz, OTR/L, FAOTA and Mary Sands, MSED, OTR, FAOTA for their editorial consultant work;
- The many OTA students who reviewed chapters;
- Yolanda Griffiths, MHR, OTR/L for the moving poem that appears at the beginning of the book;
- Kai Galyen, OTR/L; Penni Jean Lavoot, MS, COTA; Barbara Jo Rodrigues, OTR; and Ada Boone, BS, COTA for their contributions to the Appendix;
- The elders who graciously agreed to appear in the photographs;
- Kevin Callahan for his photographic skill;
- Amy Dubin Christopher, Martha Sasser, Linda McKinley, Julie Zipfel, Liz Fett, and Don Carlisle at Mosby–Year Book, Inc;
- Ursula Hopkins for her invaluable assistance in preparing the manuscript;
- The administrators and faculty of the Department of Occupational Therapy, School of Pharmacy and Allied Health Professions, Creighton University for their encouragement;
- The Associate Dean and OTA Program Director, Allied Health Division, Mt. Hood Community College in Gresham, Oregon, for their support.

HELENE LOHMAN, MA, OTR/L
RENÉ L. PADILLA, MS, OTR/L
SUE BYERS-CONNON, BA, COTA/L, ROH

Foreword

The unprecedented number of older people in our society creates incredible challenges. Because of physiology, life experiences, environment, financial and cultural influences, and a vast array of other reasons, people become less alike rather than more alike as they age. This dissimilarity creates a variety of issues for practitioners who are interacting with older people.

A central concern that affects this population explosion is the older person's increased need for health care services. As this demand continues so does the need for occupational therapy and, as the editors share with us in the preface, particularly the services of the certified occupational therapy assistant (COTA).

The changes in physical, sensory, and cognitive functioning that occur as a result of the aging process affect elders despite their living and treatment settings. The editors of *Occupational Therapy With Elders: Strategies for the COTA* have brought together a knowledgeable group of authors that present the pertinent issues the COTA must consider when working with older adults.

This text includes the basic concepts of aging, including theories, trends, and policies. Concepts of wellness and disease prevention are emphasized. Sexuality of elders is discussed. The biologic, psychologic, emotional, and cultural issues that influence the function of the individual and interaction with caregivers are reviewed. Practice settings, including hospice, are reviewed.

Strategies for treating people individually and in groups are identified. The effects of motivation on behavior and the ethical aspects of working with elders are discussed. The use of medications is considered, and eating and nutrition concerns are addressed. Occupational therapy interventions for people with physical, sensory, and cognitive changes are discussed.

Occupational Therapy With Elders: Strategies for the COTA has brought together an array of concerns and interventions and presents them in a forthright logical sequence. The contributions of the authors have been organized so the text flows in a logical and purposeful manner. It is extremely practical in its approach, with numerous case studies to illustrate the topical area.

Because of this organization, the text can be used effectively by student and practitioner alike.

The inclusion of the many issues that must be considered in working with the older client are extremely helpful to the student. No doubt the text will be referenced repeatedly as new clients, with previously unseen diagnoses and problems, come under the COTA's care. For the COTA who has not worked with older clients, this text provides a thorough overview of the challenges in working with this population. For the COTA used to working with elders, the text is a ready reference for new techniques to apply to current caseloads.

For developing programs, this text is helpful for Occupational Therapy Assistant program faculty members who are designing the curriculum to prepare students to meet the multiple needs of the older population. For established programs, it provides the most recent thinking in working with elders. *Occupational Therapy With Elders: Strategies for the COTA* is a helpful addition for baccalaureate or advanced degree programs that prepare students to work successfully with COTAs.

For the clinic that is hiring COTAs for the first time, this text provides a wonderful overview of the roles of the COTA. It may be of similar help for the OTR who has not previously worked with COTAs but will be doing so in the future. A better understanding of roles can provide the opportunity for collaboration between the OTR and COTA that is ideal for delivery of occupational therapy services.

In the preface the editors convey their collective desires for *Occupational Therapy With Elders: Strategies for the COTA* to be a text that will "acknowledge the reality of life experience of elders and be respectful of them as whole human beings." It is a pleasure to realize the editors have accomplished their task.

MARGARET CHRISTENSON, MPH, OTR, FAOTA
President
Lifease, Inc.
New Brighton, Minnesota

Preface

Certified Occupational Therapy Assistants (COTAs) comprise the greater part of the occupational therapy workforce treating elders. Two-thirds of all COTAs work with elders 65 years of age and older (Steib, 1996). In addition, skilled nursing/intermediate care facilities have been the number one practice setting for COTAs since 1990 (AOTA, 1990). These statistics underscore the need for COTAs to possess a strong knowledge base that will allow them to provide the best possible service to elders, thus representing the profession with confidence. The purpose of this text is to contribute to the COTA's knowledge base in this important practice area.

This text has a purposeful organization. The first section, *Concepts of Aging*, presents foundational concepts related to the importance of understanding the life experiences of elders. A general discussion of aging trends, concepts, and theories is followed by a more specific discussion of occupational therapy (OT) professional concepts as they relate to elders. The second section, *Occupational Therapy Intervention with Elders*, presents specific applications of OT strategies that should be considered in light of the broader concepts of Section I. Chapter topics in this section include cultural diversity of the aging population, application of OT theories with elders, ethical aspects, documentation, and working with families and caregivers. We have addressed specific OT applications for elders whose conditions or impairments are psychiatric, orthopedic, and neurologic.

As we prepared to put this text together, there were several goals that guided the process:

- We wanted the project to acknowledge the reality of life experiences of elders and to be respectful of them as whole human beings. Our goal is to dispel myths about aging. Therefore we chose the term *elder* to avoid reducing these elders to the stereotypic role of helpless patients.
- We wanted the feature of collaboration between the Occupational Therapist, Registered (OTR) and

COTA as a team to be a salient point throughout the text. As an editorial team we have experienced firsthand the richness of working this way. Many of the chapters were also authored by OTR and COTA teams, and several of the authors were COTAs before becoming OTRs.
- We wanted to produce a comprehensive text for both OTA students and practicing COTAs. There has been a void for a text specifically designed for this purpose. As this project progressed, it became evident that the information covered would be useful not only to COTAs but to OTRs as well.
- We wanted to produce a text that would capture the essence of COTA practice and help COTAs feel proud of their significant contributions.
- We wanted to ground the strategies of care suggested in this text in traditional OT theory and practice.
- We wanted to illustrate the situations in which COTAs may work with elders by using narratives that promote unique ways of identifying problems and solutions. Some of the stories were very personal to the chapter authors.
- We wanted to emphasize basic clinical reasoning that should be part of any OT intervention regardless of professional level.

It is our hope that this text will instill a desire in the readers to further their understanding of elders and of OT practice.

HELENE LOHMAN, MA, OTR/L
RENÉ L. PADILLA, MS, OTR/L
SUE BYERS-CONNON, BA, COTA/L, ROH

REFERENCES

American Occupational Therapy Association: Research Information and Evaluation Division: *1990 member data survey*, Rockville, Md, 1990, The Association.
Steib P: Skilled nursing facilities: Top employment setting for COTAs, *OT Week* November 21: 16, 1996.

Contents

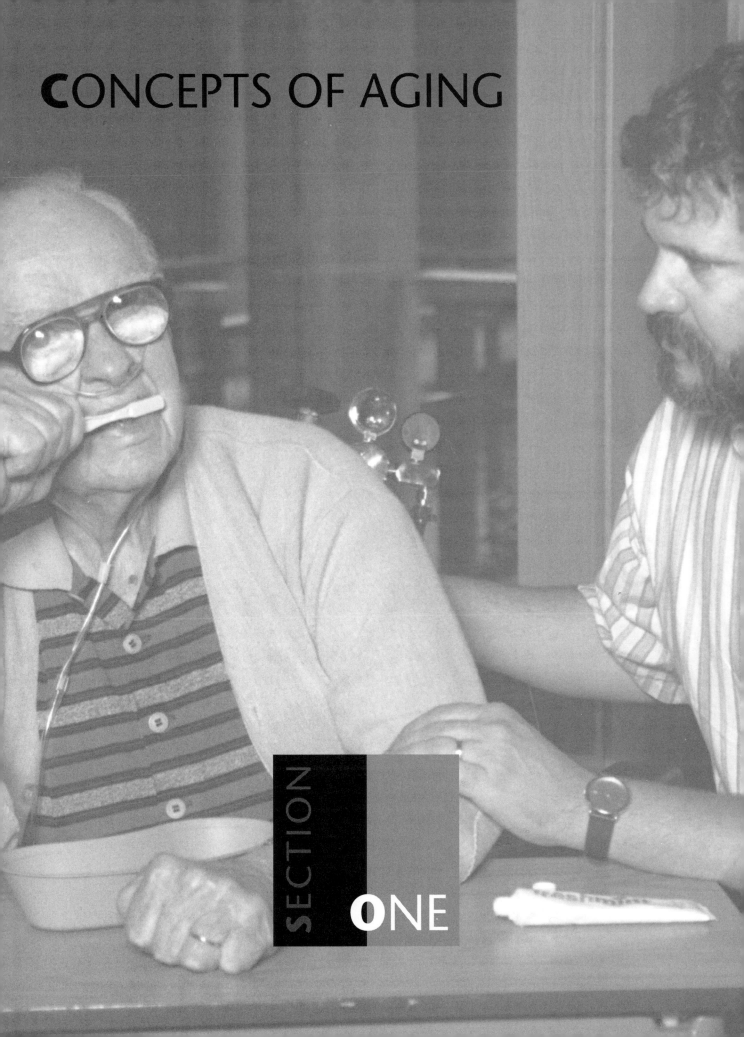

CONCEPTS OF AGING

Aging Trends and Concepts

HELENE LOHMAN AND ELLEN SPERGEL

KEY TERMS

gerontology, geriatrics, cohort, health, illness, chronic illness, young old, mid old,
old old, demography, intergenerational, ageism

CHAPTER OBJECTIVES

1. Define relevant terminology regarding the elderly.
2. Describe the relationship between aging and illness.
3. Discuss components of health and chronic illness.
4. Explain the "dismissal approach" and the "collaborative approach" and their effects on elder care.
5. Describe the three stages of aging and define their differences.
6. Describe the effects of growth of the elder population on society.
7. Discuss the effects of an increasingly large number of elder females on society.
8. Describe the problems and needs of the oldest old population, which consists of elders 85 years of age and older.
9. Describe usual living arrangements of most elders.
10. Discuss the significance of economic trends for the elderly.
11. Relate implications of demographical data for occupational therapy practice.
12. Describe the importance of intergenerational contact for occupational therapy treatment.
13. Describe the concept of "ageism" in today's society and the effect of the views of the American youth culture on aging.

John is a 30-year-old certified occupational therapy assistant (COTA) practicing in a skilled nursing home facility. He provides daily occupational therapy (OT) treatment five days a week to elders. Most of the elders are in some stage of recovery from an acute illness and are going through OT to regain their functional abilities. On weekends, John visits his grandparents, both of whom are 75 years of age and very independent, active members in the community. John often thinks about the differences between his grandparents and the nursing home resi-

dents. He wonders whether his active grandparents are exceptions to most elders or examples of typical elders.

Tammy is a 20-year-old occupational therapy assistant (OTA) student in an OTA program with a coed population between the ages of 20 and 50. Tammy has noted differences in interests between students her age and those in their 40s. The classmates in their 40s share common generational life experiences in class discussions. These life experiences are different from those of the younger students.

Tammy has a strong desire to go into geriatric practice. She can remember helping her grandmother after she had a stroke. When she studied the geriatric content of her course work, Tammy was surprised to learn of the diversity among the elder population. She realized that just as her OTA class represents diversity among age groups, so does the elder population. She also recognized misconceptions she had about the elder generation. Some were based on clinical observations at a nursing home and informal observations from visits to her grandmother. One misconception was that all elders were sick and frail like her grandmother. Another misconception was that most elders had cognitive impairments. Tammy learned that many elders are quite healthy and active, especially the younger generation of elders, who are 65 to 75 years of age. Tammy also learned that cognitive impairment affects a small portion of the elder population, mostly the oldest of the old (those 85 years of age and older) (Suzman, 1995).

COTAs may easily acquire a skewed picture of the elder population, especially in a nursing home setting. Elders in nursing homes tend to be representative of the sicker and more frail elder population. In truth, only 5% of all elders at any one time reside in nursing homes (American Association of Retired Persons [AARP], 1995). COTAs must have a broader perspective about geriatrics to work effectively with a diverse, continuously changing elder population. This chapter provides relevant background information as it relates to OT practice and to the overall elder population.

The term **gerontology** comes from the Greek terms *geron* and *lojas*, which mean "study of old men." Gerontology is often thought of as the study of the aged and can include the aging process in humans and animals. The field of gerontology is very broad and includes the historic, philosophical, religious, political, psychological, anthropological, and sociological issues of the elder population. The term **geriatrics** is often used to describe

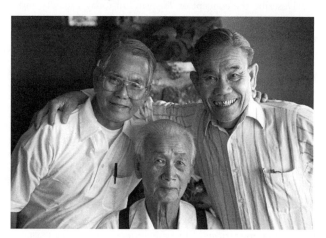

FIGURE 1-1 This group of cohorts enjoys spending time together.

medical interventions with the elderly. In OT practice, *geriatrics* is referred to as an area of clinical specialty. The term **cohort** refers to "a collection or sampling of individuals who share a common characteristic, such as members of the same age or sex group" (Anderson, Anderson, Glanze, 1994). In gerontological literature, the elder generation may also be referred to as the *elder*, or *aged*, *cohort* as compared with younger cohorts (Figure 1-1). Different terms used in this book refer to the geriatric population as the *aged*, *older*, or *the elder population*.

HEALTH, ILLNESS, AND WELL-BEING

Although **health**, **illness**, and *well-being* are familiar terms, they require expanded definitions for OT practice in geriatrics. One definition of health is the absence of disease (Flexner, 1987). Very few elders would be considered healthy with this general definition. However, a theory of well-being can be developed if health is considered the optimal level of functioning for a person's age and condition. Many individuals have chronic illnesses to which they have adjusted and are able to live optimally. These people could be considered to be in a state of well-being. For example, to live optimally, individuals with lifelong disabilities such as cerebral palsy and multiple sclerosis need health care system services such as OT home evaluations for environmental adaptations even though they are not ill. These individuals do not think of themselves as ill and may resent being labeled as "patients" and placed in the sick role by health care professionals.

The biological systems of elders can change. Some changes that result in disease or dysfunction may be treated by medication or surgery. Other biological changes such as decreased balance can be handled with environmental adaptations such as installing brighter lights in stairwells and removing loose rugs and electrical cords from traffic areas in the home. Some sensory changes can be partially resolved with glasses and hearing aids. These biological and sensory changes should not be thought of as illnesses. They are changes that elders adjust to and incorporate into their activities of daily living (ADLs).

Most elders suffer from a minimum of one or more chronic conditions such as arthritis (49%), hypertension (35%), heart disease (31%), hearing impairments (31%), orthopedic impairments (18%), cataracts (15%), sinusitis (15%), diabetes (10%), tinnitus (10%), and visual impairments (10%) (AARP, 1995). The following example illustrates the way an elder learns to adapt to a chronic illness.

Henry suffers from osteoarthritis and needs assistance with some ADL functions. He continues to maintain his apartment and values his independence. He takes frequent breaks to rest while housekeeping. Because of his poor endurance, he uses a lightweight upright vacuum, which also helps to reduce upper extremity (UE) strain.

Henry has an active social life outside his home. He maintains mobility in the community by taking a bus to activities. Henry has osteoarthritis, a disease that cannot be cured. However, most COTAs would say that Henry is not sick.

Chronic Illness

Many medical conditions of elders are chronic. That is, they cannot be cured, but they can be managed. The physician may not cure heart disease, but the pain and debilitating consequences can be managed for years with medications, diet, exercise, surgery, and technology. The health professional would likely say that the disease has not been cured, but the elder's life has been extended in a qualitatively meaningful way.

Some health care practitioners dismiss an elder's complaints with comments such as "It's your age; it's your problem; what do you expect from me? I can't cure you." They are likely to overlook important ways to treat and reduce symptoms that may increase the length and quality of that elder's life. Generally, health professionals are educated to cure illness, and many may be less knowledgeable about illness management. Some health care practitioners feel uncomfortable treating elders and they develop this dismissal approach in response.

The alternative to the dismissal approach is the collaborative approach. In this approach, health practitioners may make comments such as "How can we work together to help improve the quality of your life?" and "What are your symptoms and how can we help you with function?" Elders are central to the management of their own health. OT practitioners evaluate the elder person's ability to function as independently as possible in the environment and recommend and initiate treatments and design accomodations for any problems.

COTAs are in an ideal position to carry out the OT plan for elders. The following example illustrates the role the occupational therapist (OTR) and COTA team plays to help enhance an elder's quality of life.

Sadie is an 86-year-old widow with arthritis living in senior citizen housing. Her daily life is a balance of self-maintenance, simple meal preparations, visits with neighbors in the community recreation room, telephone calls to family members, and watching television. Sadie has complained to her health maintenance organization (HMO) primary care physician of decreasing vision, weakness, and joint pain. General anxiety and depression also appear to be features of her condition. She comments to her physician "I think that I belong in a nursing home. I'm old and I'm having difficulty taking care of myself."

Placing Sadie in a nursing home may manage a medically complex problem. However, the physician can also evaluate additional supports to maintain independent living, adjust drug dosages for management of Sadie's arthritis, and order OT evaluation and treatment.

The OTR and COTA next gather information about Sadie. They collaborate to develop the following treatment recommendations:

1. A referral to Meals on Wheels
2. A lighted magnifier to improve visual function
3. A large-button remote control for the TV
4. An updated telephone with voice recognition dialing or programmed numbers
5. Light activities to maintain joint mobility
6. Arthritis education that includes joint protection and mobilization, energy conservation, work simplification, and adaptive devices
7. Home evaluation for independent function

Collaboration addresses the elder's chronic conditions, interests, and desires. Elders with multiple chronic diagnoses that often accompany acute conditions or changes in functional status are not unusual. When managed properly, all treatments work smoothly to improve the elder's independent status or occupational well-being. The elder may need to adjust to a different status of functioning with different occupational roles. The OT treatment interventions suggested in the example may result in improved functional abilities in many areas of life and decreased anxiety about independent living. Accumulation of medical conditions does not necessarily lead to decreased function and increased disability. Despite the "graying of America," elder citizens are experiencing less disability and living longer and better.

THE STAGES OF AGING

What age constitutes "old age"? The federally mandated age to collect social security is 65. The age that most retirement communities set as the minimum for their residents is 55. At age 50, one can join the AARP. At age 40, Americans are protected by the Age Discrimination in Employment Act (ADEA). The third stage of aging, called *senescence*, which social gerontologists define as a stage of biological decline, begins at age 30.

One definition of old age classifies 65 to 75 years of age as young old, 75 to 85 as mid old, and 85 and above as old old. This may help COTAs to think of old age in terms of occupational role performance and expectations. However, COTAs should use this classification as a guideline because every person ages differently and every elder does not fit neatly into one of these three categories. Socioeconomic factors and personality considerations can largely influence the way each elder approaches aging. Elders who are members of a minority group are more likely to live in poverty and suffer from chronic illness than elders who are white (Rubenstein, Kramer, 1994). These minority elders may not enjoy some of the same benefits.

Young Old (65 to 75 years of age): Elders who are **young old** may be recently retired and enjoying the results of their years of employment, their essential role as grandparents, and their continuing role as parents in the growth of their adult children (Figure 1-2). They have increased leisure time to pursue interests and develop new ones. They may choose to do volunteer work with community service, return to school, and travel. The young old must often cope with chronic conditions such as osteoarthritis, hypertension, and cardiovascular disease. However, these chronic conditions are often managed medically and usually do not represent a major barrier to functioning or satisfactory occupational role performance.

Mid Old (75 to 85 years of age): In the **mid old** period of life, more changes are evident. Mid old elders make modifications in their occupational role performance. They often reduce or simplify their lives in various ways, including resting during the day, volunteering less, traveling less, and limiting distance of trips. They rely more on social systems such as Meals on Wheels and public transportation and family for some assistance with ADLs (Figure 1-3). COTAs may provide interventions when necessary. The frequent loss of significant others brings affective stressors and additional role changes.

Old Old (85 years of age and above): During the **old old** period of life, elders may reflect on the meaning of their lives, the quality of their relationships, and their contributions to society (Figure 1-4). They may think about the losses they are experiencing and about their own deaths. This may be a time of peace and generosity; elders in the old old period of life may find it meaningful to give valued objects to loved ones who will treasure them. On the other hand, it can be a period of fear and anger resulting from unresolved conflicts. Resolution of these conflicts can make this period the most spiritual and fulfilling experience for elders. Personal growth and reflection continue throughout life.

This time in an elder's life is usually a period of further systemic change affecting the sensory, motor, cardiac, and pulmonary systems. Chronic conditions impair self-maintenance capacities, and elders in the old old stage may need personal assistance with bathing, mobility, dressing, and money management that COTAs can provide. If these elders live independently, they may manage best when caring family, friends, and neighbors "look in after them" (Suzman, 1995).

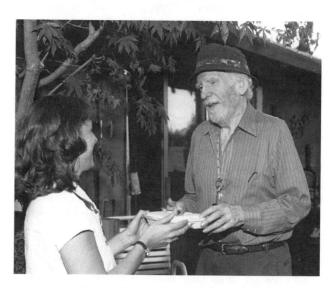

FIGURE **1-3** Some elders may use Meals on Wheels to maintain nutrition and remain in their own homes.

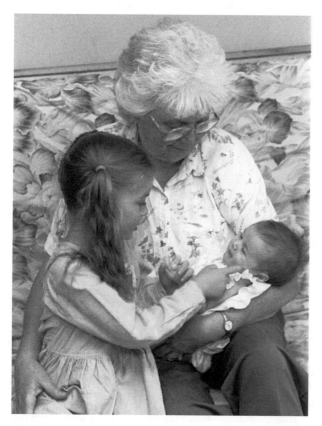

FIGURE **1-2** This newly retired elder enjoys time with her grandchildren.

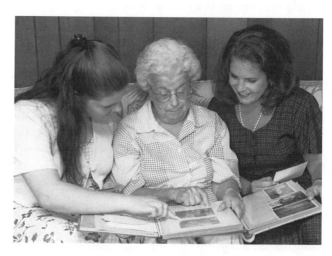

FIGURE **1-4** Elders may enjoy reflecting on life with other generations.

A national demonstration project, Program for All Inclusive Care of the Elderly (PACE), is based on a managed care model and was designed for the frail urban elderly (Shen, Iversen, 1992). The project focuses on keeping frail elders who would otherwise be in skilled nursing facilities in their homes (Branch, Coulam, Zimmerman, 1995). In general, the goal of the project is to demonstrate that elders remain independent longer when their health care delivery system is sensitive and responsive to their medical, rehabilitative, social, and emotional needs. This project provides alternative models of long-term care such as adult day care, primary health care, rehabilitation, home care, transportation, housing, social services, and hospitalization. An interdisciplinary team handles case management. This may be one answer to the ethical and economic dilemmas regarding ways to meet the increasing needs of elders as they live longer in a health care climate of declining resources and advancing technology.

DEMOGRAPHICAL DATA AND THE GROWTH OF THE AGED POPULATION

Demography is "the study of human populations, particularly the size, distribution, and characteristics of members of population groups" (Anderson, Anderson, Glanz, 1994). Demographical data clearly suggest that the aged population is growing. This growth is often referred to in the literature as "the graying of America" (McLean, 1988). The portion of the elder population that consists of those 65 years or older comprises 12.7% of the total U.S. population. This population is expected to continue growing, with the "most rapid increase expected between the years 2010 and 2030 when the 'baby boom' generation will reach age 65" (AARP, 1995). The elder generation is projected to be 20% of the total population by the year 2030 (AARP, 1995). Based on projections, the elder population may slowly decline in size after a peak in the year 2041 because the younger population has a declining birth rate (Horn, Meer, 1987; Rogers, Rogers, Belanger, 1990). Minority elder populations are also growing rapidly and are projected to represent 25% of the elder population by the year 2030 as compared with 13% of the elder population in 1990 (AARP, 1995). Many factors contribute to this significant population growth, including a declining mortality rate, advances in medicine and sanitation, improved diet, and improved technology. Figure 1-5 illustrates the growth of the elder population.

Accompanying the "graying of America" is a growth of the female aged population. For every 100 men over 65 years of age, there are 146 women. This ratio increases with age. There are 122 women for every 100 men in the 65 to 69 age group and 259 women for every 100 men in the 85 and older age group (AARP, 1995). Although women live longer than men, many function in their later years in a dependent ADL status, which demonstrates a need for COTA intervention (Rogers, Rogers, Belanger, 1990).

About 50% of older women over age 65 are widows, and there are almost 5 times as many widows as widowers (AARP, 1995), a statistic that has broad sociocultural implications (Figure 1-6). A major consequence for some elder women on the loss of a spouse is an increased risk for poverty. The U.S. Senate Special Committee on Aging statistics show that almost three out of four poor elders are women (O'Grady-LeShane, 1990).

The Aging of the Aged Population

The fastest growing segment of the elder population is the 85 years and over cohort. By the year 2000, approximately 12% of the elder population over age 65 will be in the 85 years and over group (Jette, Bottomley, 1987). Between 1990 and 2060 the number of elders between 80 and 89 years of age will increase threefold and the number over 90 years of age will increase sevenfold (Rogers, Rogers, Belanger, 1990).

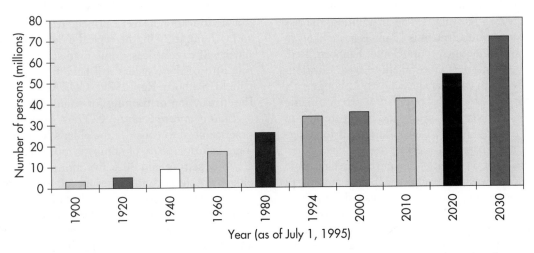

FIGURE 1-5 Number of persons 65 years of age and older: 1900 to 2030. (Adapted and reprinted with permission from the American Association of Retired Persons, 1995.)

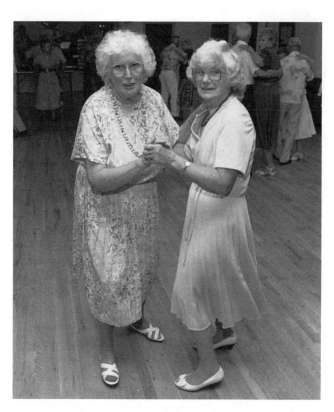

FIGURE 1-6 There are almost five times as many widows as widowers.

The 85 years and older cohorts have their own unique needs. The increased number of frail, dependent elders uses a larger amount of health, financial, and social services than other age cohorts (Rogers, Rogers, Belanger, 1990). This age group is at increased risk for disabilities and other health problems such as cardiovascular disease and vision and hearing problems. In the year preceding death, individuals of this age group experience significant disability (Guralink et al, 1991). The risk for serious injuries from falling increases as aging progresses (Horn, Meer, 1987; Thornby, 1995). In addition, the risk for severe cognitive impairment is 15 times more likely in the 85 years and older age group (Bould, Sanborn, Reif, 1989). This age cohort is more likely to be institutionalized compared with younger age cohorts. Although only 5% of the 65 years and older population are in nursing homes, 24% of those 85 years and older reside in institutional settings (AARP, 1995). The need for long-term care is anticipated to increase as this age group grows, especially for those with no living children or those living alone (Zedlewski, McBride, 1992). The number of elders requiring nursing home care is expected to increase from 1.5 million to 5.3 million by the year 2030. (Pepper Commission, 1990). However, increases in home health and other alternative living situations may ease this projected need for more nursing homes (Glantz, 1996).

Although there are more elders among the 85 years and older population than any age cohort that lives in nursing homes, the majority still live in the community. Living in the community presents challenges because the need for assistance with ADL functions dramatically increases with age. "ADLs include bathing, dressing, eating, transferring from bed or chair, walking, going outside, and using the toilet. Instrumental activities of daily living (IADL) include preparing meals, shopping, managing money, using a telephone, and doing housework" (AARP, 1995). In recent years, some researchers have discussed the concept of "active life expectancies," or the expected duration in years of functional well-being of the elder population (Rogers, Rogers, Belanger, 1990). Those elders 85 years and older are most influenced by decreased ability to perform ADL functions.

Many elders require a support system to have assistance with ADLs. Presently more than half of those 85 years and older live in households without a spouse and more than half live in their own homes. Many members of this age cohort are also living with family members such as adult children who provide assistance with ADL functions (Bould, Sanborn, Reif, 1989; Horn, Meyer, 1987). The majority of care provided in the community is by female family members.

Assistance for elder men is generally provided by spouses, whereas assistance for elder women is more likely provided by adult children. There are also gender differences in the type of care provided. Daughters are most likely to provide assistance with personal care, health care, and household tasks. Sons are more likely to provide assistance with financial tasks and household repairs. Elders and their relatives prefer such care to institutionalization and strongly resist nursing home placement (Olson, 1994).

Another important factor for COTAs to consider is that most members of the old old age group have relatively minimal formal education (Bould, Sanborn, Reif, 1989). Many of them have not completed eighth grade. Educational level is projected to gradually increase, so by the year 2000, the typical elder who is 85 years or older will have at least some high school education, and one fifth of these elders will have finished eighth grade (Bould, Sanborn, Reif, 1989). COTAs may need to adjust the instruction or training for some elders.

Living arrangements. COTAs working in geriatric practice need to consider the elder's home environment. The majority (68%) of noninstitutionalized elders live in a family setting and 30% live alone (AARP, 1995). For elders with few economic resources, low-income housing is available. However, the number of units is limited and there may be long waiting lists or lottery systems for applicants. Continuing Care Residential Communities and Life-Care Community Housing are other alternatives for elders with low income. In some cases, residents are required to contribute all their assets. Residents have contracts for housing, supportive services, and often a continuum of services including health and nursing homes.

Board and care homes, personal care, adult day care, adult foster care, family care, and adult congregate living facilities are other alternative care options in the community. Board and care homes service elders many of whom have been deinstitutionalized. Adult day care is a community-based group program designed to meet the needs of functionally impaired elders. This structured, comprehensive program provides a variety of health, social, and related support services in a protective setting during any part of the day but provides less than 24-hour care. Adult foster homes are family homes or other facilities that provide residential care for elderly or physically disabled residents not related to the provider by blood or marriage. Adult congregate living facilities provide seniors in high-rise living accomodations with innovative service-delivery options such as team laundry, cleaning, shopping, congregate meals, and home-delivered meals. Home health services also are available but are usually restricted to more acute episodic needs and require some level of homebound restrictions for reimbursement (Glantz, Richman, 1996).

For those elders with assets, retirement communities include a variety of services such as leisure activities, congregate meals, laundry, transportation, and possibly health care. Costs have escalated in retirement communities, in some cases forcing residents to find alternative housing (Olson, 1994). In these communities, COTAs can act as activity directors, using their skills to select, analyze, and adapt activities to the abilities and interests of the residents (Glantz, Richman, 1995).

Recent data on community elders showed that 23% of all elders living in the community had difficulty with one or more ADL, and 28% had difficulty with one or more IADL (AARP, 1995). The number of older people requiring help with basic tasks is expected to be 13.8 million by the year 2030 (Pepper Commission, 1990).

Economic demographics. The economic status of the elder population has not been clearly presented in literature. During the 1960s and 1970s the elder population was depicted as economically deprived. In current literature, however, the elder population is presented as economically advantaged (Gunyea, 1994). The reality, based on demographic facts, is that the economic status of elders is somewhere in between. The poverty rate for the elder population is 11.7%, which is very close to the rate of 11.9% for those 18 to 64 years of age in the general population (AARP, 1995).

The economic status of elder men and women differs as a result of many factors. When they were younger, the women in the present elder generation were generally housewives or worked occasionally at paid employment. This resulted in less Social Security benefits and smaller or no pensions. Elder widows in particular are at risk for poverty because of the significant pension benefits lost with the death of a spouse (Bould, Sanborn, Rief, 1989; Horn, Meer, 1987). A wide economic disparity exists between elder whites and elder minorities. Approximately 10% of elder whites are poor, compared with 27% of elder blacks and 23% of elder Hispanics (AARP, 1995).

Public policy continues to influence the elder population's economic status. In the year 2010 the young old, or those elders born between 1941 and 1945, should see a growth in retirement income. However, after 2010, there will be a slow decrease in the economic growth of retirement income, which will most affect the aged cohort born in the early 1960s (Zedlewski, McBride, 1992). According to Zedlewski and McBride (1992) this cohort may be the first to feel the full effects of the 1983 Social Security Amendments, which increased the age for those qualified to receive full retirement benefits. The current retirement age of 65 years will eventually increase to 67 years. This change, which will be gradually phased in, is applicable to workers who will be 62 years of age in the year 2000 (McBride, 1996). Changes in Medicare and Medicaid policy will also continue to affect the economic status of the elder population, especially if elders are required to pay more money for health care.

Implications for OT Practice

Because of continued growth with elders, the need for OT practitioners in this area will continue to grow. The effects of other issues related to this population's growth on OT remain to be seen. However, it can be assumed that in the future, dilemmas related to limited resources will affect the practice arena. As Manton (1991) states, when the baby boom cohorts reach 85 years of age between the years 2032 and 2048, "it will produce a major policy challenge to provide community and institutional long term care (LTC) services to a significant portion of the U.S. population." At this time, no one can predict whether there will be adequate funding and social services to meet the needs of a growing elder population and whether there will be enough health care resources to address this population's health care needs. OT personnel will continue to be challenged to provide quality treatment in a cost-constrained environment. New models of OT geriatric care must evolve in the future, and all OT practitioners should be on the front end of this evolution.

INTERGENERATIONAL CONCEPTS

In today's society, same-age cohorts socialize for the most part among themselves and have minimal **intergenerational** contact. When they are not in the clinical

Fill in the following lifelines with significant historical and personal events about yourself, someone from the generation 10 years older than you, one of your parents, and one of your grandparents. After filling in the lifeline, answer the questions below.
Refer to the following example:

Grandparent:

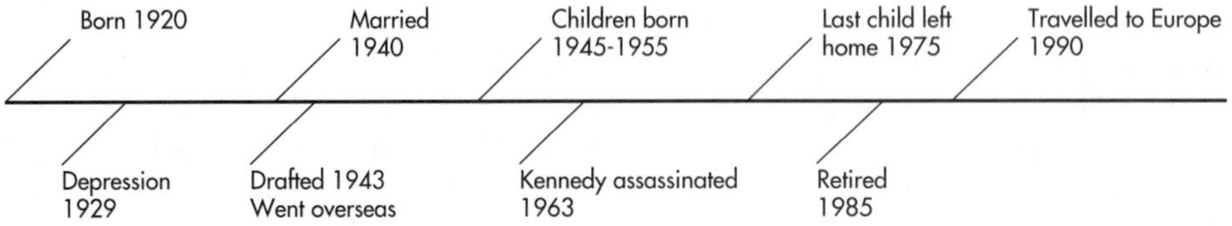

| Born 1920 | Married 1940 | Children born 1945-1955 | Last child left home 1975 | Travelled to Europe 1990 |

| Depression 1929 | Drafted 1943 Went overseas | Kennedy assassinated 1963 | Retired 1985 |

Yourself:

Born

Someone 10 years older than you:

Born

Your parent (choose one):

Born

Your grandparent (choose one):

Born

Answer the following questions:
What significant intergenerational differences did you notice between your generation, parents' generation, grandparents' generation, and even the generation 10 years older than you?
What are some of the significant values of each generation and how were they influenced by historical events?
How might these similarities and differences between generations affect clinical treatment?

FIGURE **1-7** Lifeline exercise. (Adapted from Davis LJ, Kirkland M, editors: *ROTE: the role of occupational therapy with the elderly: faculty guide*, Rockville, Md, 1986, American Occupational Therapy Association. Reprinted with permission.)

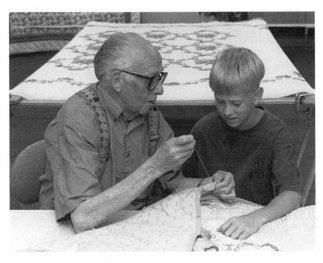

FIGURE **1-8**   Older generations can give support and advice to younger generations.

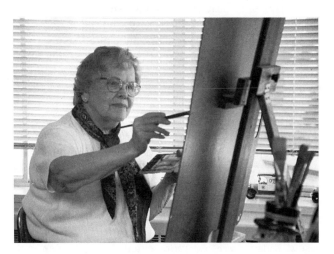

FIGURE **1-9**   Contrary to myth, this elder has embraced a new occupation.

setting, COTAs may have little daily interaction with well elders in the community. In clinical treatment, COTAs work with elders who are often two or three generations removed.

COTAs must be aware of generational values to better understand some elders' perceptions of treatment interventions. Some elder patients may refuse to purchase adaptive equipment because of a generational value regarding thrift that evolved from the depression era. The exercise in Figure 1-7 demonstrates that each generation has certain values and attitudes that are influenced by similar generational experiences and historic events (Davis, 1986). It can be completed as a group or an independent exercise.

COTAs must have meaningful contact, either informally or formally, with both well and frail elderly to work effectively with the elder population. Many benefits are mentioned in the literature about formal intergenerational programs. Some of these benefits include a better understanding (on the part of the younger generation) of the different developmental phases of the life cycle, the opportunity for the older generation to give support and advice to the younger generation, a decrease in isolation of the elderly, an increase in self-esteem of elders, dispelling of myths, and review of values and experiences (Ventura-Merke, Friedman, 1988) (Figure 1-8).

AGEISM, MYTHS, AND STEREOTYPES ABOUT THE AGED

"If you are a man and you are prejudiced against women, you will never know how a woman feels. If you are white and you are prejudiced against blacks, you will never know how a black person feels. But if you are young and you are prejudiced against the old, you are indeed prejudiced against yourself, because you, too, will have the honor of being old someday" (Lewis, 1989).

"Ageism is an attitude that discriminates, separates, stigmatizes, or otherwise disadvantages older adults on the basis of chronological age" (Anderson, Anderson, Glanze, 1994). **Ageism** is a form of prejudice because it promotes general assumptions, or stereotypes, about a group of people. These assumptions are not true for all members of that group. Following are some stereotypes of ageism:

- Elders are useless because they can't see, hear, or remember.
- Elders are slow when they move about.
- Elders are in ill health.
- Elders cannot learn new things.
- Elders drain the economy rather than contribute to it; they are unproductive.
- Elders cannot perform or enjoy sexual activity.
- Elders prefer being with and talking with other elders.
- Elders are depressed and complain about all that is new.
- Elders are rich (or) elders are poor.

Many of these statements have been challenged by research. With any stereotype, there may be a small amount of truth for some members of the group. For example, it is true that elders frequently need glasses as aging progresses; however, the need for glasses does not render an elder useless. An unfortunate result of these myths is that some elders may believe them. For example, whereas young persons may joke about becoming forgetful, elders may seriously question their cognitive abilities as a result of the stereotype that elders have trouble remembering (Figure 1-9).

These stereotypes develop as a result of fear of the unknown. American culture often focuses on youth.

Youth is seen as beautiful, as something to aspire to and maintain at any cost. Young is sexy, and old is not.

The current medical system in the United States is also focused on youth. The goal of this system seems to be finding a cure for all illnesses. This goal has prompted significant contributions to the world's health care; however, the belief in a cure for all ills may conflict with the care elder citizens need. With America's present technological knowledge, some chronic illnesses of old age can only be managed, not cured. In some ways America's health care system has been short-sighted about the health care needs of elders. For example, when the Medicare law was established in 1965, it excluded coverage for continual treatment of chronic conditions unless there was a change in the patient's status. As a result, today there are more elders living longer with chronic conditions that are not covered by Medicare. People working in the health care field may unintentionally be short-sighted and condescending when they refer to elders as "dear," "darling," or "sweetie" (French, 1990). In the health care system, references to ageism often occur as a response to a medical diagnoses. OT documentation that begins, "This 91-year-old female was admitted with the diagnosis of total hip replacement," may trigger preconceived ideas based on age bias, such as feelings that the client is too old for treatment. Readers of this type of documentation may question the reason for risking surgery or OT treatment with this elder client.

Many aspects of American society, including housing, employment, and recreational resources, are geared toward youth. However, that picture is slowly changing with the emergence of the senior citizen as a powerful political and economic force and with the growth of the aged population.

CHAPTER REVIEW QUESTIONS

1 Define the terms *gerontology*, *geriatrics*, and *cohort*.
2 What is the relationship between aging and illness?
3 What are the dismissal and collaborative approaches, and how might they affect client care?
4 What considerations should be taken for managing clients with chronic illnesses?
5 What factors are related to the significant population growth of the elder generation?
6 What is a result of more widows than widowers among the elder population?
7 What are some of the needs of the 85 years and older generation?
8 What does the COTA need to know about the educational level of the 85 years and older generation for treatment interventions?
9 What age group has the highest poverty rate and why?
10 How has public policy influenced the economic status of elders?
11 What are some implications of the demographical data for future occupational therapy practice?
12 What is ageism? Provide examples of it in today's culture.
13 What are misconceptions you had about growth of the aged population, minority elders, the old old (85 years and over), economic demographics, and living arrangements before reading this chapter?

REFERENCES

American Association of Retired Persons: *A profile of older Americans*, 1995, The Association.
Anderson KN, Anderson LE, Glanze WD, editors: *Mosby's medical, nursing, and allied health dictionary*, ed 4, St. Louis, 1994, Mosby.
Bould S, Sanborn B, Reif L: *Eighty-five plus: the oldest old*, Belmont, Calif, 1989, Wadsworth.
Branch LG, Coulam RF, Zimmerman YA: The PACE evaluation: initial findings, *Gerontologist* 35:349, 1995.
Davis LJ: Gerontology in theory and practice. In Davis LJ, Kirkland M, editors: *ROTE: the role of occupational therapy with the elderly*, Rockville, Md, 1989, American Occupational Therapy Association.
Davis LJ, Kirkland M, editors: *ROTE: the role of occupational therapy with the elderly: faculty guide*, Rockville, Md, 1986, American Occupational Therapy Association.
Flexner SB, editor: *The Random House dictionary of the English language*, ed 2, New York, 1987, Random House.
French S: Ageism, *Physiother* 76:3, 1989.
Glantz C: Personal communication, Aug 1996.
Glantz C, Richman N: Personal comunication, Oct 1995.
Gunyea JG: The paradox of the advantaged elder and the feminization of poverty, *Soc Work* 39:35, 1994.
Guralink JM et al: Morbidity and disability in older persons in the years prior to death, *Am J Pub Health* 81:443, 1991.
Horn JC, Meer J: The vintage years, *Psychol Today* 21:76, 1987.
Jette AM, Bottomley JM: *Phys Ther* 67:1537, 1987.
Lewis C: How the myths of aging impact rehabilitative care for the older person, *Occup Ther Forum* 10, 1989.
Manton KG: The dynamics of population aging: demography and policy analysis, *Milbank Q* 69:309, 1991.
McBride TD: Personal communication, Aug 1996.
McLean C: The graying of America, *Oregon Starter* 11, 1988.
O'Grady-LeShane R: Older women and poverty, *Soc Work* 35:422, 1990.
Olson LK, editor: Public policy and privatization. In *The graying of the world: who will care for the frail elderly?* New York, 1994, Hawthorne Press.
Pepper Commission: *U.S. bipartisan commission on comprehensive health care: a call for action: final report*, Washington, DC, 1990, US Government Printing Office.
Rogers RG, Rogers A, Belanger A: Active life among the elderly in the United States: multi-state life table estimates and population projections, *Milbank Q* 67:370, 1989.
Rubenstein LZ, Kramer BJ: Health problems in old age: cross population comparisons, *Gerontol Geriatr Educ* 15:23, 1996.
Suzman RM: Oldest old. In Atchley RC et al, editors: *The encyclopedia of aging: a comprehensive resource in gerontology and geriatrics*, ed 2, New York, 1995, Springer.

Shen J, Iversen A: PACE: a capitate model towards long-term care, *Henry Ford Hosp Med J* 40:41, 1992.

Thornby MA: Balance and falls in the frail older person: a review of the literature, *Top Geriatr Rehabil* 11:33, 1995.

Ventura-Merkel C, Freedman M: Helping at-risk youth through intergenerational programming, *Child Today* 17:10, 1988.

Zedlewski SR, McBride TD: The changing profile of the elderly: effects on future long-term care needs and financing, *Milbank Q* 70:247, 1992.

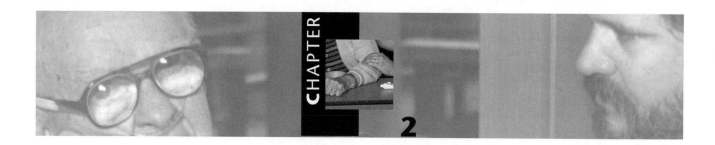

CHAPTER 2

Social and Biological Theories of Aging

MARLENE J. AITKEN

KEY TERMS

genetic aging, nongenetic aging, successful aging, developmental stages

CHAPTER OBJECTIVES

1. Identify the purpose and use of current theories of aging.
2. Discuss the biological theories of aging, including genetic and nongenetic.
3. Discuss the psychosocial theories of aging.
4. Understand the ways to apply the theories of aging to the care of elders.

Michelle is a COTA on a subacute unit in a nursing home. Her daily work involves treating clients that have a variety of diagnoses. Michelle has observed that although all the clients have some type of problem that requires rehabilitation, each reacts differently to illness and the aging process. At least once a week Michelle meets Kelly, an OTR, for a supervision session, during which time they thoroughly discuss each client receiving OT. Michelle feels very comfortable discussing almost any concern with Kelly.

After reviewing the caseload during one particular session, Michelle and Kelly began a lively discussion about the complexities of aging. Michelle noted that some of the clients on her caseload seemed very active and vigorous, whereas others seemed very withdrawn and had low energy to do therapeutic tasks. She also commented that some of the clients seemed older than their actual age, whereas others seemed their age or younger. Kelly encouraged Michelle to review some theories about aging to form a context in which to think about the clients. The following week, Michelle and Kelly discussed the appli-

cation of the theories to their work with clients on their caseloads.

Questions like Michelle's regarding reasons for aging and the differences in aging are unanswered because aging research consists of many different studies and perspectives. COTAs need to understand the content of many theories because they help provide the scientific basis for treatment and explain, describe, and predict behavior (Hopkins, 1988). The biological theories may answer questions about the reasons for aging. Social theorists are concerned with the social consequences of aging and provide insight on the ways persons age successfully. This chapter uses the format of current biological, social, and psychological theories to provide insight on social aspects of aging. (The physical and psychological changes that occur with the aging process are described in later chapters.)

BIOLOGICAL THEORIES OF AGING

The population of people over 65 years of age is growing rapidly. These people begin to face illnesses that become more prevalent as the aging process continues. However, most studies of human aging find that no uniform rate of aging exists.

Individuals of the same age demonstrate differences in age-related variables such as vital capacity and glomerular filtration rate in the kidneys (Schneider, Reed, 1985). The major current theories that attempt to explain this differential aging fit into one of two categories: **genetic aging**, which presumes that aging is predetermined, and **nongenetic aging**, which presumes that aging events occur randomly and accumulate with time (Abrams, Beers, Berkow, 1995). The four genetic aging theories are programmed aging, somatic mutation, free radical, and cybernetic. The nongenetic theory is the wear and tear theory.

Genetic Theories

Programmed aging. The premise of the programmed aging theories is that the human body has an inherited internal "genetic clock" that determines the beginning of the aging process. This genetic clock may manifest as a predetermined number of cell divisions that can occur for some individuals (Hayflick, 1987). Studies of living cells in the laboratory have shown that some cells lose the ability to replicate or divide with time. Cells are thought to become more specialized with each turnover cycle until they can no longer replicate effectively. Some scientists believe that aging may be caused by an impairment of cells in the translation of necessary ribonucleic acid (RNA) as a result of the ineffective communication with deoxyribonucleic acid (DNA). Although the essential messages may be transcribed at all ages, the translation of these messages into functional proteins may be restricted in elders (Brookbank, 1990). The cell may stop exchanging genetic information with DNA, and without genetic guidance the cell may become senescent, or old (Hayflick, 1968).

The significance of this theory continues to be debated. Studies have established that either some segments of DNA become depleted with advancing age or selected cellular structures seem to change with age so that the transcription of certain DNA is restricted. However, if aging were attributable to this alteration in the program of cellular development, a more regular and predictable sequence of organ system failures might be expected than occurs (Brookbank, 1990).

Somatic mutation theory. According to the somatic mutation theory, spontaneous unexpected chromosomal changes occur as a result of miscoding, translation errors, chemical reactions, irradiation, and spontaneous replication of errors. Mutations can occur in the tissues of aging animals. Cumulative mistakes occur not only in DNA but in RNA and enzyme synthesis. These mistakes result in progressive loss of function or feedback to the cell.

Many health problems in elders are related to immune system dysfunction, including late onset diabetes and cancer. The somatic mutation theory relates aging to the way the immune system increasingly makes mistakes by identifying the body's own cells as foreign and reacting against them. This theory may explain the higher frequency of cancer in the elderly or the aging of the immune system ascribed to the elderly (Brookbank, 1990).

Free radical theory. The free radical theory of large molecular injury looks at the products of oxygen utilization within cells. Oxidation of lipids, proteins, fats, and carbohydrates (large molecules) can result in the formation of oxygen compounds with an extra electron charge or "free radical." Additional free radicals are formed whenever metallic ions, enzymes, or cellular materials combine with oxygen. Proponents of this theory believe that low-level free radical damage accumulates over time, resulting in age-associated decline of function in major organs such as the kidneys (Abrams, Beers, Berkow, 1995). Environmental contaminants such as air pollutants are also related to free radical production. Free radicals act at the cell membrane level, thus interfering with the function of cells (Crastes-de-Paulet, 1990). Antioxidants to protect against aging are eagerly sought by the public and form the basis for the continued financial success of products such as vitamin e and beta carotene. Proof that physiological aging is altered by antioxidants, however, is still lacking.

Cybernetic theory. The neuroendocrine theory of cybernetics suggests that the central nervous system is the aging pacemaker of the body (Cristofalo, 1988). According to this theory, changes in the endocrine system and hypothalamus result in some of the end organ changes seen with aging such as the rate of thyroid hormone and adrenocortical steroid production. Functional changes in this system are accompanied by a decline in functional capacity of all systems. Additionally, alteration of brain dopamine levels may increase potential development of age-associated diseases such as Parkinson's Disease.

Nongenetic Theories

Wear and tear theory. The wear and tear theory proposes that cumulative damage to vital parts of the body leads to the death of cells, tissues, organs, and finally, the organism. Numerous theories ascribe aging to secondary damage from toxins, cosmic rays, gravity, and so forth. These theories demonstrate the change in the length of life span for humans under different environmental situations (Abrams, Beers, Berkow, 1995). Studies of identical twins indicate a genetic basis for longevity. Cases in which the time of death varies between twins indicate that environmental factors may be as important as genetic factors in determining life span (Bank, Jarvik, 1978).

Exposure to environmental and dietary compounds can cause changes in the characteristics of major body organ tissues such as collagen and elastin. These tissues become less pliable and less elastic, resulting in some of the gross changes associated with aging in skin, arterial blood vessel walls, the musculoskeletal system, and the lens of the eye (Cristofalo, 1988).

SOCIAL THEORIES OF AGING

Longer life spans and an increased number of elders in American society have resulted in greater attention to the aging process. Quality of life and successful aging are becoming important areas of study. The disengagement, activity, and continuity social theories each present a different process of aging and focus on different aspects of **successful aging**. The next three social theories, which consist of Erikson's and Peck's stages of psychological development and the life course, place more emphasis on the **developmental stages** of aging. The last social theory of aging, the theory of exchange, examines perceptions regarding the value of interactions and the ways these perceptions affect elders' relationships.

Researchers on the major social theories of aging, activity theory, disengagement theory, and continuity theory have not consistently demonstrated accuracy in identifying behaviors at various stages.

Disengagement Theory

Disengagement occurs when people withdraw from roles or activities and reduce their activity levels or involvement. While completing an interest checklist, an elder may indicate to the COTA former activities with various social clubs or organizations. When asked for the reason for withdrawal from these activities, the elder may state that it was because of age. Based on their research in Kansas City in the 1950's, Cumming and Henry (1961) theorized that the turning inward typical of aging people produces a natural and normal withdrawal from social roles and activities, an increasing preoccupation with self, and decreasing involvement with others. Cumming and Henry perceived individual disengagement as primarily a psychological process involving withdrawal of interest and commitment. Social withdrawal was a consequence of individual disengagement, coupled with society's withdrawal of opportunities and interest in elder's contributions.

This disengagement theory resulted in increased research. The proposition of withdrawal being normal challenged the conventional wisdom that keeping active was the best way to deal with aging. Streib and Schneider (1971) suggested that differential disengagement was more likely to occur than total disengagement. For example, people may withdraw from some activities but increase or maintain their involvement in others. Troll (1971) found that elders often disengage into the family; that is, elders often cope with lost roles by increasing involvement with their families. People are seldom completely engaged or disengaged. Rather, they strike a balance between the two states that reflects their individual preferences, often mediated by social encouragement or discouragement from others.

The major criticism of the disengagement theory is that it does not give enough weight to the role of society's determination and initiation of disengagement. Patterns of declining interactions have been uncovered by researchers studying societal disengagement (Newell, 1961; Havighurst, Neugarten, Tobin, 1963; Williams, Wirths, 1965). However, the decline of opportunity may not be a result of either individual disengagement or societal disengagement but a combination of both (Atchley, 1991). The frequency of disengagement is very much the product of the opportunity for continued engagement. For example, elders may wish to continue many activities, but because they believe that other people may think they are "too old," they withdraw.

Activity Theory

About the same time the disengagement theory was described, others proposed an alternative way of describing the psychosocial process of aging. Havighurst, Neugarten, and Tobin (1963) articulated an activity theory of aging, which held that unless constrained by poor health or disability, elders have the same psychological and social needs as people of middle age. This theory emphasizes the importance of ongoing social interactions; as a result of this activity, elders maintain positive self-concepts (Cavan, 1962). This theory assumes that social activity is beneficial for elders and that it contributes to the their achievement of life satisfaction. The activity theory also assumes that elders need and desire high levels of social activity and that they interpret different types of activity in the same ways as younger people. In addition, some researchers have noted that the relationship between activity and well-being among elders depends on the type of activity in which they are engaged (Lemon, Bengtson, Peterson, 1972).

A further component of the activity theory considers the preferences of elders and the extent to which they wish to be active. Setting aside time for quiet reflection may be equally as important as more active pursuits for some elders. COTAs should remember this when attempting to get everyone involved in an activity. Some elders may welcome participation in physical activities such as bowling and walking, and others may be content with listening to quiet music and reading (Figures 2-1 through 2-3).

Continuity Theory

The premise of the continuity theory is that elders adapt to changes by using strategies to maintain continuity in their lives. Continuity is both internal and external. *Internal continuity* refers to the strategy of forming personal links between new experiences and

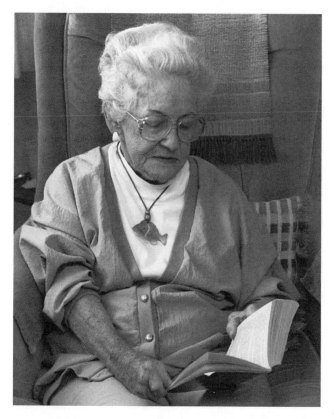

FIGURE 2-1 This elder enjoys a sedentary activity.

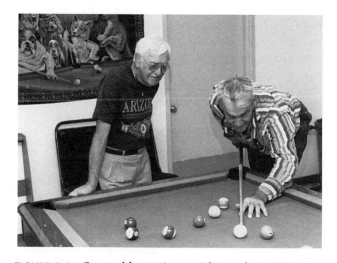

FIGURE 2-2 Some elders enjoy socializing during an active leisure activity.

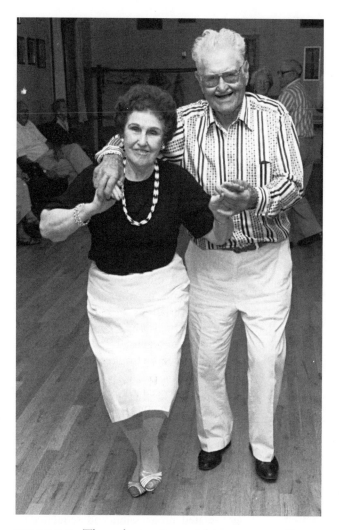

FIGURE 2-3 Through ongoing social interactions, elders can maintain a positive self-concept.

memories of previous ones (Cohler, 1982). *External continuity* refers to interacting with familiar people and living in familiar environments (Atchley, 1991). According to this theory, elders should continue to live in their own homes as long as possible. If this is not possible, the family should attempt to locate housing for the elder in the same general area to maintain friendships and familiar

environments. Many elders continue to be independent as long as they are in familiar surroundings. Some families have noted that once they moved their elder family member from a familiar area, the elder was confused and disoriented.

Continuity of activities and environments helps the individual concentrate energies in familiar areas of activity. Practice of activities can often prevent, offset, or minimize the effects of aging. Atchley (1991) states that by maintaining the same lifestyle and residence, an older person is able to meet instrumental activities of daily living (IADL) needs. Continuity of roles and activities is effective in maintaining the capacity to meet social and emotional needs for interaction and social support. Maintaining independence is important for continued good self-esteem. Continuity does not mean that nothing changes; it means that new life experiences occur and the elder must adapt to them with familiar, persistent processes and attributes. New information is likely to produce less stress when an elder has memories of similar experiences. This may be one reason new information does not have the same weight for both younger and older generations and may help explain the reason some elders seem more conservative than others. For example, an elder may reject learning to use a reacher in spite of difficulty reaching items on a high shelf because the activity involves a new way of performing a task.

Life Span/Life Course Theory

The life span, or life course, perspective is a recent approach of human development by theorists interested in the social and behavioral processes of aging (Box 2-1). *Life course* is defined by Atchley (1991) "as an ideal sequence of events that people are expected to experience and positions that they are expected to occupy as they mature and move through life." This theory was influenced by the age stratification model, which emphasizes the significant variations in elders depending on the characteristics of their birth cohort. Some researchers believe this is not actually a theory, but a conceptual framework for conducting research and interpreting data.

Most elders who experienced the Great Depression seem to have a different perception of the meaning of "poor." Many elders reject offers of help because they compare what little they had in the past with what they currently have, which seems sufficient. In addition, some elders who are eligible for Social Security insurance (SSI) may not accept it.

Neugarten and associates (1965) found considerable consensus on age-related progression and sequence of roles and group memberships that individuals are expected to follow as they mature and move through life. The stages of the adult life course as defined by this group are middle age, later maturity, and old age. Unlike the Erikson and Peck stages, life course stages are related to specific chronological ages. Age norms generally define what people within a given life stage are "allowed" to do and be at certain ages. Many norms are established by long traditions. Others are often the result of compromise and negotiation. In addition, a series of assumptions related to the capabilities of the people in a given life stage underlies age norms. Thus opportunities may be limited for some elders because others assume they are not strong enough or lack education or experience (Atchley, 1991). Elders who achieve greatness beyond expectations for their life stages are perceived as unique or different. Their accomplishments elicit comments about their endeavors being met by a person of "their age." Many older elders are considered pioneers because few prescribed behaviors or age norms exist for them. Havighurst (1972) suggested that people 60 years of age and older needed to adjust to declining health, a life of retirement, death of spouse and friends, changing living arrangements, and increased leisure time if they wanted to experience life satisfaction.

Erikson's Theory of Human Development

Erik Erikson's theory of human development over the life span is one of the most influential descriptions of psychological change (Erikson, 1985). Erickson's stages of ego development are familiar to most students of psychology (Table 2-1).

Erikson's framework addresses the developmental tasks at each stage of the life cycle. The stage most commonly identified with aging is that of integrity versus despair. In this stage the elder comes to terms with the gradual deterioration of the body but at the same time may reflect on the acquisition of wisdom associated with life experiences. Ego integrity involves the elder's ability to see life as meaningful and to accept both positive and negative personality traits without feeling threatened. Integrity provides a basis for approaching the end of life with a feeling of having done the best possible under the

---

BOX 2-1

Key Elements of the Life Span Framework
▪ Aging occurs from birth to death. ▪ Aging involves biological, social, and psychological processes. ▪ Experiences in aging are shaped by historical factors.

(From Passuth P, Bengston V: Sociological theories of aging: current perspectives and future directions. In Birren J, Bengtson V, editors: *Emergent theories of aging*, New York, 1988, Springer.)

TABLE 2-1

Erik Erikson's Stages of Ego Development

Time period	Stage
Early infancy	Trust versus distrust
Later infancy	Autonomy versus shame and doubt
Early childhood	Initiative versus guilt
Childhood middle years	Industry versus inferiority
Adolescence	Ego identity versus role confusion
Early adulthood	Intimacy versus isolation
Middle adulthood	Generativity versus stagnation
Late adulthood	Ego integrity versus ego despair

From Erikson E: *Childhood and society*, New York, 1985, Norton.

circumstances. Despair is the elder's rejection of self and life experiences and includes the realization that there is insufficient time to alter this assessment. The despairing elder is prone to depression and afraid to die. COTAs can play a vital role in assisting elders to master this developmental stage. Helping elders develop self-empathy, the ability to bounce back from change, and a focus on the completeness of their lives supports elders' efforts to deal with this life stage.

Erikson originally proposed eight stages of psychosocial development. As Erikson himself reached later life, he noted that the predominant image of old age was quite different from when he had first formulated his theory (Erikson, 1982; Erikson, Erikson, Kivnick, 1986). Newman and Newman (1991) responded to the changing patterns of biological and cultural development by redefining late-life psychosocial development. They added descriptions of three additional stages, including the stage of very old age.

As increasing numbers of people reach very old age, tasks and other aspects of psychosocial development that were not systematically described in Erikson's original formulations are emerging. Newman and Newman (1991) have labeled the crisis of the old-old years (age 75 years and beyond) as immortality versus extinction. The positive resolution of this crisis is the elder's confidence in the continuity of a personal contribution beyond death. For example, an elder who handcrafts rocking chairs may pass on those skills to children, who may pass them on to their children. Tasks of this stage include coping with the inevitable physical changes that accompany aging. The elder may be increasingly obliged to turn attention from the more interesting aspects of life to the demands of the body. In addition, the very old may have to shape new patterns for adapting to late life because few norms for behavior and few responsibilities are established for elders

who reach very old age. Numerous articles on persons over 100 years of age show a fascination with the many activities of this fastest growing age group. Most of these elders attribute their longevity to keeping their minds, not their bodies, stimulated (Stern, 1996)(Figure 2-4).

Kishton (1994) added another task of late life, that of developing a historical perspective of the psychological events of life such as mistakes and disappointments. Kishton described this task as a process of integration of the past, present, and future. Integration of the past usually involves reconciling prior mistakes or disappointments. Reminiscence groups conducted as part of a treatment program by COTAs can be very effective in helping elders work through this developmental task.

Peck's Stages of Psychological Development

Robert Peck (1968) felt that Erikson's eighth stage, integrity versus despair, was intended to "represent in a global, nonspecific way all of the psychological crises and crisis-solutions of the last forty or fifty years of life" (p. 88). He suggested that it might be more accurate and useful to take a closer look at the second half of life and divide it into several different psychological stages and adjustments (Table 2-2).

Peck proposed four stages that occur in middle age and three in old age. He avoided establishing a chronological period for these stages, suggesting instead that they might occur in different time sequences for different individuals.

The first stage of old age is ego differentiation versus work-role preoccupation. The effect of retirement, particularly for men in their late sixties, is the issue at this

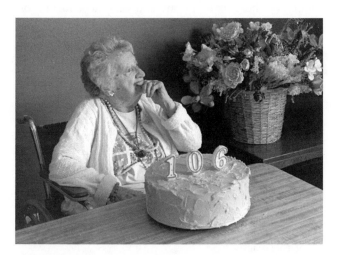

FIGURE 2-4 Persons over 100 years of age make up the fastest-growing age group.

TABLE 2-2

Robert Peck's Psychological Stages in the Second Half of Life	
Time period	**Stage**
Middle age—first stage	Wisdom versus physical powers
Middle age—second stage	Socializing versus sexualizing
Middle age—third stage	Cathectic flexibility versus cathectic impoverishment
Middle age—fourth stage	Mental flexibility versus mental rigidity
Old age—first stage	Ego differentiation versus work-role preoccupation
Old age—second stage	Body transcedence versus body preoccupation
Old age—third stage	Ego transcendence versus ego preoccupation

From Peck R: Psychological developments in the second half of life. In Neugarten B, editor: *Middle age and aging*, Chicago, 1968, University of Chicago Press.

stage. In the American culture, identity tends to be tied to the individual's work role. Retiring individuals must reappraise and redefine their worth in a broader range of role activities. Retirement also affects women, regardless of whether their careers were outside the home. The housewife's work role changes drastically when the husband retires and is suddenly always in "her" domain.

Peck states that a critical requisite for successful adaptation to this stage may be the establishment of varied sets of valued activities and self-attributes. These activities and attributes allow the individual to have satisfying and worthwhile alternatives to pursue. Participation in voluntary organizations can provide recreational activities and political action. The American Association of Retired Persons (AARP) can be initiated as early as 50 years of age and continued after the formal work role has ended.

Peck's second stage of old age is body transcendence versus body preoccupation. Physical decline, along with a marked decline in recuperative powers and increased body aches and pains, occurs in many elders in this stage. To those who especially value physical well-being, this may be the most difficult period of adjustment. For some elders this adjustment means a growing preoccupation with their bodily functions. However, others have learned to define comfort and happiness in human relationships or creative mental activities. For them, only complete physical destruction can deter these feelings.

The third stage is ego transcendence versus ego preoccupation. With this stage of old age comes the certain prospect of death. Successful adaptation is not compatible with passive resignation or ego denial. It requires deep, active effort on the part of the elder to make life more secure, meaningful, and happy for those who will live after the elder's death. These elders experience a gratifying absorption in the future and are interested in doing all that is possible to make the world better for familial or cultural descendants.

Exchange Theory

In clinical practice the OT practitioner may find it more rewarding to work with an elder who is motivated and has a "fun" personality than with an elder who does not relate well with others. COTAs may observe that the client who displays a winning personality receives more attention from everyone. This is an example of exchange theory (Figure 2-5).

Exchange theory, as originally developed by Homans (1961), assumes that people attempt to maximize their rewards and minimize their costs in interactions with others. The major attempts to use exchange theory in work with elders are attributed to Dowd (1975, 1980). Elders are viewed from the perspective of their ongoing interactions with a number of persons. Continuing interaction is based on what the elder perceives as rewarding or costly. Elders tend to continue with interactions that are beneficial and withdraw from those

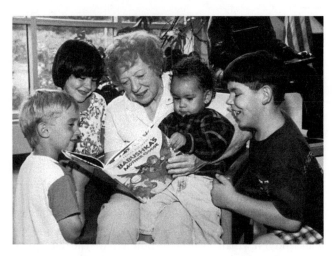

FIGURE 2-5   This elder enjoys interacting with young children.

perceived as having no benefit. Rewards may be defined in material or nonmaterial terms and could include such components as assistance, money, information, affection, approval, property, skill, respect, compliance, and conformity. Costs are defined as an expenditure of any of these.

In American culture, more emphasis is often placed on resources a person is assumed to have rather than on the actual exchange resources. The concept of ageism includes assumptions about elders, such as that elders have less current information, outdated skills, and inadequate physical strength or endurance. If elders are perceived as having few resources to contribute to a relationship, an issue over power can result, with the elder at a distinct disadvantage. Elders may be seen as powerless actors who are forced into a position of compliance and dependence because they have nothing of value to withhold to get better treatment (Atchley, 1991). Many elders accept the validity of these assumptions and fear dependency on others more than death (Aitken, 1982).

CHAPTER REVIEW QUESTIONS

1 Scenario one: Ethel Shanas, a very famous gerontologist, once said that if you want to live a long time, you should choose your grandparents carefully. Which aging theory or theories support Dr. Shanas' suggestion?

2 Scenario two: Michelle, the COTA introduced at the beginning of the chapter, decided to include reminiscence and life review as part of her therapeutic interventions with elders in the nursing home. Which aging theory supports the selection of these activities?

3 Scenario three: The family of one of Michelle's elderly clients is upset because the client insists on planning her own funeral and asking for specific

clothes in which to be buried. In addition, she has made a list of all her furniture and other property and has designated which of her children or grandchildren are to inherit these items. Although this client has accepted her terminal illness, her family has not. Which aging theory would Michelle use to explain to the family what is happening with their relative?

4 The risk of being diagnosed with cancer increases significantly as people grow older. Use an aging theory to explain the possible reason for this.

5 Many elder men become extremely depressed once they retire. What could you suggest, other than antidepressant medications, that may improve their outlook on life? Discuss the theory that supports your suggestion.

6 An 80-year-old man recently made headlines because he entered the Boston marathon. Why did this make the news? How do cultural age norms influence the persistence of ageism?

7 An 85-year-old woman has requested that during her ADL session the COTA help her dress herself and put on makeup. Her doctor has suggested that she is "too old for rehab" and is thinking of discontinuing her OT. How can you justify her treatment with a theory and convince the doctor that it is important?

8 According to exchange theory, why does an elder feel dependent on her relatives?

9 Give an example of disengagement theory.

10 Give an example of activity theory.

REFERENCES

Abrams W, Beers M, Berkow R: *The Merck manual of geriatrics,* Whitehouse Station, NJ, 1995, Merck.

Aitken M: Self concept and functional independence in the hospitalized elderly, *Am J Occup Ther* 36:243, 1982.

Atchley R: *Social forces and aging,* Belmont, Ca, 1991, Wadsworth.

Bank L, Jarvik L: A longitudinal study of aging human twins. In Schneider E, editor: *The genetics of aging,* New York, 1978, Plenum Press.

Brookbank J: *The biology of aging,* New York, 1990, Harper & Row.

Cavan R: Self and role in adjustment during old age. In Rose A, editor: *Human behavior and social processes,* Boston, 1962, Houghton Mifflin.

Cohler B: Person narrative and life course. In Baltes P, Brim O, editors: *Life-span development and behavior,* New York, 1982, Academic Press.

Crastes de Paulet A: Free radicals and aging, *Ann Biolog Clin Paris* 48:323, 1990.

Cristofalo V: An overview of the theories of biological aging. In Birren J, Bengtson V, editors: *Emergent theories of aging,* New York, 1988, Springer.

Cumming E, Henry W: *Growing old,* New York, 1961, Basic Books.

Dowd J: Aging as exchange: a preface to theory, *J Gerontol* 30:584, 1975.

Dowd J: Exchange rates and old people, *J Gerontol* 35:596, 1980.

Erikson E: *Childhood and society,* New York, 1985, Norton.

Erikson E: *The life cycle completed,* New York, 1982, Norton.

Erikson E, Erikson J, Kivnick H: *Vital involvement in old age,* New York, 1986, Norton.

Havighurst R: *Developmental tasks and education,* New York, 1972, David McKay.

Havighurst R, Neugarten B, Tobin S: Disengagement, personality, and life satisfaction. In Hansen P, editor: *Age with a future,* Copenhagen, 1963, Munksgaard.

Hayflick L: Human cells and aging, *Sci Am* 218:32, 1968.

Hayflick L: Biological theories of aging. In Maddox G, editor: *The encyclopedia of aging,* New York, 1987, Springer.

Homans G: *Social behavior: its elementary forms,* New York, 1961, Harcourt Brace Jovanovich.

Hopkins H: Current basis for theory and philosophy in occupational therapy. In Hopkins H, Smith H, editors: *Willard and Spackman's occupational therapy,* Philadelphia, 1988, JB Lippincott.

Kishton J: Contemporary Eriksonian theory: a psychobiographical illustration, *Gerontol Geriatr Educ* 14:81, 1994.

Lemon B, Bengtson V, Peterson J: An exploration of the activity theory of aging: activity types and life satisfaction among in-movers to a retirement community, *J Gerontol* 27:511, 1972.

Neugarten B, Moore J, Lowe J: Age norms, age constraints, and adult socialization, *Am J Sociol* 70:710, 1965.

Newell D: Social structural evidence for disengagement. In Cumming E, Henry W, editors: *Growing old,* New York, 1961, Basic Books.

Newman B, Newman P: *Understanding adulthood,* New York, 1991, Holt, Rinehart & Winston.

Passuth P, Bengtson V: Sociological theories of aging: current perspectives and future directions. In Birren J, Bengtson V, editors: *Emergent theories of aging,* New York, 1988, Springer.

Peck R: Psychological developments in the second half of life. In Neugarten B, editor: *Middle age and aging,* Chicago, 1968, University of Chicago Press.

Schneider E, Reed J: Modulations of aging processes. In Finch C, Schneider E, editors: *Handbook of the biology of aging,* New York, 1985, Van Nostrand Reinhold.

Stern C: Who is old? *Parade* Jan 21:4, 1996.

Streib G, Schneider C: *Retirement in American society,* Ithaca, New York, 1971, Cornell University Press.

Troll L: The family of later life, *J Marriage Fam* 33:263, 1971.

Williams R, Wirths C: *Lives through the years,* New York, 1965, Atherton Press.

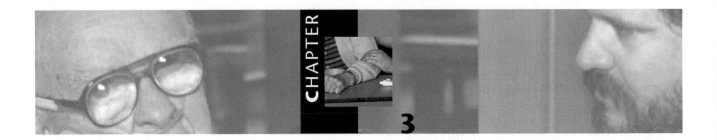

CHAPTER

3

Aging Process

CLAUDELLE **A.H.** CARRUTHERS AND JODI LANE

KEY TERMS

function, dysfunction, primary aging, secondary aging

CHAPTER OBJECTIVES

1. Describe the aging process.
2. Explain the concepts of function and dysfunction.
3. Define and distinguish between the concepts of primary aging and secondary aging.
4. Discuss the terms *normal* and *abnormal* within the context of the aging process.

5. Apply the concepts of normal and abnormal to each of the aging changes found in cognition and in the cardiopulmonary, skeletal, muscular, skin, and sensory systems.

Attempting to understand the aging process is one of the challenges of medicine. The aging process of a simple organism may be observed in a single sitting at a microscope; however, identifying the precise process in a human being is extremely difficult (Kane, Ouslander, Abrass, 1989). Although aging is universal, it varies among people. One elder at 74 years of age may be physically fit and an avid golfer, whereas another elder of the same age may have very limited function and find daily activities challenging. Numerous theories explain the process of aging, which leads to the conclusion that the aging process is multicausal (Blair, 1990).

Factors that affect aging include heredity, lifestyle, environment, and illness. Regardless of the causes and changes experienced, people of all ages want to be functional and independent. **Function** refers to the physical ability to live in a person's own environment

(Kane, Ouslander, Abrass, 1989). It requires the ability to perform activities of daily living (ADLs) and to accurately perceive and interact with the environment. **Dysfunction** refers to the inability to live the way a person wants and possibly to an impairment that prevents independent performance of ADLs (Trombly, 1995). COTAs can intervene and enhance an individual's function and independence with ADLs.

AGING CHANGES

The concepts of **primary aging** and **secondary aging** help clarify function and dysfunction for a given individual at any age. Primary aging changes result from the aging process determined by an individual's genetic make-up. These changes do not necessarily result in dysfunction or impairment. Conversely, secondary aging changes are caused by a disease process, an impairment, or a dysfunction (Lewis, 1979). Researchers have developed criteria to distinguish a primary, or normal, aging change from a secondary, or abnormal, change.

One criteria published by Hall (1976) was named *CUPID*, which is an acronym denoting five possible characteristics of an aging change: *c*umulative, *u*niversal, *p*rogressive, *i*ntrinsic, and *d*eleterious. A particular aging change characterized by each standard is considered a primary change. A change that cannot be categorized within each standard is a secondary aging change.

A different criteria describes primary aging changes with the "1% rule" (Kane, Ouslander, Abrass, 1989). Most organ systems seem to gradually lose function at a rate of approximately 1% per year after the age of 30.

Understanding the differences between primary and secondary aging enables both elders and COTAs to recognize a normal aging change as opposed to a disease process. This helps COTAs perform appropriate interventions and applications for meaningful client care (Dubin, 1992).

Cognition

Cognitive aging changes relate to varied abilities and occur at different rates depending on a variety of personal characteristics. Fluid abilities are information-processing skills passively acquired through incidental learning, inductive reasoning, and daily life experiences. An elder who uses problem-solving and reasoning skills to open a cake mix box without written or verbal instructions demonstrates fluid ability. Crystallized ability is knowledge acquired formally through experience and education such as internships and classes. Crystallized ability tends to decline earlier than fluid or passive ability (Schaie, 1989). Research has indicated that cognitive decline for most elders is selective, often ability-specific, and global rather than catastrophic (Schaie, 1984). An elder who can no longer maintain an accurate checkbook balance because of visual loss and decreased short-term memory demonstrates a global cognitive decline. This loss is gradual and encompasses several cognitive processes.

Catastrophic declines occur with sudden onset. An elder with an infection such as a urinary tract infection (UTI) may suddenly display cognitive loss. This elder may appear confused and suddenly be unable to perform routine ADLs. COTAs should communicate with the elder and family members to determine the causes of this sudden cognitive loss. Factors that may cause a sudden cognitive decline include illness, medication side effects, and neurological infarcts. When working with elders who display catastrophic declines, COTAs should inform appropriate team members of their observations.

Both primary and secondary cognitive aging changes can be reduced. Participating in an intellectually stimu-

lating environment, having a flexible personality style, and possessing a high cognitive status may inhibit and even reverse some primary aging effects (Gribbin, Schaie, Parham, 1980; Schaie, 1984, 1993; Schaie, Willis, 1986) (Figure 3-1). Secondary aging changes in cognition can be reduced if cardiovascular and other similar chronic diseases are prevented (Hertzog, Schaie, Gibbin, 1978).

Skin

Several primary aging changes involve the skin. Wrinkles, which are one of the most noticeable changes, are often attributed to decreased blood supply and changes in collagen and elastic fiber resulting in a loss of elasticity and resilience (Vitto, 1986). Layers of subcutaneous tissue (tissue under the skin) insulate and cushion the skin against trauma. As aging progresses, the subcutaneous tissues undergo atrophic changes resulting in thinner layers of skin (Castelo-Branco et al, 1994). When these tissues atrophy, the body may have difficulty regulating temperature. Loss of subcutaneous fat and

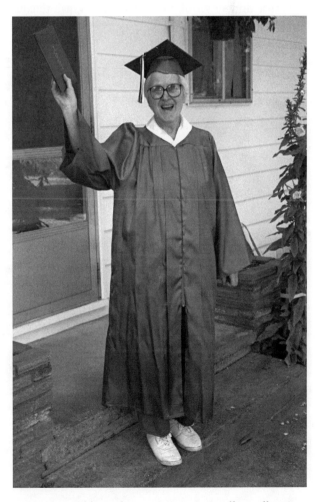

FIGURE 3-1 Elders who participate in intellectually stimulating environments may forestall some primary aging events.

muscle may cause the face to appear thinner, eyes to appear sunken, and lips to appear larger (Buono, McKenzie, Kasch, 1991). In the epidermis (the surface of the skin), cell replacement slows to about 50% between 30 and 70 years of age (Lyden, McGinley, Grove, 1978). The sebaceous, or seborrheic, glands tend to decrease in function, which may lead to dry areas on the scalp and skin (Buono, McKenzie, Kasch, 1991; Dubin, 1992).

The skin shows evidence of aging with blotches, bruising, spots, and discoloration. As the skin undergoes atrophic processes, brown and yellow discolorations occur as a result of an overall decrease in vascularity (Dubin, 1992). Red blotches on the skin are usually caused by changes in the blood vessels beneath the skin (Lyden, McGinley, Grove, 1978). Capillaries lose the protection provided by surrounding fat, thereby possibly causing more bruising and small hemorrhagic spots in the lower extremities (Dubin, 1992) (Figure 3-2).

Other changes occur in the tongue, gums, hair, nails, and sweat glands. The tongue and gums undergo atrophic changes and redden. Gum shrinkage around the teeth may cause difficulty with eating and dental maintenance.

Hair is thickest in adulthood and decreases in diameter by as much as 20% by 70 years of age. Hair becomes thin and fine, and the color changes to gray or white because of a loss of pigmented cells. Besides thinning on the scalp, the hair tends to grow in a more sparse pattern. The sebaceous glands attached to the hair follicles enlarge and the muscles lose their attachments to the follicles; thus pigmented hairs are more easily lost (Buono, McKenzie, Kasch, 1991; Dubin, 1992) (Figure 3-3). Atrophy of nail tissues causes the nails to gradually become more brittle and grow more slowly. The ability to sweat decreases as the sweat and oil glands atrophy and decrease in size and number (Dubin, 1992). As aging progresses, men and women experience changes in hormones. In men a loss of testosterone leads to a general loss of body hair. In women a decrease in estrogen production leads to increased facial hair (Buono, McKenzie, Kasch, 1991).

Secondary aging changes to the skin may occur from exposure to the sun's ultraviolet rays and the inability to sweat. Regular exercise may retard the decrease in peripheral sweat gland production (Buono, McKenzie, Kasch, 1991). Two 70-year-old individuals may have very different skin textures, which may be partially attributed to different work environments during preretirement years. Ultraviolet rays damage the elastic fibers beneath the skin surface and are responsible for wrinkled, dried, and tough skin textures. COTAs may suggest applying creams and lanolin, which replace natural oils and thus reduce the drying effect (Buono, McKenzie, Kasch, 1991; Dubin, 1992).

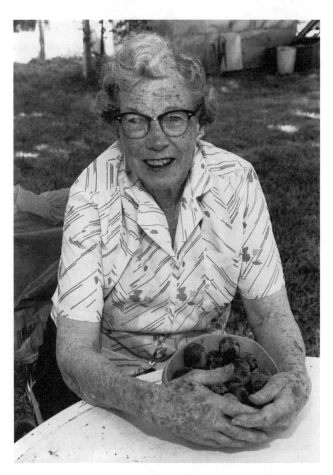

FIGURE 3-2 As people age, changes in skin such as wrinkles and bruises become evident.

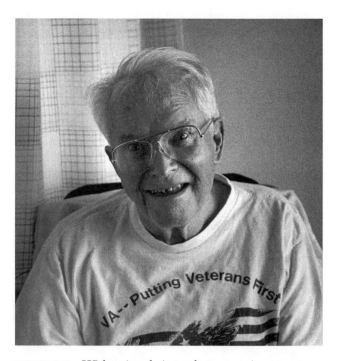

FIGURE 3-3 With aging, hair tends to grow in a more sparse pattern.

Cardiopulmonary System

Primary aging changes of the cardiac system result in reduced cardiac output. The endocardium, which is the inner lining of the heart, thickens because of increased fat deposits that accumulate over time, possibly creating a condition known as *atherosclerosis* (Gasho, Fanelli, Zelis, 1989). This thickened, fibrous formation around the heart causes changes to the heart's electrical system resulting in arrhythmias, or abnormal heart beats. The myocardium, or heart muscle, becomes less elastic; hence contraction and dilation of the cardiac muscle becomes more difficult. Inside the heart, thickening occurs in the wall between the lower chambers (Kitzman et al, 1988). The combination of a decrease in heart rate and an increase in prolonged contraction (systole) prevents elders from tolerating activity involving increased heart rates, which may result in congestive heart failure. Cardiac output declines with age as a result of changes in heart rate, peripheral vascular resistance, and coronary disease (Dubin, 1992).

Primary changes in the arterial system lead to diminished performance. General calcification within the arteries results in a diminished stress response to activities (Pierce et al, 1993). The aortic branches dilate, become twisted, and are less able to accommodate the changes in arterial pressure (Dubin, 1992). As vessel compliance decreases, the vessels in the extremities progressively increase resistance to blood flow (peripheral resistance), which increases systolic blood pressure (Kitzman et al, 1988). Therefore the response to stress is less efficient, more oxygen is needed, and the heart requires a longer period to slow down after physical stress (Blair, 1990). This diminished response could also be related to decreased cardiac output and lack of physical conditioning (Dubin, 1992).

Secondary changes include the development of atherosclerosis (lipid deposits), which makes it difficult for blood to be pumped through blood vessels (DeVries, 1970). Regular exercise and reduction in fat intake can minimize these effects (Seals et al, 1984).

One primary pulmonary change is a gradual decline in body fluid composition. By 70 years of age, body fluid composition may be 50% water compared with 80% water at birth. This dehydration affects the moist mucous membranes that line the nose, pharynx, trachea, bronchi, and bronchioles. Mucus may become thick and plug the tracheobronchial tree, which may lead to infections.

Other changes decrease the available oxygen supply to the body. Calcification of rib cartilage and a decline in lung tissue elasticity result in reduced compliance of the thorax. This reduced compliance causes poor gas exchange and a large anteroposterior diameter (Dubin, 1992; Kuhn, McGovern, 1992). Muscles that support lung function lose elasticity. Therefore the maximum volume of oxygen that can be brought into the lungs with one deep breath decreases. Cilia, which are hairlike structures in the airways, decline in number and become less effective in removing foreign matter, thus diminishing the amount of oxygen available in the lungs and consequently raising the individual's susceptibility to secondary changes (Rockstein, Sussman, 1979).

Disease, environment, and lack of physical activity may all contribute to secondary pulmonary changes. Osteoporosis and kyphosis alter the shape of the thorax and reduce lung expansion, which may result in anatomic emphysema in elders. In addition, declining chest muscle strength impairs the effectiveness of a cough and therefore can increase susceptibility to pneumonia and chronic bronchitis. The respiratory system suffers more from exposure to environmental pollutants and infections than any other cause (Rockstein, Sussman, 1979). Serious loss of lung function can be prevented with physical activity.

Skeletal System

The primary aging changes within the skeletal system include a reduction in height, degenerative changes to joints, and a decrease in bone mass (Castelo-Branco et al, 1994). Reduction in height is caused by atrophy of the intervertebral disks and ligaments along the vertebral column. The joints of the body undergo erosion and ossification of cartilaginous joint surfaces as well as degenerative changes of the synovium. These processes lead to stiff joints and decreased spinal mobility (Einkauf et al, 1987). An increase in bone porousness causes loss of skeletal bone and elasticity.

Substantial increases in bone porousness lead to a secondary condition known as *osteoporosis*. Approximately 44% of white women and 34% of white men that are 65 to 74 years of age have measurable osteoporosis. Osteoporosis is an increase in bone porousness that may be precipitated by a hormonal change such as a decrease in estrogen levels in postmenopausal women. Specifically, bones become less firm and more compressed and therefore more prone to fracture (Dubin, 1992).

Possible secondary changes related to poor posture during the life span are calcification and eventual ossification of the ligaments (Dubin, 1992). Proper nutrition, good posture, and exercise can minimize these changes.

Muscular System

The primary change in the muscular system is a gradual decline of physical strength beginning around 30 years of age. In the average adult, muscle mass constitutes 43% of total body weight, whereas in elders the figure drops to 25%. As the muscle fibers degenerate, they are replaced by fat cells so by 70 years of age, fat cells may constitute one third of a muscle. Some evidence of increasing proximal muscle weakness also exists. Acetylcholine acts as a neurotransmitter, relaying messages between nerves that can result in movement of the muscles. With aging the interactions between acetylcholine and the nerve endings are reduced, resulting in muscle weakness, atrophy, and hypotonia (Dubin, 1992; Hasselkus, 1974). Muscle strength is also reduced by the decreased number of capillaries per muscle fiber.

The ability to perform light and moderate work is maintained. However, the ability to perform heavy work declines because a decrease in maximum lung capacity for oxygen occurs (Frolkis, Martynenko, Zamostyan, 1976). A gradual loss of glycogen storage in muscles reduces a person's capacity to respond to emergency situations. In addition, the metabolic differences between fast (less oxygenated) and slow (more oxygenated) muscles begin to lessen during the aging process (Frolkis, Martynenko, Zamostyan, 1976).

These primary changes of the muscular system can be observed in functional tasks. Muscle weakness may be evident in an elder's shorter-than-average step length, wider walking base, and proportionally longer time spent in the support phase versus the swing phase of the walking cycle (Dubin, 1992). As walking speed increases, forces on the musculoskeletal system increase, and faster speeds may create levels of force that place an elder at risk of injury. Because the likelihood of injury increases with the level of force, the reduction of walking speed and length of steps reduces injury (Dubin, 1992). In addition, a general slowing in reaction time and the speed of performance for completing tasks occurs (Spirduso et al, 1988; Welford, 1977). One secondary change in the muscular system is a decrease in muscle strength caused directly by lack of muscle use or exercise. In the aging individual, decreased muscle endurance and strength related to lack of use can be improved through activity (Fisher, Pendergast, Calkins, 1991). By remaining active, elders are usually able to maintain performance of functional tasks (Carruthers, 1995).

Neurological System

Primary aging changes affect the neurological system, which consists of the brain and spinal cord (central nervous system) and the peripheral nerves that supply the rest of the body. The brain decreases in weight by 5% to 17%; the brain volume and number of neurons also decrease (Boss, 1991; Dubin, 1992). Dubin (1992) found a decrease in the number of nerve cells in the frontal and temporal lobes. These areas influence personality, motor activity, speech, and hearing. In addition, 50% of neurons can be lost in the visual area of the occipital cortex and 33% can be lost in the sensory area of the parietal cortex without functional impairment (Blair, 1990).

Hasselkus (1974) cites changes that include a thickening of the dura mater, the material that covers the brain, excessive subarachnoid fluid under the dura, and reduction in the size of the brainstem. In addition, shortening of the spinal cord may occur, and on transection, a greatly reduced contrast in color between the white and gray matter may be evident. In a more recent study, researchers found that white matter does not decrease. (Lim et al, 1992). Therefore the primary changes that result from decreased brain matter are caused specifically by a loss of gray matter.

Additional primary changes include a widening of sulci and fissures (spaces between the convolutions of the brain). The ventricles, or cavities, holding cerebrospinal fluid, which helps to cushion the brain, also widen (Boss, 1991).

These primary changes of the neurological system can be observed in an elder's performance of functional tasks. A decrease in reaction time related to muscular changes occurs with aging. Neurologically, a decrease in reaction time is a result of visual impairment, a decrease in the number of axons in the nerves, and a reduction of synthesis at nerve terminals (Boss, 1991; Dubin, 1992). In addition, sleep cycles may change such that less time is used for sleeping, with more time in light sleep and less in deep sleep (Blair, 1990; Dubin, 1992).

Secondary neurological aging changes may include a severe decrease in a neurotransmitter relaying information about an elder's surroundings. This may result in increased falls (Hasselkus, 1974). These secondary changes are related to losses in proprioceptive (position of body parts in space), kinesthetic (position and balance), and visual mechanisms (Boss, 1991). If neurotransmitters that relay information are significantly decreased, a person may also experience decreases in motor control, ability to process information, postural balance, and muscle tone (Boss, 1991).

COTAs can help elders enhance short-term memory by encouraging visual and auditory stimulation and memory associations. The elder can and does process new and old information. The neurological system is very complex; therefore delineating between primary and secondary aging changes may be difficult (Blair, 1990).

COTAs working with elders may observe neurological changes during daily activities. An elder preparing a meal may have difficulty reading cooking instructions and may benefit from an enlarged-print cookbook or a magnifying glass. Reaching for high and low objects may cause an elder to lose balance and fall. COTAs must help elders organize their environments for easier access and minimal confusion.

Changes may disrupt elders' normal routines because steps have been added or new techniques have been introduced to maintain safety. COTAs need to permit enough time for elders to process information. Writing a daily schedule may assist elders and their families to be consistent in changing a routine behavior.

Sensory System

The sensory system involves the processes of sensation, perception, and sensory discrimination. Sensation involves acquiring information through the sense organs. Perception is a higher sensory function, in which the information received is processed in the brain. Sensory discrimination is the minimal difference necessary for a person to distinguish between two or more sensations. Because the ability to sense is processed through the brain, the sensory systems are closely related. A general decline in the sensory system occurs in primary aging (Hooyman, Kiyak, 1988).

The senses used for handling and discriminating information include auditory, visual, tactile, olfactory, gustatory, and kinesthetic. These sensory mechanisms enable a person to gather information and interact with the environment. (The primary aging changes related to vision and hearing are discussed in Chapters 17 and 18, respectively.)

Gustatory. Gustation involves the ability to discriminate and perceive the four taste qualities: sweet, sour, salty, and bitter. Two primary aging changes are decreased salivation and a lessened ability to discriminate taste. By 50 years of age, most people have lost 50% of their taste buds at the front of the tongue. Sweet and salty taste buds atrophy first. Consequently many elders think their food tastes bitter or sour (Blair, 1990; Christianson, 1990). A diminished sense of taste may result in a decline in adequate dietary intake. COTAs may focus treatment on planning and preparing meals, encouraging elders to try good-tasting foods and maintain a nutritional diet.

Olfactory. Olfactory function declines approximately 40% with aging. Olfactory receptors are located in the upper portion of the nasal cavity. Although these receptors show some deterioration with age, a reduction in ability to smell does not necessarily occur. However, elders have difficulty distinguishing between pleasant and unpleasant odors.

COTA interventions may focus on ensuring home safety and making elders aware of their declining abilities to smell smoke, gas, and spoiling foods. Elders should be instructed to change batteries in smoke detectors regularly and check appliances visually. The "on" and "off" positions on appliances should be clearly marked. Regularly cleaning the refrigerator and marking dates on leftovers may help prevent elders from consuming spoiled food. Another area of concern may be personal hygiene. A diminished olfactory sense may cause elders to be unaware of body odors. COTAs can help elders create a schedule of laundering and bathing days.

Tactile. Reduction in tactile sensitivity in the fingertips, palms, and lower extremities is common (Verillo, 1980). According to recent research the relationship between increasing age and a decrease in tactile discrimination apparently cannot be attributed to mechanical changes of the skin but may be a result of changes in the nervous system affecting speed, quantity, or quality of information processing (Woodard, 1993). An elder may experience a general inability to perceive heat, cold, and touch.

COTAs must address any safety issues that arise from decreased sensation. COTAs can use activities such as cooking to demonstrate safety with sharp objects, stove use, and water temperature. Depending on severity of sensation loss, elders can use a temperature gauge to prevent burns with liquids.

Kinesthetic. Kinesthesia is the sense of movement and balance. It involves the ability to perceive changes in body position and orientation. This ability decreases with age. Neurological and neuromuscular aging changes lead to disturbances in kinesthesia (Dubin, 1992). An elder experiencing kinesthetic changes has a decreased ability to determine when and in what direction the head is moving and therefore may experience a sensation of falling (Christianson, 1990; Hasselkus, 1974). The sense of vibration in the extremities may also be lost (Whanger, 1974).

Because kinesthetic decline may contribute to falls, COTAs should instruct elders, caregivers, and family members to remove rugs and clutter from walking areas and keep rooms well lit. (Chapter 16 provides more details on mobility and safety issues.)

CASE STUDY

Agnes is an 80-year-old woman who was recently discharged from an acute care hospital after a short stay. She has had recurring admissions as a result of complications from diabetes. Kim is a COTA working for a home care agency. She provides OT services for Agnes. In addition to Agnes' medical condition, the normal aging process has limited her ability to live safely and independently.

Several adaptations have been made to Agnes' home. Her phone has been amplified for clarity of conversations. The telephone also has large numbers to facilitate making calls. Frequently used telephone numbers have been preprogrammed into the phone for quicker access in emergencies. The home has been cleared of clutter and a few grab bars have been added to the shower. Kim (the COTA) further adapted the bathroom by adding a grab bar next to the toilet. Agnes' family purchased a shower chair, and Kim trained them to assist Agnes with bathing. Agnes' daughter comes by periodically to help with cleaning, laundry, and shopping.

Kim plans to begin working with Agnes on kitchen safety. Agnes has had a small kitchen fire and the family has noticed several burnt pans, suggesting that Agnes forgets about items on the stove or to turn off burners. Kim will probably refer Agnes to Meals on Wheels and recommend cooking food in a microwave oven rather than on the stove.

Agnes enjoys spending time working in her garden. While Agnes demonstrated this activity, Kim noticed that the deck and stairs were in disrepair and that a handrail was needed. Kim referred Agnes to the Senior Job Center for repair services at low or no cost. Finally, with Agnes' agreement, Kim arranged for a social worker to visit and discuss other available community services that may help Agnes keep living in her own home.

CHAPTER REVIEW QUESTIONS

1 Based on the case study, name the primary losses of aging Agnes has experienced and the interventions that Kim provided for them.

2 In what ways did Kim involve Agnes' family in her therapy?

3 Explain the differences between primary and secondary aging.

4 Summarize primary and secondary changes and describe possible functional implications of these changes for each of the following: cognition and skin, cardiopulmonary, skeletal, muscular, neurological, and sensory systems.

REFERENCES

Blair K: Aging: physiological aspects and clinical implications, *Nurse Pract* 15:14, 1990.

Boss B: Normal aging in the nervous system: implications for SCI nurses, *SCI Nurs* 8:42, 1991.

Buono M, McKenzie B, Kasch F: Effects on aging and physical training on the peripheral sweat gland, *Age Ageing* 20:439, 1991.

Carruthers C: *Functional movement themes of the elderly to transfer on and off the bed.* unpublished doctoral dissertation, Minneapolis, 1995, University of Minnesota.

Castelo-Branco C et al: Relationship between skin collagen and bone changes during aging, *Maturitas* 18:199, 1994.

Chtristianson M: Aging in the designed environment, *Phys Occup Ther Geriatrics* 8:1, 1990.

DeVries H: Physiological effects of an exercise training regimen upon men aged 52-88, *J Gerontol* 25:325, 1970.

Dubin S: The physiologic changes of aging, *Orthopaed Nurs*, 11:45, 1992.

Einkauf D et al: Changes in spinal mobility with increasing age in women, *Phys Ther* 67:370, 1987.

Fisher N, Pendergast D, Calkins E: Muscle rehabilitation in impaired elderly nursing home residents, *Arch Phys Med Rehabil* 72:181, 1991.

Frolkis V, Martynenko O, Zamostyan V: Aging of the neuromuscular apparatus, *Gerontol* 22: 244, 1976.

Gasho J, Fanelli C, Zelis R: Aging reduces distensibility and the venodilatory response to nitroglycerin in normal subjects, *Am J Cardiol* 63:1267, 1989.

Gribbin K, Schaie K, Parham I: Complexities of the life style and maintenance of intellectual abilities, *J Soc Iss* 36:47, 1980.

Hall D: *The aging of connective tissue*, Orlando, 1976, Academic Press.

Hasselkus B, Shambes G: Aging and postural sway in women, *J Gerontol* 30:661, 1975.

Hertzog C, Schiae K, Gibbon K: Cardiovascular disease and changes in intellectual functioning from middle to old age, *J Gerontol* 33: 872, 1978.

Hooyman N, Kiyak H: *Social gerontology: a multi-disciplinary perspective*, Needham, MA, 1988, Allyn and Bacon.

Kane R, Ouslander J, Abrass I: *Essentials of clinical geriatrics*, New York, 1989, McGraw-Hill.

Kitzman D et al: Age-related changes in normal human hearts during the first 10 decades of life, Part II (Maturity): a quantitative anatomic study of 765 specimens from 20 to 99 years old, *Mayo Clin Proc* 63:137, 1988.

Kuhn J, McGovern M: Respiratory assessment of the elderly, *J Gerontol Nurs* 18:40, 1992.

Lewis S: *The mature years: a geriatric occupational therapy text*, Thorofare, NJ, 1979, Slack.

Lim K, Zipursky R, Watts M, Pfefferbaum A: Decrease gray matter in normal aging: an in vivo magnetic resonance study, *J Gerontol* 47:B26, 1992.

Lyden J, McGinley K, Grove G: Age-related differences in the rate of desquamation of skin surface cells. In Adelman RD, Roberts J, Christafalo V, editors: *Pharmacological interventions in the aging process*, New York, 1978, Plenum Press.

McFarland R, Fisher M: Alteration in dark adaptations as a function of age, *J Gerontol* 3:131, 1984.

Pierce W et al: Aortic diameter as a function of age, gender and body surface area, *Surgery*, 114:691, 1993.

Rockstein M, Sussman M: *Biology of aging*, Belmont, Ca, 1979, Wadsworth.

Schaie K: Midlife influences upon intellectual functioning in old age, *Int J Behav Dev* 7:463, 1984.

Schaie K: The hazards of cognitive aging, *Gerontologist* 29:484, 1989.

Schaie K: The Seattle longitudinal studies of adult intelligence, *Am Psychol Soc* 2:171, 1993.

Schaie K, Willis S: Can intellectual decline in the elderly be reversed? *Dev Psychol* 22:223, 1986.

Seals D et al: Endurance training in older men and women, *J App Physiol* 57:1024, 1984.

Spirduso W et al: Exercise effects on aged motor function, *Ann N Y Acad Sci* 575:363,1988.

Trombly C: *Occupational therapy for physical dysfunction*, ed 4, Baltimore, 1995, Williams & Wilkins.

Verillo R: Age-related changes in the sensitivity to vibration, *J Gerontol* 35:185, 1980.

Vitto J: Connective tissue biochemistry of the aging dermis: Age-related alterations in collagen and elastin, *Dermatol Clin* 4:433, 1986.

Welford A: Causes of slowing performance with age, *Interdisc Top Gerontol* 11:43, 1977.

Whanger A, Wang H: Clinical correlates of the vibratory sense in elderly psychiatric patients, *J Gerontol* 29:39, 1974.

Woodward K: The relationship between skin compliance, age gender and tactile discriminative thresholds in humans, *Somatosens Mot Res* 10:63, 1993.

Psychological Aspects of Aging

YOLANDA GRIFFITHS

KEY TERMS

stressors, loss, coping skills, adaptations, learned helplessness

CHAPTER OBJECTIVES

1. Identify myths and facts about psychological aspects of aging.
2. Identify common stressors, changes, and losses to which elders must adapt.
3. Discuss common emotional problems that may accompany losses.
4. Discuss coping skills and interventions that promote healthy transition with age.

Physical milestones measure a person's age in years, but indications of mental aging are less clear. Learning about the psychological aspects of aging enhances the COTA's ability to deal effectively and empathetically with elders. This chapter explores several key concepts about the psychology of aging and includes discussion of what it feels like to be old and lose hope.

MYTHS AND FACTS ABOUT AGING

The way elders are perceived significantly affects the way they are treated. Stereotypes are rigid concepts, exaggerated images, and inaccurate judgments used to make generalizations about groups of people. Positive and negative stereotypes create false images of aging.

Western civilization often produces negative views of aging (Butler, Lewis, Sunderland, 1991). Advertisements often focus on and emphasize youth and characterize elders as frail, nonproductive, agitated, and forgetful. Following are some myths of the psychological aspects of aging.

MYTH 1
CHRONOLOGICAL AGE DETERMINES THE WAY AN ELDER ACTS AND FEELS

Melissa, a COTA, receives a referral to see Mr. Jann, who is 89 years of age. Melissa has images of an elderly, cranky man sitting in a chair with his head bowed, responding in a belligerent way about receiving treatment. Melissa enters the room of the nursing home that Mr. Jann shares with Mr. Barrow. The room is filled with sports mementos from both their respective grandchildren. Mr. Barrow taps Melissa's shoulder and says, "If you're looking for Mr. Jann, he's in the sun room teaching dance lessons. You have to get up pretty early to catch up with Mr. Jann or he'll leave you in the dust!"

Natural responses to actual losses, expected reactions to one's own aging process and death, and predictable emotional reactions to physical illness are separate aspects of aging. Some elders do believe that their minds will deteriorate along with their bodies. The biological aspects of aging can be predicted; however, the aging process varies. The truth is that elders are in a time of transition.

MYTH 2
YOU CAN'T TEACH AN OLD DOG NEW TRICKS

The applause is thunderous as the graduates walk across the stage. It is a very special day for both Jennifer and Marion Meyer as they receive their Master of Science degrees in counseling. Marion Myer is 77 years of age. Jennifer is her 32-year-old granddaughter. Jennifer was a COTA for several years and assisted her grandmother with lifestyle changes after Marion experienced a heart attack. Marion often expressed regret about not going to college. Jennifer encouraged Marion to follow her dreams of furthering her education.

The ability to learn does not decline with age (Figure 4-1). According to Erp and Freeman (1971), adults learn differently than children because of physical characteristics, learning styles, reaction time, interests, motivation, attitudes, and values. Elders do not perform as well as children when a learning task requires speed of performance and fine motor coordination. However, elders may perform better than children when the learning task requires judgment, vocabulary, or understanding, which are all based on experience.

Biological changes may also affect learning. For example, elders may be unable to sit for long periods because of back or hip problems. Elders may tire quickly and demonstrate decreased physical stamina. As a result of poor vision or hearing skills, elders may not accurately process all sensory information. Elders may need additional time to organize and process new information. People may quickly assume that an elder is confused when the information recalled seems jumbled or inaccurate. However, the elder may not know that the information processing was erroneous.

Elders who feel threatened by new situations may have poor self-confidence in learning situations. New situations require decision making and risk taking. Elders may avoid learning opportunities that may result in embar-

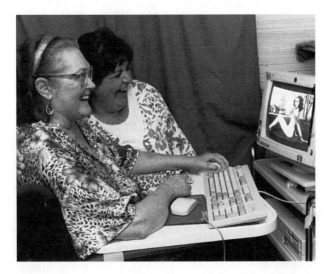

FIGURE 4-1 Learning ability does not diminish with age.

rassment, frustration, or conflict. In times of **stress,** elders may be less flexible in problem solving and rely on set ways of dealing with situations. Ultimately the elder must want to learn, be willing to recognize any limitations, and want to try other learning techniques. Some elders view retirement as a time to try new things.

MYTH 3
AS YOU AGE, YOU NATURALLY BECOME OLDER AND WISER

It was most disturbing to Ellen that she could not remember what she was doing sometimes. After all, Ellen was a former professor of chemistry. Now her body seemed slower and her mind so forgetful. Her forgetfulness started with little things like losing her keys and progressed to forgetting the road home after driving to the store. Finally one day Ellen broke down in tears in the grocery store parking lot, unable to recall the kind of car she owned. What was happening? Her husband feared that Ellen was suffering from early stages of Alzheimer's disease. Neither Ellen nor her husband could understand the reason this was happening, especially because Ellen had always been so active. Ellen was only 65 years of age. She was an accomplished author and lecturer and prided herself on her intellectual abilities.

Positive stereotyping can be as detrimental as negative stereotyping. In old age, adaptation and learning take place against a backdrop of experience (Erp, Freeman, 1971). Unrealistic expectations that elders can and should continue to perform as they did when they were younger may cause an elder to feel like a failure.

Intelligence does not decline with age. Studies done in the 1920s by Bayley and Bradway indicate that IQ scores increase until the twenties, then level off and remain unchanged until late in life (Butler, Lewis, Sunderland, 1991). The concepts of crystallized and fluid intelligence were introduced by Horn and Cattell (1966). Crystallized intelligence is a result of experience and increases throughout a person's life. Fluid intelligence is biological and subjective to the process of aging.

Stating that all elders will be wiser or that all elders will become senile is impossible. These contradictory statements prove that elders cannot be lumped into one homogeneous group. Brain cells do not replicate; however, continued intellectual stimulation inhibits the decline in intellectual abilities with aging.

MYTH 4
ELDERS ARE NOT PRODUCTIVE, ESPECIALLY AT WORK

Initially, all the young employees at the local burger place called the new employment program "adopt a geezer." Jim, the manager and owner of a thriving fast food restaurant located across from the high school, often came home and complained to his wife about the unreliability of many of the youth he hired to fill the shifts. Jim said that "it was as if the kids just wanted the paycheck and had no real concern about the quality of their work."

Jim's wife, Candace, a COTA who worked 3 days a week at the senior citizen center, suggested a mutually beneficial program that would financially help elders who were interested and capable of fulfilling a part-time position. Jim would be able to fill shifts open during the school day with steady, reliable help.

To the amazement of the young employees, the elder employees were efficient and demonstrated stamina. In fact, the young employees often remarked, "They're cool!"

According to Erp and Freeman (1971), a work ethic often shapes people's feelings about themselves in terms of usefulness, productivity, personal satisfaction, and social interaction. Retirement creates changes in a person's life. The psychological adaptation to the new role of retiree can be either dreaded or embraced. For some elders, retirement is anticipated as a withdrawal from traditional, stressful workday events. After retirement, elders often seek new areas of employment. They are capable of learning new skills and effectively solving problems in new situations (Figures 4-2 and 4-3).

Retirement is sometimes a paradox when elders may have time and energy but lack financial means to be active. On the other hand, they may have the financial means but feel less physically energetic to engage in new activities.

In addition, contact with familiar friends through work may lessen. COTAs can help retired elders create a plan for managing added leisure hours (Figure 4-4).

MYTH 5
ELDERS BECOME MORE CONSERVATIVE AS THEY AGE

Organizing a neighborhood petition to get an overpass built over the busy street next to the elementary school was the last thing Meg thought she would be doing on her 80th birthday. But here she was in the midst of neighbors and community workers stacking flyers, affixing petition forms to clipboards, and filling out a shift schedule. For years, Meg had observed many close calls when children crossing the street were almost hit by automobiles. Meg thought, "I could never forgive myself if one of those kids got hurt and I just sat here and watched from my front window."

Contrary to myth, many elders are receptive to new ideas. In fact, many elders become more politically active and even seek political office to initiate social change (Figure 4-5). Adaptation to change depends on the level of success a person has had with previous life changes. Personality traits contribute to the ability to adapt and learn new things (Erp, Freeman, 1971). Developmental psychologists note that personality continues to develop as individuals deal with crisis points in each phase of life. If crisis situations are effectively resolved, persons add to their repertoires of adaptive skills.

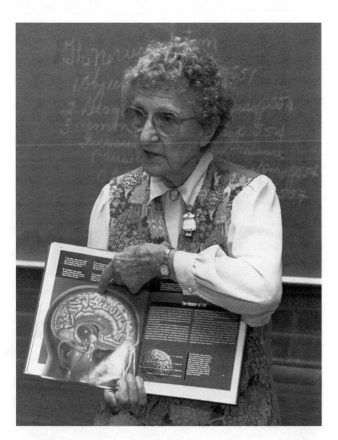

FIGURE 4-2   Elders often seek new areas of employment.

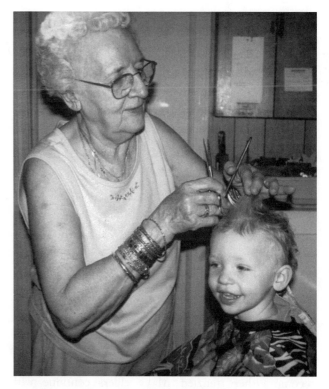

FIGURE 4-3   Some elders remain productive at work. (Courtesy Helene Lohman, Omaha, Neb.)

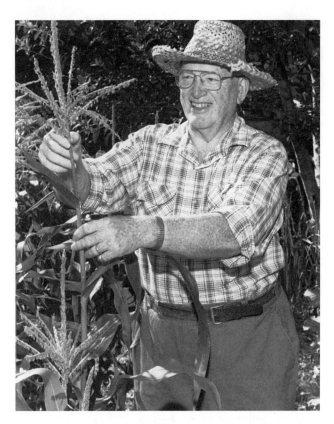

FIGURE **4-4** With added leisure hours elders must consider a new plan for managing time.

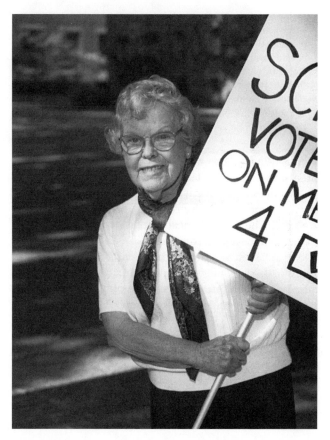

FIGURE **4-5** Many elders become politically active to initiate social change.

MYTH 6
ELDERS PREFER QUIET AND TRANQUIL DAILY LIVES

Tina looked around the reception area of Applewood Manor on her first day of work as a COTA. Only the sounds of a television murmuring the chant of a daily game show and the shuffling of residents down the hall broke the silence. The head nurse, Mrs. Kessler, walked up to Tina and said, "Isn't it wonderful how quiet and peaceful it is here? We work very hard to preserve a sense of tranquility in the sunset years of one's life."

Tina interviewed all the residents during the week to determine activities she could develop based on their interests. Not surprisingly, more than half the residents wanted less sedentary activities than they currently experienced. Some even wanted organized sports like tennis. Other residents wanted a piano and perhaps a jazz hour scheduled (Figure 4-6).

Another incorrect generalization is that all elders prefer a sedentary lifestyle. An elder who has experienced a rather staid and uneventful life before retirement will not necessarily continue that type of lifestyle. Elders often move in with their children's families, and their lives may become rather frenzied. Many elders continue with vibrant lifestyles and do not sit awaiting death. Staying active is a key to healthy psychological aging.

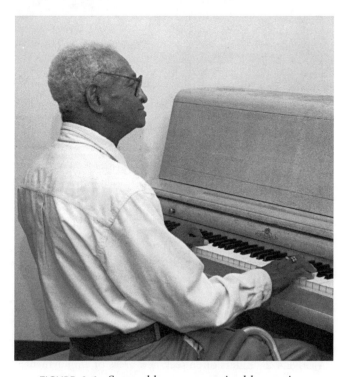

FIGURE **4-6** Some elders are energized by music.

MYTH 7
ALL ELDERS BECOME SENILE

Harry has always been a proud, independent man. He was decorated twice in World War II. After experiencing a heart attack, Harry adjusted to the many lifestyle changes that were suggested by the health care team. Today Harry sighed as he walked with multiple pieces of paper toward the receptionist in the Occupational Therapy department. This was the third stop in a confusing, mazelike journey inside the Veterans' Administration Hospital. The hospital was under another reorganization, and procedures for appointments had changed. Previously, Harry always called for an appointment, showed up characteristically 10 minutes early, and cheerfully greeted the young COTA who assisted with the treatments. Today a young man at the front desk rattled off multiple instructions about the new procedures and handed Harry a photocopied map of the building along with the new forms to be completed. Harry was still trying to understand where he was supposed to go according to the map. He asked the young man to slowly repeat the instructions, but the young man only repeated himself in a louder tone and pointed Harry in the direction of the elevators. The young man muttered, "These senile old guys . . . . ."

When elders appear confused or require more time to understand directions, misunderstandings often result. Getting older is not synonymous with feeble-mindedness or imbecility.

Brain damage may be evident as a result of physical illness. However, *senility* is a label often used inaccurately to describe specific psychosocial diagnoses with which elders may be dealing, such as depression, grief, anxiety, dementia, and Alzheimer's disease. People age at different rates. Butler, Lewis, and Sunderland (1991) indicated that people become more diverse with age rather than more similar.

STRESSORS, LOSSES, AND EMOTIONS ASSOCIATED WITH AGING

Elders often must deal with major life crises such as retirement, **loss** of spouse, economic changes, residence relocation, physical illness, loss of friends, and the reality of mortality. Lieberman and Tobin (1983) found that "events that lead to loss and require a major disruption to customary modes of behavior seem to be the most stressful for elders." Hayslip (1983) identified the following personal factors that may influence stressors: flexibility, recognition of personal needs and limits, internal locus of control, perceived family support, and willingness to acknowledge feelings about death and dying (Box 4-1).

Christiansen (1991) indicated that certain life events are more stressful and contribute more than others to poor health. The Holmes and Rahe Social Readjustment Scale identifies life events ranked in terms of relative stress to an individual. Life events affect individuals differently depending on circumstance, duration, and previous **coping skills** among other factors. More recent

---

BOX 4-1

Stressors that Affect Elders

Social stressors
Death of a loved one
Ill spouse-caretaking
Family members moving away
Move to live with family members
Retirement
Relocation to a nursing home because of illness
Loss of worker role

Physical stressors
Serious illness
Cumulative sensory losses
Sexual problems
Chronic conditions that reduce mobility or self-care

Cultural stressors
Negative stereotyping of elders
Health care policy management

Personal stressors
Diminished finances
Grief
Loneliness
Anger
Guilt
Depression
Anxiety
Reality of own death

Data from MacDonald KC, Davis LJ: Psychopathology and aging. In Davis L, Kirkland M, editors: *The role of occupational therapy with the elderly (ROTE)*, Rockville, Md, 1988, The American Occupational Therapy Association.

---

studies have attempted to measure other aspects of life events and stress levels. COTAs must consider the ways various life events affect elders to understand what motivates certain behaviors.

The support an elder receives with the death of a loved one often diminishes to a large extent after the burial. The reality of the loss may not occur until later, when the elder is alone. The survivor may grieve over the loss of finances and possible change in residence, social status, or role associated with the death of the loved one. The grieving elder may also experience a form of guilt known as "death survival guilt" (Chodoff, 1963).

Loneliness is a form of emotional isolation. Elders may experience increased social isolation with retirement, as family members relocate, or as friends move or die. Social interactions with pets, weekly church services, grocery shopping trips, or occasional visits from family members may not be emotionally fulfilling enough for an elder (Figure 4-7). COTAs can assist in exploring

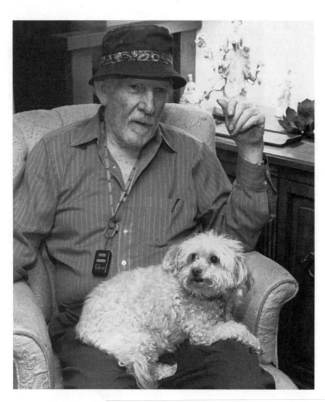

FIGURE 4-7 Interaction with pets only may not be emotionally fulfilling for some elders.

BOX 4-2

Stressors Associated with Physical Illness Common to Elders

- Threat to life
- Loss of body integrity
- Change in self-concept
- Threat to future plans
- Change in social roles
- Change in routine activities
- Loss of autonomy

- Need to make critical decisions rapidly
- Loss of emotional equilibrium
- Physical discomfort
- Monotony and boredom
- Fear of medical procedures

Adapted from Davis L: Coping with illness. In Davis L, Kirkland M, editors: *The role of occupational therapy with the elderly (ROTE)*, Rockville, Md, 1988a, The American Occupational Therapy Association.

and structuring additional social interaction experiences in the community.

Elders may become reclusive and socially paralyzed with anxiety as a result of increasing neighborhood violence. Increasing anger is a common emotional problem experienced by many elders as they feel a loss of control over their lives. Elders may be viewed as cantankerous or verbally aggressive when in fact they may be expressing feelings of helplessness with angry words.

Elders may need to cope with a chronic disease or a serious physical illness. Davis (1988) notes that unexpected illness is a catastrophic stressor. The unexpected illness may be debilitating to the elder in terms of independence and self-care. A chronic illness is no less stressful; however, the elder may have adapted to the illness more gradually. (Box 4-2 lists stressors associated with common physical illnesses of elders.)

An elder person copes with physical illness through a psychosocial process. A negative perception of the situation and a hopeless attitude will adversely affect the way a person deals with the illness. Cohen and Larazus pointed out that those elders who view a physical illness as a challenge cope better than those who view it as a punishment (Davis, 1988).

A grief process in dealing with any illness is to be expected. Elisabeth Kübler-Ross (1969) identified five stages to the grief process: denial, anger, depression, bargaining, and acceptance. This grief process may not be linear; that is, the elder may become depressed and then become angry or deny the situation again before accepting the illness.

An elder's ability to **adapt** is contingent on physical health, personality, life experiences, and level of social support (Butler, Lewis, Sunderland, 1991). Several important adaptive tasks an elder must accomplish to successfully deal with a chronic condition are as follows:

- Recognize permanent changes such as diet, lifestyle, work habits, or exercise that may promote recovery
- Mentally deal with losses caused by the illness
- Accept a new self-image
- Identify and express feelings such as anger, fear, and guilt
- Seek out and maintain social support from family and friends

COTAs can help an elder deal with a chronic illness in the following ways:

- Reduce the fears about the illness through education
- Listen and be sensitive to the feelings expressed verbally and nonverbally
- Provide encouragement
- Assist in the development of creative yet realistic ways for elders to gain more control over their illnesses or losses associated with an illness
- Identify ways to reduce stress and promote social support
- Surround the elder who has moved to a nursing care facility as a result of the illness with familiar objects, which may help maintain a sense of continuity, provide comfort and security, and aid memory

Learned Helplessness

When elders perceive that they have no control over a particular outcome, they may give up hope (Solomon, 1982). Health care workers and family members often contribute to this state of **learned helplessness** in the following ways:

- Expecting elders to be unable to do for themselves and completing tasks for them, thereby promoting dependence
- Imposing routines on elders for the sake of convenience, such as giving them a bath at 2:00 PM
- Showing a negative attitude by making condescending remarks about physical appearance or handling the elder callously with transfers
- Perpetuating the sick role

Learned helplessness often results when the elder becomes depressed and feels a marked lack of self-esteem. Elders who have already experienced multiple physical losses may feel a lack of control over their bodies and environments (Teitelman, 1990). Elders may be passive, apathetic, and depressed and demonstrate a lack of motivation for tasks. Increased feelings of vulnerability also contribute to learned helplessness (Foy, Mitchell, 1990). COTAs must encourage independence and self-care activities. As elders regain a feeling of competence, learned helplessness can be reversed.

CONCLUSION

Old age can be a happy time of self-reflection and exploration of new interests. It can also be a time of dealing with great losses and severe stress. Changes occur throughout the lifespan, and the way a person copes with changes and adapts to transitions ultimately determines the ability to psychologically cope with aging. By gaining awareness of the different stressors and losses associated with aging and understanding the ways elders cope with serious illnesses, COTAs can help elders enhance their aging experiences.

CASE STUDY

Mrs. Brown is a 68-year-old woman who recently became a widow after almost 50 years of marriage. Mr. Brown had been the primary financial support for the couple. Mrs. Brown never worked outside the home; being a wife and mother was her whole life.

Mr. Brown had been diagnosed and treated for pancreatic cancer before his death. Much of their life savings were depleted by health costs and major home repairs. Mrs. Brown spent the last year taking care of her husband. Her daughter lives 6 hours away, but her son, who is married, lives in the same town. Mrs. Brown and her daughter-in-law have a turbulent relationship. Her son and daughter-in-law are expecting their third child in a few months.

Mrs. Brown worries about finances and wonders whether she will be able to continue living in her current neighborhood, which has become more unsafe in the last few years. She has been experiencing shortness of breath and is concerned about who will care for her if she should become seriously ill.

Mrs. Brown does not drive and depends on a neighbor to take her grocery shopping. The Browns had two sets of close friends, but they moved away to be near their grandchildren. Mrs. Brown's son invited his mother to move in with his family, but Mrs. Brown adamantly refused.

Consider Mrs. Brown's case and answer the following questions:

1. Identify the losses Mrs. Brown has experienced.
2. Describe the stressors or emotional problems that may be related to these losses.
3. Identify interventions the COTA could use to help Mrs. Brown deal with these losses.

EXERCISES

INTO AGING

This is a commercially available game that focuses on building empathy for those who are growing old. The manual describes the game as a way for players to increase awareness of elders' problems by simulating experiences with similar problems, such as loss, isolation, powerlessness, dependency on others, and ageism. This game is available through Slack Incorporated, 6900 Grove Road, Thorofare, New Jersey, 08086.

ROLE PLAYING

This is a useful activity for groups to understand aging-related issues. In preparation for the activity, each of the myths of aging discussed in this chapter should be written on index cards. Each small group will be given a set of index cards. Members of each group then role play some of the myths and stereotypes associated with the psychological aspects of aging. Each role play should be followed with a discussion of feelings and thoughts about the stereotype or myth.

STEREOTYPE EXERCISE

Each member of a group should list the first six or seven images that immediately come to mind with the word *elder*. Group members should think about advertisements, movies, and personal experiences that influence their perceptions of elders. Each member should share the images with the group and explain the reasons the images are so vivid. All group members should discuss whether the images are realistic or stereotypical. Group members should brainstorm different ways to change stereotypical images to make them more realistic.

FIELD TRIP IMAGERY

Place yourself comfortably in a quiet room. You may sit in a comfortable chair or lie down. Take three deep breaths. As you exhale, clear your mind of any concerns and concentrate on the directions. Give yourself permission to use the next 10 to 15 minutes to explore what it would feel like to be 75 years old.

Pretend that you are looking into a large mirror. Imagine your physical appearance at age 75. What physical changes have taken place? Do you need any assistance with self-care? What emotions are you experiencing as a result of these changes?

What changes have occurred in your living arrangements? Do you live alone? Identify any changes in lifestyle as a result of finances.

What have you accomplished in your life thus far? Do you regret any events? Do you regret not achieving certain goals? Are you satisfied with your life?

Remember what you have just experienced with the visual imagery. Now slowly count to 10. As you get closer to 10, you will become more awake and tuned to the sounds of the room you are in. When you reach 10, gently open your eyes.

Free write for the next 5 minutes. It may be poetry, prose, or just phrases of what you remember of your visual imagery trip to age 75.

◼ CHAPTER REVIEW QUESTIONS

1 Does chronological aging determine psychological aging? Discuss your position.

2 Identify aspects of aging that may affect learning for elders.

3 Coping with a serious illness can be especially stressful for an elder. Discuss why and how COTAs can assist.

4 What is learned helplessness and what can COTAs do to reverse it?

REFERENCES

Butler R, Lewis M, Sunderland T: *Aging and mental health*, New York, 1991, McMillan.

Christiansen C: Performance deficits as sources of stress. In Christiansen C, Baum C, editors: *Occupational therapy: overcoming human performance deficits*, Thorofare, NJ, 1991, SLACK.

Chodoff P: Late effects of the concentration camp syndrome, *Arch Gen Psychiatry* 9:323, 1963.

Davis L: Coping with illness. In Davis L, Kirkland M, editors: *The role of occupational therapy with the elderly (ROTE)*, Rockville, Md, 1988, The American Occupational Therapy Association.

Erp SH, Freeman JD: *Aging: psychological changes*, Corvallis, Ore, 1971, Continuing Education Publications.

Foy SS, Mitchell MM: Factors contributing to learned helplessness, *Phys Occup Ther Geriatr* 9(2):1, 1990.

Hayslip B: *The aged patient: a sourcebook for the allied health professional*, St. Louis, 1983, Mosby–Year Book.

Horn JL, Cattell RB: Age differences in primary mental ability factors, *J Gerontol* 21:210, 1966.

Kübler-Ross E: *On death and dying*, New York, 1969, Macmillan.

Lieberman MA, Tobin SS: *The experience of old age*, New York, 1983, Basic Books.

MacDonald K, Davis L: Psychopathology and aging. In Davis L, Kirkland M, editors: *The role of occupational therapy with the elderly (ROTE)*, Rockville, Md, 1988, The American Occupational Therapy Association.

Solomon K: Social antecedents of learned helplessness in the health care setting, *Gerontologist* 22(3):282, 1982.

Teitelman JL: Eliminating learned helplessness in older rehabilitation patients, *Phys Occup Ther Geriatr* 9(2):43, 1990.

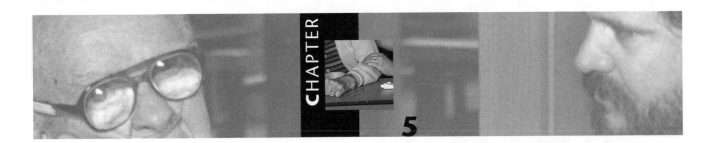

Aging Well: The COTA as Change Agent in Health Promotion and Disease Prevention

CLAUDIA GAYE PEYTON

KEY TERMS

health, occupation, wellness, occupational form, occupational performance, health promotion, disuse syndrome, prevention, primary prevention, secondary prevention, health and risk screening, tertiary prevention

CHAPTER OBJECTIVES

1. Discuss the value of health and wellness promotion and disease prevention to OT practice with well and institutionalized elders.
2. Identify methods of screening and assessment used in promoting health among elders.
3. Describe health promotion activities that can be incorporated into practice with elders.
4. Describe theoretic models that emphasize the importance of occupational form to the integration of healthy life patterns and performance.

5. Explain the reasons and demonstrate the ways health promotion and disease and disability prevention are instrumental in changing the future of OT practice at all levels.
6. Discuss the ways disuse syndrome contributes to the incidence and prevalence of preventable diseases and disabilities common to elderly populations.
7. Identify factors that contribute most to influencing elders to participate in wellness-focused activities.

> *"Grow young along with me!*
> *The best is yet to be,*
> *The last of life for which*
> *The first is made."*
> (Adapted from Robert Browning by Ashley Montagu, 1981)

Al is an 87-year-old man who hopes to live to see the turn of the century or maybe even to be 100; his wife Irene is 77 years of age and is content to have a few quiet hours each day to read and write letters. Al and Irene have been

married for 56 years and have three adult children. They moved into a retirement housing area last year to ensure a safe living arrangement for whichever of the two lived longer. Al and Irene moved from their home of over 40 years to this new environment with the help of a family friend.

After moving into their new home, Al and Irene often complained of feeling tired. Over the next few months, they organized their lives in their new setting. They laughed and talked about getting to know some of their

37

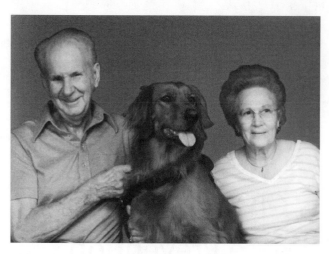

FIGURE 5-1   Al, Chelsea, and Irene. (Courtesy Olan Mills.)

new neighbors. Overall the move went well, and Al and Irene experienced the usual trials of adjusting to change.

These two people are some of America's fortunate well elders. They are not without challenges, however. Al has been totally blind since 22 years of age. He had a cranial subdural hematoma removed from the left side of his brain and was recently treated with radiation therapy for prostate cancer. Irene had several surgeries over the past 15 years, including a heart double bypass, cataract surgery, a hip replacement, a rotator cuff repair, and gallbladder removal.

These two elders enjoy a remarkable level of independence, given their ages and medical histories. Some of this level of independence and relatively good health is a result of genetic endowment. In addition, lifestyle changes or other factors contributing to good health such as regular exercise and a balanced, low-fat diet have influenced independence. Historically, Al and Irene have not lived without health risk. Both smoked for some time but eventually quit; he at 55 years and she at 52 years. They agreed to adjust their diets based on some research Al had read about the positive effects of reducing fat intake. Their dietary habits changed approximately 28 years ago. About that same time, Al began walking regularly. Initially, he experienced pain from angina, which required him to stop walking, rest, and take nitroglycerin tablets prescribed by his doctor. After several weeks of daily walking and taking the prescribed medication, Al could finally complete a trip around the block without interruption. He increased the daily walks to eventually complete 2 miles each day, which he continues to maintain. At the age of 84 he went to guide-dog training school for 3 weeks to be suited with a new guide dog because his previous dog died. His new guide dog, Chelsea, helps Al stay independent and mobile. Irene often accompanies Al and Chelsea on their daily walk (Figure 5-1).

This story could be about anyone. The story itself depends to some extent on the health care choices that are

made. As health care providers, COTAs and OTRs can offer important health information and alternatives to elders. Society will increasingly look to health care providers for guidance and to model healthful ways of living. This chapter describes techniques for health promotion and disease or disability prevention with elders to enhance the COTA's understanding of the importance of promoting good health at all ages.

CONCEPTS OF HEALTH PROMOTION AND WELLNESS IN OCCUPATIONAL THERAPY PRACTICE

The historic roots of OT philosophy and practice demonstrate the profession's long-standing belief in the value of occupation in promoting health and preventing functional loss caused by disease. Nelson and Stucky (1992) reviewed important OT values over the decades and wrote, "The potency of occupation in promoting health has long been recognized; this recognition is the basis for the existence of the profession of occupational therapy." Since the inception of OT as a profession in 1917, its premise has been to promote a healthy balance of activities for those persons who seek treatment. Activities perceived by an individual to be meaningful occupations are believed to influence the state of actual or possible health and well-being. Gilfoyle (1986) stated, "The therapeutic use of occupation to promote fullness of life is the basic value at the heart of our (professional) culture." The concepts of **health** and **occupation** are interrelated. In spite of the various definitions and societal influences, the concept of occupation has remained centered on the value of activity to maintain enthusiasm about living. In essence, humans find meaning in what they do (Gilfoyle, 1986) (Figure 5-2).

The value of occupation and the meaning of health are explicitly interrelated (Yerxa, 1993; Nelson, Stucky, 1992; Riccio, Nelson, Bush, 1990; Speake, 1987; Johnson, 1986). As Nelson and Stucky (1992) described, "activation of function (occupation) is a main method of health promotion and disease prevention." Yerxa (1993) further described this relationship between occupation and health in her working definition of occupation:

> Occupations are units of activity which are classified and named by the culture according to the purposes they serve in enabling people to meet environmental challenges successfully.... Some essential characteristics of occupation are that it is self-initiated, goal directed (even if the goal is fun or pleasure), experiential as well as behavioral, socially valued or recognized, constructed of adaptive skills or repertoires, organized, essential to the quality of life experienced and possesses the capacity to influence health.

Filner and Williams (1992) suggested that *health* might be defined as "the ability to live and function effectively in society and to exercise self-reliance and autonomy to the maximum extent feasible, but not necessarily as total freedom from disease." Activity has profound positive

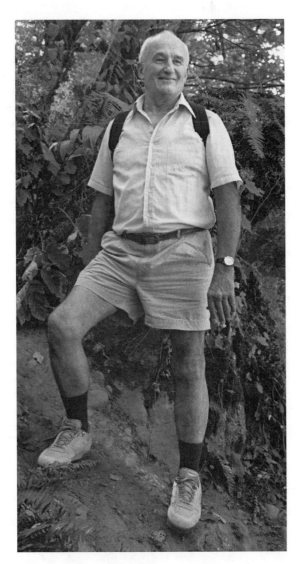

FIGURE 5-2 Activities perceived by an individual to be meaningful occupations are believed to influence the state of actual or perceived health.

effects on the lives of elders who are well and live in the community in addition to those who are frail and live in institutions. Habitual activities, those which are performed with consistency, have a profound influence on health. These activities limit both the occurrence and the progression of most disabling conditions. However, many elders have been typecast by society and health care professionals as being unable to improve their health. This myth is detrimental to the health and well-being of the elder population.

COTAs have a wonderful opportunity to influence change in the quality of the lives of elders by implementing activities. The use of activities has been the preferred method of health promotion and disease prevention for centuries. Greek societies, for example, believed deeply in the value and influence of active participation on health, and their religious celebrations were combined with participation in physical activities. Over the centuries these celebrations became known as the Olympics. Looking toward the 21st century, the need for health care reform, the urgency to reduce cost for care, and the necessity of returning the responsibility for health to the individual are evident. The time has come for OT practitioners to demonstrate leadership in planning health-promoting activities. Society is prepared to move from the medical model to a more health-centered, cost-effective approach to health care. In the medical model the disease state has taken priority over the person as a whole being. Thus people are often treated as an illness or a disability. For example, a hospital staff member may refer to an elder as "the total hip in room 420" rather than "Mrs. Smith." Not only has the medical model reduced the value of the human spirit to the cellular or disease level, it has also contributed dramatically to the cost of health care as a result of specialization. In contrast, **wellness** approaches and holistic theories consider people in the context of their lives.

Assisting people at all ages to participate actively in their health care is not unique to OT, but it has been central to OT practice concerns since the profession began. Political, economic, and practice environments need health professionals who understand that health can be enhanced and disease can be prevented through occupation. Mary Reilly stated in her Eleanor Clark Slagle Lecture in 1961 that "man through the use of his hands as energized by mind and will, can influence the state of his own health."

Health Risks and Their Effects On Occupational Performance

Substantial research evidence supports the need for increased health promotion and disease prevention activities for elders. Hickey and Stilwell (1991) maintain that the primary goal of health promotion programs for elders should be focused on prevention of "the progression of disease and the risks of disability and death . . . that health promotion should be designed to help older persons maintain their functional independence and autonomy for as long as possible."

As Fidler and Fidler once said, "As we do so we become. Through occupations, we adapt in healthy ways, or, through our occupations we maladapt in unhealthy ways" (Nelson, Stucky, 1992). In daily practice settings, COTAs and OTRs meet elders who have made choices to improve their health. Some elders do not recognize that the quality of their lives can change with even minor adjustments in their lifestyles. During daily therapeutic interactions, COTAs have an opportunity to influence their clients' considerations of healthy lifestyles and improve the quality of these elders' lives. Encouraging exploration of health-promoting activities and providing educational information to elders and their families may help motivate an elder to take actions that promote health and limit the potential debilitation associated with current habits. Elders are frequently uninformed or believe that changes later in life may offer few benefits. Helping elders understand the tremendous potential for physical regeneration that may come with even small amounts of change to routines can make the difference between future independence and debilitated dependence.

Nelson and Stucky (1992) suggested that "one's occupational patterns of self-care and interests comprise . . . occupational situations (occupational forms) that are health promoting and disease preventing." The **occupational form** Nelson and Stucky refer to is the environment the individual occupies, sometimes also referred to as a *context*. The context is composed of physical and sociocultural characteristics that stimulate the individual to choose **occupational performance.** For example, an elder who lives in a retirement village may choose to play golf (occupational form) because there is a golf course on the grounds (physical characteristic) and this is where most people at that village socialize (sociocultural characteristic). The value that the person places on the occupational form gives meaning and purpose to the individual's actions. This sense of purposefulness is the motivator or stimulus that results in participation in activities such as playing golf. Playing golf on Thursday mornings may involve many habitual occupational performance skills such as socialization, preparation of refreshments for guests, and the actual performance of playing golf. This involves motor performance, cognition, and other complex functions. Activation of an interest in and performance of a cherished occupation helps the person establish a positive continuous cycle or habit pattern. Fidler and Fidler theorized the existence of a link between imagery and purpose. In their view, action leading to achievement can be thought of as the product of a mental image that sets a goal (Nelson, Stucky, 1992). Thus mental imagery adds purpose to occupations. These mental images are constructed before taking the action and facilitate the person's participation (Figures 5-3 and 5-4).

The actual enjoyment of participation in chosen occupations or activities is referred to as *intrinsic motivation* (Florey, 1976). Baking a pie, walking a dog, and gardening are all activities that elicit intrinsic motivation. These actions provide feedback that inspires continued participation in that activity or other activities. Feedback may take the form of wonderful tomatoes from a well-nurtured garden or excitement from the completion of a small but meaningful project. Also, many external rewards result from other peoples' recognition and enjoyment. Each interaction sets up the potential for additional involvement in occupations that ultimately contribute to growth, development, self-confidence, and improved self esteem. Conversely, negative feedback or experiences may result in a cycle of feelings of helplessness, humiliation, and failure (Nelson, Stucky, 1992).

The outcome of effective **health promotion** is enhancement or maintenance of function in activities of daily living (ADL). The need for elders to maintain functional capacity has been demonstrated by research findings suggesting that losses occur in the ability to perform ADL functions as a result of the disabling effects of **disuse syndrome** and other common physical and cognitive disabilities. Approximately 23% of elders living in the community experience difficulty completing one or more ADLs because of health-related problems. Approxi-

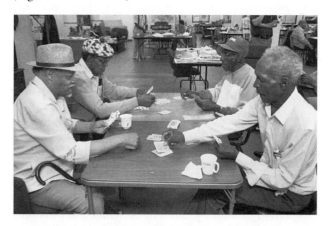

FIGURE 5-3 Purposefulness stimulates participation in activities such as the hobby of playing cards.

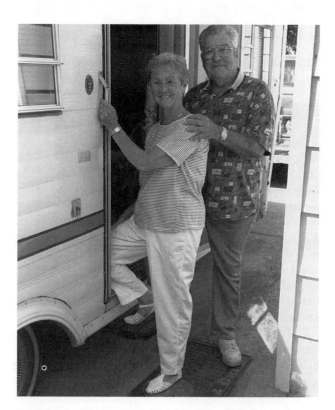

FIGURE 5-4 This couple finds pleasure in visiting new places.

mately 28% of elders report difficulties with instrumental activities of daily living (IADL), and 14% require assistance to complete IADL tasks. Research shows that the need for assistance increases with age (American Association of Retired Persons [AARP], 1995).

McMurdo and Rennie (1993) reported that elders in nursing homes who participated in a seated exercise group for 8 weeks showed significant improvement in grip strength, chair-to-stand time and ADLs, and experienced decreased depression. "Even very elderly residents of nursing homes can benefit from participation in regular seated exercise and can improve in functional capacity" (McMurdo, Rennie, 1993) (Figure 5-5).

The benefit of health promotion and disease **prevention** programs may be best understood by considering the most common risks to the health of elders. Physical and psychological risks to health and well-being, which are common to postretirement elders, are numerous. These risks include cardiovascular problems, hypertension, arthritis, osteoporosis, cancer, inadequate nutrition, lower levels of musculoskeletal flexibility and strength, diabetes, stroke, fall potential, and discomfort associated with anxiety and depression (Shephard, 1990). The AARP (1995) cites the following chronic conditions as those that most frequently "contribute to difficulty in independently performing activities of daily living (ADL) and instrumental activities of daily living (IADL) functions": arthritis, hypertension, heart disease, hearing impairment, cataracts, diabetes, tinnitus, and visual impairment.

Other authors suggest that the decline seen in aging

may not be caused by age but by a condition referred to as *disuse syndrome*. This term alludes to the detrimental effects of sedentary living and limited use of capabilities on the development of chronic and debilitating conditions. Approximately 50% of symptoms currently associated with aging such as increases in body fat and decreases in endurance, lean body mass, and strength and flexibility are actually a result of hypokinesia, a disease of disuse (Drinkwater, 1985; Smith, 1981; Shuster, 1995). Experimental immobilization has been noted to cause decreases in musculoskeletal, cardiovascular, and metabolic functions similar to those seen with aging. Thus a portion of the loss of physiological integrity in elders may be attributable to disuse syndrome (Fiatarone, Evans, 1990) (Box 5-1).

Prevention and Health Promotion Among Elders

COTAs who work with elders should be familiar with categories of prevention. Many health problems of elders

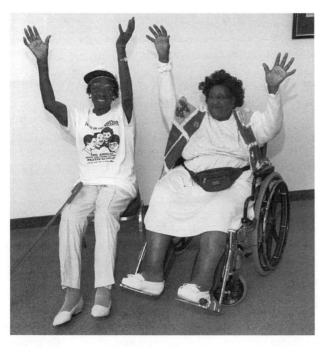

FIGURE 5-5 Elders can benefit from regular seated exercise.

BOX 5-1

Common Characteristics of Physiologic Aging and Disuse Syndrome

Decreases
- Total body water
- Bone mass
- Exercise capacity
- Muscle fiber (number and size)
- Muscle strength and flexibility
- Connective tissue elasticity
- Strength of bone
- Nerve conduction speed
- Visual acuity (near vision)
- Appetite
- Metabolic rate
- Glucose tolerance
- Insulin sensitivity
- Calcium uptake
- Lymphocyte response

Increases
- Fat mass
- Resting heart rate
- Venous pooling
- Intramuscular fat
- Anxiety
- Insomnia
- Depression
- Apathy and fatigue
- Sensitivity to temperature
- Levels of blood cholesterol

Data from Fiatarone MA, Evans JE: Exercise in the oldest old, *Top Geriatr Rehab* 5(2):63, 1990.

TABLE 5-1

Levels of Prevention

Definition	Strategies
Primary	
Includes general health promotion and specific disease protection	Immunization
	Accident prevention
	Exercise programs
Precedes disease or dysfunction and is applied to a population generally considered both physically and emotionally healthy	Nutritional education
	Smoking and alcohol cessation
	Exploration of leisure interests such as hobbies
Is performed to maintain health and prevent disease or the occurcence of disability*	
Secondary	
Emphasizes early detection and treatment to return the person to a healthy state as early as possible	Health screening
	Hypertension screening through monitoring blood pressure and nutritional evaluation
Averts or delays the consequences of advanced disease†	Identification of vision and hearing impairments
	Screening for colon, breast, cervical, and prostate cancer
	Observation for adverse medication effects (iatrogenic)
	Screening for excessive alcohol intake
	Screening for changes in cognition
Tertiary	
Prevents complete disability	Functional assessment and rehabilitation efforts
Returns client to maximum function within disability constraints	Typical focus on enhancement of occupational performance and ADL and IADL functions
Occurs when a defect is permanent and irreversible	

*From Green LW, Kreuter MW: *Health promotion planning: an educational and environmental approach*, Mountain View, Calif, 1992, Mayfield.
†From Rothman J, Levine R: *Prevention practice: studies for physical therapy and occupational therapy*, Philadelphia, 1992, WB Saunders.

are especially suited for prevention planning, including impaired mobility, injury from falls, sensory loss, adverse medication reactions, disuse syndrome, depression, malnutrition, alcohol abuse, hypertension, and osteoporosis. These conditions can be prevented or postponed through prevention-focused health education efforts (Webster, 1992).

Prevention strategies are generally organized into three categories: primary, secondary, and tertiary (Webster, 1992; Garner, Young, 1993) (Table 5-1). Primary prevention focuses on reducing the risk of disease before its onset. Primary preventive efforts with elders may consist of facilitation of lifestyle changes and use of necessary medications to reduce potential for life-threatening conditions such as cardiovascular disease and stroke. Primary prevention programs include immunization, accident prevention, exercise, nutritional counseling, and smoking and alcohol cessation (Webster, 1992). A critical primary prevention effort should be focused on prevention of falls in elders because traumatic injuries are the fifth leading cause of death among persons over 65 years of age (Garner, Young, 1993).

Primary prevention. COTAs may represent the first line of **primary prevention** for well, homebound, or institutionalized elders. In this capacity, COTAs have an opportunity to influence change in elders' awareness of health risks. By assisting elders to develop or return to interests that stimulate increased activity and mobility, COTAs may help reduce ill effects of a sedentary lifestyle or disuse syndrome. Many disabilities of elders start with disuse and are preventable. Studies have demonstrated the long-reaching effects of regular exercise in the prevention of weakness and fatigue, which interfere with independence in ADL functions (Fiatarone, Evans, 1990; Glantz, Richman, 1996; Schuster, Petrosa, Petrosa, 1995; McMurdo, Rennie, 1993). Exercise has also helped prevent obesity and consequent hypertension and diabetes. A daily or three-times-weekly exercise program or regular participation in an activity such as walking or chair aerobics can significantly reduce fall potential, a serious threat to the health and well-being of elder clients (Figures 5-6 and 5-7).

A noteworthy difference exists between clients involved in rote exercise and those participating in intrinsically motivated activities. Rote exercise involves the repetition of a particular movement to develop strength, endurance, or skill, such as lifting a 10-pound dumbbell 10 times. Intrinsic motivation describes the characteristic of activities that have a purpose in and of themselves, such as picking up a 10-pound infant. Yoder, Nelson, and Smith (1989) found that elderly women engaged in significantly more exercise repetitions with intrinsic activities such as food preparation than with a rote exercise program. Riccio, Nelson, and Bush (1990) later found that the use of imagery as a cue facilitated more exercise repetitions than a rote exercise program. In this study, elders imagined that they were using first the right and then the left arm to pick apples and place them in a basket. A number of other studies have investigated the effects of purpose in facilitating movement beyond the benefits of rote exercise (Bloch, Smith, Nelson, 1989; Heck, 1988, Kircher, 1984; Miller, Nelson, 1987; Yoder, Nelson, Smith, 1989). These studies validate OT beliefs regarding the health-enhancing value of occupation. Meaningful activities important to the client help generate motivation and excitement that rote exercise cannot. Thus clients gain more from exercises that are "embedded in meaningful, purposeful occupations" (Nelson, Stucky, 1992) than from a rote regimen of exercise.

Fall prevention is another critical aspect of primary prevention practices COTAs can facilitate. A home or an institutional environment assessment may identify many fall hazards for elders (see Chapter 16). The *Fall Risk Factor Screening Checklist* (Carlson, 1996) can contribute significant information to fall prevention (Figure 5-8).

Secondary prevention. **Secondary prevention** efforts consist of "identification and treatment of persons with early, minimally symptomatic diseases to improve outcomes and maintain health" (Garner, Young, 1993). Early

detection of hypertension and cancers may prevent early disability and mortality. Vision and hearing deficits are also preventable at times if detected early, as are breast and cervical cancers and depressive or substance use disorders. COTAs can contribute to early detection of serious conditions and those that contribute to disability and interfere with independent ADL and IADL functions by reminding elders of the importance of annual exams such as mammograms and Papanicolaou (PAP) tests. **Health and risk screening** of elder populations is often overlooked or considered unimportant by health care workers. For example, in 1987, 73.3% of women of all ages had a PAP smear during the previous 3 years, but only 44.9% of women over 70 years of age had undergone the test.

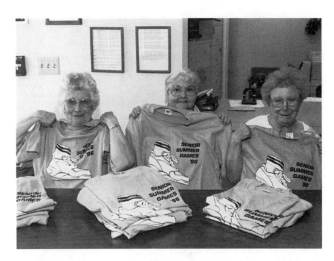

FIGURE **5-7** Participation in regular activity can significantly affect the negative results of disuse.

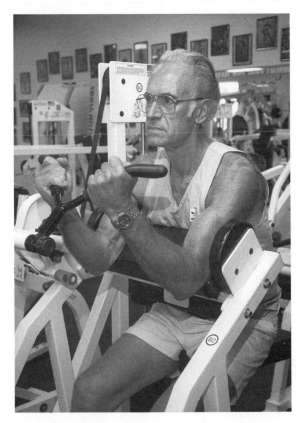

FIGURE **5-6** Regular exercise has long-reaching effects in maintaining independence.

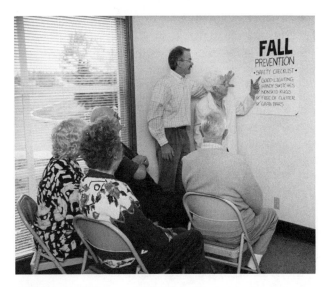

FIGURE **5-8** Fall prevention is another critical aspect of primary prevention. (Courtesy Sue-Byers Connon.)

BOX 5-2

Prevention Behavior Questionnaire

1. Name some behaviors in your life that you believe endanger or compromise your health.
2. How much control do you have to change them? (circle one)   a. some   b. little   c. none
3. Do you participate in some form of physical activity on a regular basis? (circle one)   yes   no
4. What activities do you participate in? (circle one)
   a. walking   b. swimming   c. gardening   d. other _____
5. How often in a week do you engage in these activities? (circle one)
   a. daily   b. twice   c. three times   d. other _____
6. How much time do you devote to these activities? (circle one)
   a. less than 30 min   b. 1 hour   c. 2 hours   d. other _____
7. Rate the level of stress in your life (circle one):
   a. very high   b. high   c. moderate   d. occasional   e. very low
8. What do you do to relieve stress in your life? (circle one)
   a. hobbies   b. exercise   c. drink alcohol   d. smoke   e. other (s) _____
9. How many meals do you eat each day? (circle one)
   a. three   b. two   c. one   d. less than one
10. Do you usually eat (circle one):   a. alone   b. with others
11. Do you consider your weight to be (circle one)   a. too high   b. average   c. too low
12. Do you monitor your daily fat intake? (circle one)   a. yes   b. no
13. How many servings do you have each day from the following food groups? (circle your answers)
    a. bread and cereal   1   2   3   4   more
    b. fruits and vegetables   1   2   3   4   more
    c. meat   1   2   3   4   more
    d. beans, peas, tofu   1   2   3   4   more
    e. milk   1   2   3   4   more
    f. dairy products   1   2   3   4   more
14. Is it necessary for you to monitor your blood cholesterol level? (circle one)   a. yes   b. no
15. Do you monitor your sodium intake? (circle one) a. yes b. no
16. Have you fallen (circle one)
    a. in the past week   b. in the last month   c. in the past 3 months   d. in the past 6 months
    e. in the past 9 months   f. in the past year   g. in the past 18 months
17. If so, how many times have you fallen? (circle one)   a. 1   b. 2   c. 3   d. other _____
18. Have you scalded or burned yourself recently? (circle one)
    a. in the past week   b. in the past month   c. in the past 3 months   d. in the past 6 months
    e. in the past year   c. in the past 18 months
19. Do you have arthritis? (circle one)   a. yes   b. no
20. Do you have heart disease? (circle one)   a. yes   b. no
21. Do you have cancer? (circle one)   a. yes   b. no
22. Do you have difficulty catching your breath
    a. when walking? (circle one)   a. yes   b. no
    b. when climbing stairs? (circle one)   a. yes   b. no
    c. when sitting? (circle one)   a. yes   b. no
23. Do you have asthma or emphysema? (circle one)   a. yes   b. no
24. Do you have difficulty
    a. bending over to remove items from low cabinets? (circle one)   a. yes   b. no
    b. going up or down stairs? (circle one)   a. yes   b. no
    c. getting up from a bed or chair? (circle one)   a. yes   b. no
25. Do you need assistance to walk? (circle one)   a. yes   b. no
26. What distance can you safely walk without assistance or stopping? (circle one)
    a. less than 1 block   b. 1 block   c. ¼ mile d. ½ mile e. 1 mile   f. other: _____
27. What would you like to change about your health?

Adapted from Lohman H, Peyton-Runyon C: Intergenerational experiences for occupational therapy students, *Phys Occup Ther Geriatr* (10)2:17, 1991.

Furthermore, women over 65 years of age accounted for 41% of the cervical cancer mortality rate (Smith, 1995). Elders from minority groups are often at higher risk for serious health conditions. Consequently, all health care providers must encourage and remind elder clients to schedule regular examinations.

Careful observation of functional capabilities may facilitate early detection of changes in elders' capabilities. COTAs can monitor sensory capacity for loss or change during routine interactions with elders (see Chapters 17 and 18). COTAs may also be instrumental in educating family members to pay attention to changes in the elder. Mood or cognitive functions may change rapidly and influence independence with ADL and IADL. Changes in mood or cognition are frequently associated with poor nutrition or dehydration, both of which can be remediated. Changes may also indicate too much medication, medication side effects, or more serious physiologic changes that require medical attention.

Tertiary prevention. **Tertiary prevention** refers to preventing the progression of already existing conditions. It "relates to functional assessment and rehabilitation both to reverse and to prevent progression of the burden of illness" (Webster, 1992). An example of tertiary prevention initiated by the COTA is the treatment of a homebound elder who has arthritis. The COTA can provide education about self-care activities such as joint protection and energy conservation to prevent further deterioration of arthritic joints. In addition, joint mobility can facilitated through regular participation in a hobby within the elder's range of tolerance. Performing energy conservation activities may also assist the elder to feel more control over the daily routine.

THE ROLE OF THE COTA IN WELLNESS AND HEALTH PROMOTION

COTAs play a critical role in promotion of health and prevention of disease among elders. Health education facilitates health promotion, disability reduction, and illness prevention (Pinch, 1993). Chronic illnesses that effect ADLs and IADLs are more often related to lifestyle, genetic predisposition, and environmental exposure than to age alone. Frequently, elders must change behaviors to prevent disability from developing or progressing. Professional evaluation, intervention, and educational programs implemented by COTAs can foster such life-enhancing changes. (Box 5-2 is an example of a health behavior questionnaire that COTAs can use to determine the need for intervention through health education activities.) Hickey and Stillwell (1991) stated, "The overall goal of health promotion in the elderly . . . should be to prevent the progression of disease and the risks of disability and death." Health promotion should also help elders maintain functional autonomy as long as possible (Davies, 1990). Glantz and Richman (1996) proposed guidelines

BOX 5-3

Wellness Program for Elders

Program goals
- Enhance awareness of the positive effect of wellness on health at any age
- Promote awareness of the sensory changes that occur as aging progresses
- Improve knowledge of food consumption and effects on health
- Improve decision-making skills
- Encourage self-responsibility for health
- Encourage independence and environmental mastery
- Maximize a positive focus
- Heighten awareness of behaviors that inhibit health and perpetuate disease
- Encourage independence in self-care

Possible topics
- Personal nutrition
- Exercise: sitting, standing, low-impact aerobics
- Planning of health screenings, including annual screening for cancer
- Smoking cessation
- Activities: exploring interests
- Stress and effects on the heart
- Relaxation
- Responsibility for health
- Sensory loss and safety: eliminating hazards

Adapted from Glantz CH, Richman N: The wellness model in long-term care facilities, *Quest* (7):7, 1993.

for the development of wellness programs for elders that emphasize goals of "optimum achievement and maintenance of competence and independence" (Box 5-3).

Hettinger (1996) developed the following *ABCs* of the wellness model in occupational therapy, which may assist COTAs in encouraging their elder clients to learn to improve and maintain their health:

*A*ttitude that includes actively pursuing wellness and ADLs that promote satisfaction and quality of life
*B*alancing productive activity, positive social support, emotional expression, and environmental interactions
*C*ontrolling health through education about behaviors that lead to wellness

Within this model, COTAs serve as mentors, coaches, and educators. Health education is the most common approach to prevention of disease and empowerment of elders to take increasing responsibility for their health. COTAs have many opportunities across practice domains to provide health education programs for elders. Health promotion can occur through individual or group education efforts (Boxes 5-4 and 5-5, Table 5-2). COTAs can

BOX 5-4

Cancer Prevention Exercise—Questions for Cancer Group

Nutrition

Q: Do you monitor fat intake in your diet?

Fact: High fat intake increases risk of developing breast, colon, uterine, and prostate cancer.

Q: Do you eat a diet high in fruits, vegetables, and breads and low in meat?

Fact: A high-fiber diet reduces the risk of cancer of the colon, uterus, and breast.

Q: Do you frequently eat foods that have been charcoal grilled or are prepackaged, such as hot dogs, bologna, and sausage?

Fact: Foods that are smoked or cured in nitrate or salt may increase the risk of cancer of the esophagus and stomach.

Smoking

Q: What have you done to stop smoking?

Fact: Approximately 30% of all deaths from cancer result from smoking. Smoking two or more packs of cigarettes per day increases the risk of lung cancer mortality to 15 to 25 times that of nonsmokers.

Q: Is there a health benefit no matter when you stop smoking?

Fact: After 10 years of not smoking, exsmokers have the same rate of lung cancer as nonsmokers.

Breast examination

Q: Do you examine your breasts monthly?

Fact: Breast cancer is the second leading cause of death among women.

Q: Have you had a mammogram every year since the age of 40?

Fact: After age 40, women should have a regularly scheduled mammogram.

Pap tests

Q: Do you have an annual Pap test and pelvic examination?

Fact: Pap and pelvic examinations should be performed regularly once child-bearing years begin. Age or sexual inactivity should not change the occurrence of this annual screening.

Colorectal examination

Q: Do you have a regular annual screening for colorectal cancer?

Fact: Early diagnosis of colon cancer improves survival for 5 years by 91%. Three types of examinations are recommended: digital rectal exam (after age 40) and stool blood tests and proctosigmoidoscopy (every 3 to 5 years after age 50).

Data from Franenknecht M: Cancer prevalence and prevention: demonstrating the role of personal responsibility, *J Health Educ* (26)4:240, 1995.

BOX 5-5

Group Activity: Cancer Prevention

According to the U.S. Department of Health and Human Services (1992), cancer is the leading cause of death among adults age 25 through 64 years. In addition, 1 of every 3 Americans will have cancer at some point (Franenknecht, 1995). Because of this fact and the lack of routine cancer screening offered to elders, COTAs must provide elder clients with prevention programs.

Rationale

- To heighten group awareness regarding the national statistic that one in three persons in the United States will have cancer at some point
- To heighten awareness that screening and active behavioral change are effective methods of reducing cancer risks

Process

- Group members are numbered 1, 2, and 3. After all members are numbered, the number 3 group is told of their diagnosis of cancer.
- Members in groups 1 and 2 receive the information sheet (see Box 5-5).
- Members in group 3 are asked questions by members in groups 1 and 2 about actions they take to avoid exposure to cancer risks listed on their information sheets. Questions may be similar to the following:
  - "Do you participate in monthly testicular self-examinations?"
  - "Do you currently smoke?"
  - "Do you abstain from alcohol?"
  - "When was your last PAP examination?"
- As members of group 3 respond with behavioral change statements indicative of reducing cancer risk, they are merged with members from groups 1 and 2.

rely on group skills to facilitate discussion of materials. Generally, health-related topics include benefits of exercise, cardiac risk factors, arthritis, stroke prevention, immunization, osteoporosis, cancer, early detection, home safety, assistive devices, and sensory changes that occur with aging (Mount, 1991). Discussion topics educate elders about leading causes of functional limitation, disability, and death, thereby facilitating the potential to change behaviors and improve quality of life.

In their research of effects of an exercise program for older adults, Hickey and Stillwell (1991) pointed out evidence to inspire COTAs to provide health-promoting activities. "The older adult responds to exercise training in the same manner as a young adult, with a 10% to 20% increase in cardiovascular fitness and strength gain of

TABLE **5-2**

Promotional Activities Guided by COTAs

Prevention	Recommended health education content
Dietary excess and imbalance Cancer, stroke, obesity, dental disease, osteoporosis	• Total fat content of less than 20% of calories • Total saturated fat content of less than 10% of total calories • Increased consumption of whole grain products, cereals, vegetables, and fruits • Decreased sodium intake • Decreased alcohol intake • Intake of calcium and daily vitamins • Estrogen replacement • Schedule of dental screenings • Cholesterol screening and reduction • Need for special diet • Socialization as a nutritional factor • Adequate hydration
Safety and unintentional injuries Falls, burns, and auto accidents	• Method of home hazard assessment: check list • Adaptive devices (for example, hand rails and traction strips) • Readjustment of home and water temperature
Regular exercise Cardiovascular disease, osteoporosis, falls, depression, stroke, loss of ADL and IADL functions	• Reduction of glucose intolerance • Reduction of constipation • Sitting exercise groups, walking • Low impact aerobics • Exercise embedded in meaningful activities such as gardening • Standing at a table • Weight bearing to maintain bone density
Immunization Lower lobe pneumonia and influenza, tetanus	• Pneumococcal (one immunization for persons 65 years of age and over) • Influenza (annually) • Tetanus and diphtheria (every 10 years)

between 50% and 174% depending on the extent of reconditioning" (Hickey, Stillwell, 1991). Such research shows that it is never too late to begin exercising.

CONCLUSION

America is moving into an era of health care reform that focuses on improving the quality of life for the lowest cost. The OT practitioner's role in this reform is to promote personal responsibility for health through meaningful occupational performance. In addition, the belief that small adaptive changes can improve the quality of a person's life regardless of age or disability must be encouraged. As Ashley Montagu (1981) wrote in his book *Growing Young,* " . . . the youth of the chronologically young is a gift; growing young into what others call 'old age' is an

achievement, a work of art. It takes time to grow young."

CHAPTER REVIEW QUESTIONS

1 Give examples of primary, secondary, and tertiary prevention functions of COTAs working with elders.
2 Name two activity groups that could be used with each classification of prevention.
3 Explain how health and occupation are interrelated.
4 How would you define *disuse syndrome?* How does this syndrome contribute to disease and disability?
5 How can purposeful activity be characterized as health promoting?
6 Describe the role of COTAs in wellness and health promotion program implementation.

REFERENCES

American Association of Retired Persons: *A profile of older Americans*, Washington, DC, 1995, The Association.

Bloch MW, Smith DA, Nelson DL: Heart rate, activity, duration, and effect in added purpose versus single-purpose jumping activity, *Am J Occup Ther* 43:25, 1989.

Carlson A: Fall prevention in Hilo, Hawaii, *OT Week* (9)5:14, 1996.

Davies AM: Prevention in the aging. In Kane RL, Evans JG, Macfadyen D, editors: *Improving the health of older people*, New York, 1990, Oxford University.

Drinkwater BL: Exercise and aging: the female master athlete. In Puhl J, Brown C, Voy R, editors: *Sports science perspectives for women*, Chicago, 1985, Human Kinetics Books.

Fiatarone MA, Evans JE: Exercise in the oldest old, *Top Geriatr Rehabil* (5)2:63, 1990.

Filner B, Williams T: Health promotion for the elderly: reducing functional dependency. *Healthy people 2000*, Washington, DC, 1992, US Government Printing Office.

Florey L: Development through play. In Schaefer C, editor: *The therapeutic use of child's play*, New York, 1976, Jason Aronson.

Franenknecht M: Cancer prevalence and prevention: demonstrating the role of personal responsibility, *J Health Educ* (26)4:240, 1995.

Garner DJ, Young AA, editors: *Women and healthy aging: living productively in spite of it all*, New York, 1993, The Haworth Press.

Gilfoyle EM: The future of occupational therapy: an environment of opportunity. In Ryan SE, editor: *The certified occupational therapy assistant*, Thorofare, NJ, 1986, Slack.

Glantz CH, Richman N: The wellness model in long term care facilities, *Quest* 7:7, 1996.

Green LW, Kreuter MW: *Health promotion planning: an educational and environmental approach*, Mountain View, Calif, 1992, Mayfield.

Heck SH: The effect of purposeful activity on pain tolerance, *Am J Occup Ther* (42):577, 1988.

Hettinger J: The wellness connection, *OT Week* (9):12, 1996.

Hickey T, Stilwell DL: Health promotion for older people: all is not well, *Gerontologist* (31)6:822, 1991.

Johnson JA: *Wellness: a context for living*, Thorofare, NJ, 1986, Slack.

Kircher MA: Motivation as a factor of perceived exertion in purposeful versus nonpurposeful activity, *Am J Occup Ther* 38:165, 1984.

Lohman H, Peyton-Runyon C: Intergenerational experiences for occupational therapy students, *Phys Occup Ther Geriatr* (10)2:17, 1991.

McMurdo, Rennie L: A controlled trial of exercise by residents of old peoples' homes, *Age Ageing* 22:11, 1993.

Miller L, Nelson DL: Dual purpose activity versus single purpose in terms of duration on task, exertion level, and affect, *Occup Ther Ment Health* 7:55, 1987.

Montagu A: *Growing young*, New York, 1981, McGraw-Hill.

Mount J: Evaluation of a health promotion program provided at senior centers by physical therapy students, *Phys Occup Ther Geriatr* (10)1:15, 1991.

Nelson DL, Stucky C: The roles of occupational therapy in preventing further disability of elderly persons in long-term care facilities. In Levine RA, Rothman J, editors: *Prevention practice: strategies for physical therapy and occupational therapy*, Philadelphia, 1992, WB Saunders.

Pinch WJ: Health promotion and the elderly, *NSNA/Imprint* (2)3:83, 1993.

Riccio CM, Nelson DL, Bush MA: Adding purpose to the repetitive exercise of elderly women through imagery, *Am J Occup Ther* (44)8:714, 1990.

Rothman J, Levine R: *Prevention practice: strategies for physical therapy and occupational therapy*, Philadelphia, 1992, WB Saunders.

Schuster C, Petrosa R, Petrosa S: Using social cognitive theory to predict intentional exercise in post-retirement adults, *J Health Educ* (26)1:14, 1995.

Shephard RJ: The scientific basis of exercise prescribing for the very old, *J Am Geriatr Soc* 38:623, 1990.

Smith MT: Implementing annual cancer screening for elderly women, *J Gerontol Nurs* 7:12, 1995.

Smith EL: The interaction of nature and nurture. In Smith EL, Serface RC, editors: *Exercise and aging*, Chicago, 1981, Human Kinetics Books.

Speake DL: Health promotion activity in the well elderly, *Health Values* (11)6:25, 1987.

US Department of Health and Human Services, *Personnel health guide: put prevention into practice program*, Public Health Services Washington, DC, 1992, ODPHP National Health Information Center.

Webster JR: Prevention, technology, and aging in the decade ahead, *Top Geriatr Rehabil* (7)4:1, 1992.

Yerxa EJ: Occupational science: a new source of power for participants in occupational therapy, *J Occup Sci* (1)1:3, 1993.

Yoder RM, Nelson DL, Smith DA: Added-purpose verses rote exercise in female nursing home residents, *Am J Occup Ther* 43:581, 1989.

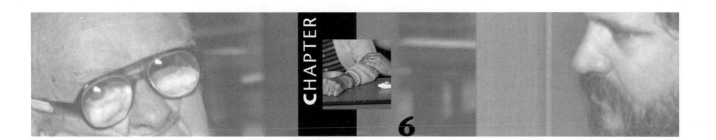

Public Policy and Aging

CORALIE H. GLANTZ AND NANCY RICHMAN

KEY TERMS

Omnibus Budget Reconciliation Act (OBRA) of 1987, Medicare, Medicaid, Older
Americans Act (OAA), managed care, Social Security Insurance (SSI), F tags, Minimum
Data Set (MDS), triggers, Resident Assessment Protocols (RAPS), care planning,
ancillary services, skilled services, unskilled services, advocacy

CHAPTER OBJECTIVES

1. Clearly define the COTA's role within OBRA regulations.
2. Learn the way the COTA's input with the resident assessment instrument is valuable in the integrated team approach.
3. Increase awareness of trends in public policy.
4. Increase knowledge about Medicare eligibility, guidelines, and regulations.
5. Understand the intent and coverage of Medicaid.
6. Understand resources for programs for elders.
7. Learn the importance of advocacy for the occupational therapy profession.

Public policy develops from legislation at the federal and state levels and represents society's values (MacClain, 1996). For example, the Medicare Act, which resulted in a national health insurance plan for elders, was enacted in 1965. Medicaid, a combined federal and state insurance that addresses the health care needs of the indigent, was enacted in 1966. Both measures were enacted at a time when the health needs of elders and the indigent were priorities.

Public policy can also affect the daily practice of COTAs. COTAs working in a skilled nursing facility need to understand the **Omnibus Budget Reconciliation Act (OBRA) of 1987** to provide appropriate care and be effective treatment team members. COTAs must also have a direct understanding of **Medicare** and **Medicaid** to ensure that treatment they provide is reimbursed by third party payers. In addition to knowledge of reimbursement sources, COTAs should know about community resources funded by public policy. For example, the COTA working in home healthcare may recommend that an elder receive Meals on Wheels or other services from the Area Office on Aging, which is funded by the **Older Americans Act (OAA).** Public policy effects on practice may be negative if funding is threatened.

Medicare, Medicaid, OBRA, and OAA are examples of public policy that can affect elder health care. This chapter discusses the influence of these acts on OT practice and concludes with suggestions for the COTA on ways to promote changes in public policy and advocate for elder rights.

HEALTH CARE TRENDS IN THE UNITED STATES

Health care policies in the United States are changing rapidly. In the past the family physician was the sole provider of health care. The physician knew individuals throughout their lives and treated them as whole people rather than as illnesses or diseases. The health care industry has undergone an extensive period of fragmented approaches to service delivery. The current trend, especially for elders, is toward comprehensive, cost-effective health care. Consumers want simplified access to a range of services with predictable costs. This has led to the emergence and growth of **managed care.**

Managed Care

Managed care is a general term for all types of integrated delivery systems such as health maintenance organization (HMOs) and preferred provider organizations (PPOs). These systems manage the care given to consumers (in contrast to traditional fee-for-service care, which is unmanaged). Managed care often involves the entire range of utilization control tools applied to manage the practice of physicians and others, regardless of practice setting.

The growth in managed care organizations (MCOs) reflects the trend of the one-stop, cost-effective care. Elders are encouraged to sign on with senior HMOs and forfeit Medicare benefits. These HMOs often advertise the inclusion of services beyond the basic Medicare plan, such as prescription and dental plans. The provision of rehabilitation services with some managed care plans is different from traditional Medicare, and elders in MCOs who require extensive rehabilitation do not have access to the level of care provided by Medicare.

Reimbursement rates to managed care providers are capitated. That is, a flat rate is agreed on and all services must be provided for that one payment per day or per incident. This payment may not be enough to include extensive therapy. A capitated system provides a financial incentive for physicians to refrain from referring clients to specialists such as OTRs. This trend toward managed care affects delivery of OT services to elders. OTRs and COTAs need to continue emphasizing the functional treatment they provide. OT practitioners anticipate an increase in the use of aides and in the use of COTAs to teach aides and other caregivers appropriate ways to deliver care.

Budgetary Issues

Financial concerns motivate the shift from entitlement programs, or government programs with specific guidelines for eligible beneficiaries, to policies based on need rather than age (Binstock, 1994). Currently **Social Security Insurance (SSI)** and Medicare benefits are structured according to age, with no restrictions based on income level. The Social Security program was established in 1935 by the U.S. government to ensure payment for survivor's insurance, contributions to state unemployment insurance, old-age assistance, and Medicare and Medicaid benefits. The trend to emphasize economic status rather than age criteria has been reflected in legislation. The Social Security Reform Act of 1983 authorized taxing of Social Security benefits for individuals and couples with a certain level of annual income. The trend for proposals to raise the eligibility age for old-age benefits is likely to continue (Binstock, 1994).

OMNIBUS BUDGET RECONCILIATION ACT

OBRA, a landmark act of Congress, is not influenced by budgetary concerns. This act focuses on elders' rights, quality of care, and quality of life in the nursing home setting. OBRA went into effect in October 1990, and was revised with final rules published in 1995. Compliance with the OBRA regulation is necessary for a nursing facility to receive reimbursement from Medicare or Medicaid.

F Tags

The federal government **"F tags"** (that is, F followed by a number) refer to specific regulations in the OBRA law. For example, F406(a) states "Provision of services: If specialized rehabilitation services such as, but not limited to physical therapy, speech-language pathology, occupational therapy, and mental health rehabilitative services for mental illness and mental retardation, are required in the resident's comprehensive plan of care, the facility must (1) Provide the required services; or (2) Obtain the required services from an outside resource from a provider of specialized rehabilitative services" (OBRA, 1995).

Scope of OBRA

OBRA was designed as a regulatory framework to recognize the importance of a comprehensive assessment, the Resident Assessment Instrument (RAI), as the foundation for planning care delivery to nursing home residents. The OBRA law focuses on not only quality care but also function and quality of life. It addresses residents' rights, including the right to " . . . services to attain or maintain the highest practicable physical, mental, and psychosocial well-being, in accordance with the comprehensive assessment and plan of care" (F309) (OBRA, 1995). This includes activities of daily living (ADLs). As stated in F310, "A resident's abilities in activities of daily living do not diminish unless circumstances of the individual's clinical condition demonstrate that diminution was unavoidable" (OBRA, 1995) and in F311, "A resident is given the appropriate treatment and services to maintain or improve his or her abilities" (OBRA, 1995). Other categories of residents' rights address freedom from restraint and opportunity to participate in social, religious, and community activities. Many categories and guidelines of residents' rights included in the OBRA law have implications for OT practice.

The Resident Assessment Instrument

To understand the COTA's role in the provision of OBRA, OT practitioners must first learn about the RAI. The RAI, which is the comprehensive assessment required by OBRA, must be completed for all residents residing longer than 14 days in specific nursing facilities. The three components of the RAI are as follows: (1) **Minimum Data Set (MDS),** (2) **Triggers,** and (3) **Resident Assessment Protocols (RAPs)** and the RAP summaries. Completion of these components leads directly to the care plan process.

The RAI first addresses the problem identification process. After a resident's problems are recognized, a **care plan** is created to identify sound clinical interventions and treatment goals. This care plan becomes each resident's unique path toward achieving or maintaining a maximal level of well-being. The RAI considers the resident as an individual with strengths in addition to functional limitations and health problems.

Federal regulations require that the RAI be conducted or coordinated with the participation of appropriate health professionals. Although not required, completion of the RAI is best accomplished by an interdisciplinary team. Team members' combined experience and knowledge enable a better understanding of the strengths, needs, and preferences of each resident, thereby ensuring the best possible quality of care. Facilities have flexibility in determining the participants in the assessment process as long as it is accurately conducted. A facility may assign responsibility for completing the RAI to a number of qualified staff members, including the COTA. In most cases, participants in the assessment process are licensed health professionals.

Minimum data set. The MDS is a screening tool in which strengths and deficits are recognized and triggered for further assessment. Many sections of the MDS address areas within the scope of OT practice, including cognition, communication, vision, mood and behavior problems, psychosocial well-being, physical functioning and structural problems, continence, various disease diagnoses and health conditions, oral and nutritional status, activity pursuits, special treatment and procedures (including therapy), and discharge potential. An OT practitioner usually fills out the section on physical functioning (Figure 6-1).

COTA involvement in completion of sections of the MDS can be very beneficial. Because the initial MDS does not have to be completed until the 14th day after admission, the resident has often been evaluated and is being treated by OT. If this is the case, COTAs can use the OT evaluation and knowledge gained in treating the resident to accurately fill out the MDS.

Even if no treatment has taken place, the data collection and resident interview may help COTAs give the necessary information. In some situations, COTAs complete the "Physical Functioning and Structural Problems" section for all newly admitted residents. COTAs may also be required to complete the same MDS section for later resident reviews. Completion of a new MDS is required when significant changes in the resident's status have occurred. (The Appendix contains information on obtaining a copy of guidelines for the MDS.)

COTAs should also be familiar with the actual OBRA Final Rules, Enforcement Requirements, Survey Procedures, and Interpretive Guidance. COTAs completing any portion of the MDS assessment must certify accuracy of the section(s) they complete by noting their credentials and the date and indicating the portion of the assessment completed. The signature of an RN is required to certify completion of the assessment.

Triggers. After completion of the MDS, those areas that have been triggered, or identified, as needing further assessment are reviewed with RAP guidelines. The triggers identify MDS responses specific to a resident. They alert the assessor to residents who either have or are at risk for developing specific functional problems and require further evaluation using the RAPs. The RAP guidelines "present comprehensive information for evaluating factors that may cause, contribute to, or exacerbate the triggered condition" (Morris, Murphy, Nonemaker, 1995). RAPs also examine guidance for further assessment and possible interventions for resolution to problems. COTAs can write meaningful RAP summaries by collecting data from the resident's records, family members, and staff members.

"If the condition is found to be a problem for the resident, the RAP Guidelines will assist the interdisciplinary team in determining if the problem can be eliminated or reversed, or if special care must be taken to maintain a resident at his or her current level of functioning" (Morris, Murphy, Nonemaker, 1995). Using the RAP guidelines, the COTA can complete this further exploration and review of the problem area with a summary that includes the following: (1) the nature of the condition (may include presence or lack of objective data and subjective complaints), (2) complication and risk factors that affect the decision to proceed to care planning, (3) factors that must be considered in developing the individualized care plan interventions, and (4) the need for referrals and further evaluation by appropriate health

SECTION G. PHYSICAL FUNCTIONING AND STRUCTURAL PROBLEMS

1. **(A)** ADL SELF-PERFORMANCE—(*Code* for resident's **PERFORMANCE OVER ALL SHIFTS during last 7 days**—*Not including setup*)

   0. *INDEPENDENT*—No help or oversight—OR—Help/oversight provided only 1 or 2 times during last 7 days

   1. *SUPERVISION*—Oversight, encouragement or cueing provided 3 or more times during last 7 days—OR—Supervision (3 or more times) plus physical assistance provided only 1 or 2 times during last 7 days

   2. *LIMITED ASSISTANCE*—Resident highly involved in activity; received physical help in guided maneuvering of limbs or other nonweight bearing assistance 3 or more times—OR—More help provided only 1 or 2 times during last 7 days

   3. *EXTENSIVE ASSISTANCE*—While resident performed part of activity, over last 7-day period, help of following type(s) provided 3 or more times:
     —Weight-bearing support
     —Full staff performance during part (but not all) of last 7 days

   4. *TOTAL DEPENDENCE*—Full staff performance of activity during entire 7 days

   8. *ACTIVITY DID NOT OCCUR* during entire 7 days

(B) ADL SUPPORT PROVIDED—(***Code for MOST SUPPORT PROVIDED OVER ALL SHIFTS during last 7 days; code regardless*** of resident's self-performance classification)

   0. No setup or physical help from staff
   1. Setup help only
   2. One person physical assist   8. ADL activity itself did not
   3. Two+ persons physical assist   occur during entire 7 days

			(A) SELF-PERF	(B) SUPPORT
a.	**BED MOBILITY**	How resident moves to and from lying position, turns side-to-side, and positions body while in bed.		
b.	**TRANSFER**	How resident moves between surfaces—to/from: bed, chair, wheelchair, standing position (EXCLUDE to/from bath/toilet).		
c.	**WALK IN ROOM**	How resident walks between locations in his/her room.		
d.	**WALK IN CORRIDOR**	How resident walks in corridor on unit.		
e.	**LOCOMO-TION ON UNIT**	How resident moves between locations in his/her room and adjacent corridor on same floor. If in wheelchair, self-sufficiency once in chair.		
f.	**LOCOMO-TION OFF UNIT**	How resident moves to and returns from off-unit locations (e.g., areas set aside for dining, activities, or treatments). **If facility has only one floor,** how resident moves to and from distant areas on the floor. If in wheelchair, self-sufficiency once in chair.		
g.	**DRESSING**	How resident puts on, fastens, and takes off all items of **street clothing,** including donning/removing prosthesis.		
h.	**EATING**	How resident eats and drinks (regardless of skill). Includes intake of nourishment by other means (e.g., tube feeding, total parenteral nutrition).		
i.	**TOILET USE**	How resident uses the toilet room (or commode, bedpan, urinal); transfer on/off toilet, cleanses, changes pad, manages ostomy or catheter, adjusts clothes.		
j.	**PERSONAL HYGIENE**	How resident maintains personal hygiene, including combing hair, brushing teeth, shaving, applying makeup, washing/drying face, hands, and perineum (EXCLUDE baths and showers).		

FIGURE 6-1 Example of the Physical Functioning and Structural Problems section of the MDS.

2.	BATHING	How resident takes full-body bath/shower, sponge bath, and transfers in/out of tub/shower (EXCLUDE washing of back and hair). **Code for most dependent** in self-performance and support.
		(A) BATHING SELF-PERFORMANCE codes appear below
		  0. Independent—No help provided
		  1. Supervision—Oversight help only
		  2. Physical help limited to transfer only
		  3. Physical help in part of bathing activity
		  4. Total dependence
		  8. Activity itself did not occur during entire 7 days
		(*Bathing support codes are as defined in* **Item 1, code B above**)
			(A) (B)

3.	**TEST FOR BALANCE**
	
	(see training manual)
		(*Code for ability during test in the* **last 7 days**)
		  0. Maintained position as required in test
		  1. Unsteady, but able to rebalance self without physical support
		  2. Partial physical support during test; or stands (sits) but does not follow directions for test
		  3. Not able to attempt test without physical help	

		a. Balance while standing	
		b. Balance while sitting—position, trunk control	

4.	**FUNCTIONAL LIMITATION IN RANGE OF MOTION**
	
	(see training manual)
		(*Code for limitations during* **last 7 days** *that interfered with daily functions or placed resident at risk of injury*)
		(A) *RANGE OF MOTION* **(B)** *VOLUNTARY MOVEMENT*
		  0. No limitation 0. No loss
		  1. Limitation on one side 1. Partial loss
		  2. Limitation on both sides 2. Full loss
			(A) (B)

		a. Neck	
		b. Arm—Including shoulder or elbow	
		c. Hand—Including wrist or fingers	
		d. Leg—Including hip or knee	
		e. Foot—Including ankle or toes	
		f. Other limitation or loss	
5.	**MODES OF LOCOMOTION**	(**Check all that apply** during **last 7 days**) Cane/walker/crutch **a.** Wheelchair primary **d.** Wheeled self **b.** mode of locomotion Other person wheeled **c.** NONE OF ABOVE **e.**	
6.	**MODES OF TRANSFER**	(**Check all that apply** during **last 7 days**) Bedfast all or most of time **a.** Lifted mechanically **d.** Bed rails used for bed mobility or transfer **b.** Transfer aid (e.g., slide board, trapeze, cane, walker, brace) **e.** Lifted manually **c.** NONE OF ABOVE **f.**	
7.	**TASK SEGMENTATION**	Some or all of ADL activities were broken into subtasks during **last 7 days** so that resident could perform them 0. No 1. Yes	
8.	**ADL FUNCTIONAL REHABILITATION POTENTIAL**	Resident believes he/she is capable of increased independence in at least some ADLs **a.** Direct care staff believe resident is capable of increased independence in at least some ADLs **b.** Resident able to perform tasks/activities but is very slow **c.** Difference in ADL Self-Performance or ADL Support, comparing mornings with evenings **d.** NONE OF ABOVE **e.**	
9.	**CHANGE IN ADL FUNCTION**	Resident's ADL self-performance status has changed as compared with status of **90 days ago** (or since last assessment if less than 90 days) 0. No change 1. Improved 2. Deteriorated	

FIGURE **6-1, cont'd.** For legend see opposite page.

BOX 6-1

COTA's Sample RAP on ADL Function and Rehabilitation Potential

Resident has exhibited problems in dressing and use of the toilet. Resident's difficulty with putting on clothing is related to weakness in the left upper extremity and possible perceptual problems. Resident needs both physical assistance and verbal instructions. Independent toileting is restricted because of unsafe transfers to the toilet and the inability to handle clothing. Resident is at risk for falls when transferring. Frustration is noted by verbal sighs when attempting to dress. Unsafe ADL techniques have been noted with dressing and transferring. Resident appears to be able and motivated to learn. These problems should be addressed in the resident's plan of care, and this resident should be referred to occupational therapy for further evaluation and treatment.

professionals. This documentation should support the decision to proceed (or not proceed) with a care plan to address the problem (Box 6-1).

Care Planning

Care planning is based on not only identified resident problems but also a resident's unique characteristics, strengths, and needs. The individual resident's characteristics are measured by using standardized MDS items and the RAP process. The care plan must be oriented toward prevention of declines in functional levels, management of risk factors, and building of strengths. It also should reflect standards of current professional practice. Care planning should also include treatment objectives with measurable outcomes and should reflect the resident's goals and wishes, especially if a resident wishes to refuse treatment and the facility's efforts to find alternative means to address the problem. The process should incorporate interdisciplinary expertise to develop a care plan to improve a resident's functional abilities and should involve residents, family members, and others close to the resident (Morris, Murphy, Nonemaker, 1995).

The COTA's role in care planning. COTAs can contribute to the care planning process by providing insight on identified resident problems. This input may include discussion of the deficits and interventions recognized in the OT evaluation process and information for other staff members about the components involved in functional deficits. COTAs can communicate their knowledge and make intervention suggestions at the care plan

conference, which is usually attended by an interdisciplinary team.

MEDICARE

Medicare, or Title 18 of the Social Security Act, was first implemented in 1966. As part of the Social Security Amendment of 1965, the Medicare program was created to establish a health insurance program to supplement the retirement, survivor's, and disability insurance benefits. Originally, Medicare covered most people 65 years of age and over. However, since then the program policy has expanded to cover other groups of people, including those entitled to disability benefits for at least 24 months, those with end-stage renal disease, and those who elect to buy into the program. Qualified disabled and working individuals who lose Medicare benefits because of a return to work are allowed to purchase Medicare Part A and Part B insurance (Lubarsky et al, 1995).

The COTA must understand Medicare rules and regulations. Because COTAs participate in the screening process to determine appropriate candidates for OT services, they may be asked to verify the client's current or potential Medicare status.

Eligibility for Medicare Part A in a Skilled Nursing Facility

Eligibility for Medicare Part A services in a skilled nursing facility (SNF) is determined by an entitled person (one who carries a Medicare card) who has stayed in the hospital for the required 3 consecutive days. The client's health condition must necessitate **skilled services** that can only be provided in a skilled care facility within 30 days of hospital discharge or within 30 days of the last covered SNF stay. Skilled service are those provided by qualified technical or professional health personnel and must be provided under the general supervision of skilled nursing or rehabilitation personnel to ensure client safety and achievement of the desired medical result. A physician must certify the necessity for skilled services, and the client must have Medicare benefit (days) available (Health Care Financing Administration, [HCFA] 1987).

Eligibility for rehabilitation services. SNF rehabilitation services are covered if the following factors are met:

1. The client requires skilled nursing services or skilled rehabilitation services.
2. The client requires these services daily.
3. Considering economy and efficiency, the daily skilled services can be provided only on an inpatient basis in an SNF.
4. These skilled services must be furnished pursuant to a physician's order.
5. The services are necessary for the treatment of a client's illness or injury and must be of reasonable duration and quantity.

Eligibility for Medicare Part A in Home Health Care

Eligibility for Medicare Part A home health services does not require a 3-day hospital stay. However, the elder must be homebound, have a physician's referral, and require skilled services. *Homebound* means the elder is unable to leave the home without considerable effort and assistance. The elder does not have to be bedridden. Visiting a physician is an example of a legitimate reason to leave the home. A client does not qualify for Part A home health services based solely on the need for OT. Nursing, physical therapy, or speech-language pathology must first open the case. However, OT may be introduced along with these other services and may continue after the other services have ended. This stipulation may change in the future.

Eligibility and Entitlement for Medicare Part B

Supplementary Medical Insurance (Part B) is a voluntary program. Part B is available to individuals (including disabled persons) entitled to Part A, U.S. residents who are legal citizens over 65 years of age, and aliens lawfully admitted for permanent residence who have resided in the United States for 5 consecutive years. The program requires enrollment and the payment of a monthly premium. In most states, elders who receive Medicaid benefits are reimbursed for the Medicare Part B premium.

Part B services include physician, outpatient, and home health services in addition to services furnished by rural clinics, ambulatory surgery centers, and comprehensive outpatient rehabilitation. Part B Medicare also covers various ancillary services such as OT. Part B coverage is provided after the 100 days of coverage under Part A are exhausted or if the client should not remain under Medicare Part A for the 100 days as determined by standard guidelines. Part B coverage can be provided to clients located in a non-Medicare certified bed within the SNF. Part B covers only 80% of the allowable changes. The remaining 20% is billed to the client or co-insurance. COTAs must be aware of this fact to educate clients about Medicare billing costs.

Ancillary services. OT is one of the ancillary services covered by Medicare Part B. Ancillary services, which are charged in addition to room and board, are covered in an SNF if the facility charges for time and services, if the services are directly identifiable to individual clients, and if the services are furnished under the direction of a physician and a result of specific medical needs. OT practitioners working in their own private practice who are certified as Medicare Part B providers may bill home health visits under Part B. They must follow all required billing and reimbursement procedures and need to bill both Medicare for 80% of the fee and the client's supplemental insurance for the 20% co-insurance.

Medicare Part B OT services include inpatient and outpatient therapy services furnished by an SNF or under contract arrangements, which means the SNF contracts for provision of therapy services. For OT practitioners to qualify for reimbursement, they must have a physician certify that the therapy services are required and have a plan for furnishing the services established by the physician and the OT practitioner, and the services are to be furnished while the client is under the physician's care. The plan of care must be developed and certified at least once every 30 days. If the physician has not seen the client within 30 days, the OT practitioner is responsible for contacting the physician and arranging for the plan of care to be signed.

Coverage Concepts: Skilled and Unskilled Therapy

The concept of skilled and unskilled therapy must be understood to obtain reimbursement from Medicare for OT treatment. Skilled care includes the concepts discussed earlier. Although a client's diagnosis is a valid factor in deciding the need for skilled services, it should never be the only factor considered. The key issue is whether the skills of a therapist are needed for the required services (HCFA, 1987) (Table 6-1).

In some cases, clients can become qualified for skilled services if a medical complication exists that requires skilled personnel to perform or supervise the service or monitor the client. For example, range-of-motion therapy by itself is usually not considered a skilled service. However, if the client has severe osteoporosis and is at risk for breaking bones, therapy should be furnished by a skilled therapist. (Table 6-2 provides examples of OT services that may be furnished by nonskilled personnel and are therefore not reimbursed.)

A screening assessment of needs to determine Medicare eligibility is performed before admission to an SNF. Clients may be eligible for Medicare reimbursement for many reasons, including the following skilled nursing services: intravenous or intramuscular medications or feedings, nasogastric feedings, and treatment for stage III or IV decubitus ulcers. If the placement is for skilled nursing services rather than skilled therapy services, the OT department may be consulted to determine whether the client also needs skilled OT services.

Justification for OT intervention. COTAs must recognize and understand criteria for OT intervention (Table 6-3). Professional therapy intervention in the SNF should be developed according to resident needs relative to the complexity and intensity of required treatment. Treatment plans should be based on function and must address integration to the total plan of care. Treatment should be reinforced by other disciplines such as skilled nursing. The resident's prior level of function, mobility, and safety in addition to self-care deficits are primary and essential indicators for professional intervention and must be reflected in assessments (Lubarsky et al, 1995).

TABLE **6-1**

Skilled OT Services

Example	Reasons
Mr. K. is a 89-year-old client who recently had a stroke. Because of hemianopsia and problem-solving difficulties, Mr. K. requires moderate assistance with ADL functions that require use of upper and lower extremities. Mr. K. is motivated to do OT treatment.	Recent condition Identifiable functional deficits in performance areas
Mrs. B. is a 72-year-old client who recently had a total hip replacement. She is unable to safely dress and requires education in hip safety precautions. The COTA provides instructions for lower extremity dressing and other ADL functions. Treatment includes teaching safety precautions.	Recent condition (hip surgery) Safety concerns Identifiable functional deficit
Mr. P. is a 92-year-old client who recently sustained a right wrist fracture. He is right-hand dominant. The client was independently performing ADL functions before his wrist was fractured. He now requires moderate assistance with ADL functions because of decreased range-of-motion (ROM) in the right upper extremity. The COTA provides a home ROM program and instruction in ADL functions.	Recent injury Functional deficits with ADL caused by difficulty with the performance component of ROM Prior level of independence Skilled expertise of COTA needed to teach home ROM program

TABLE **6-2**

Nonskilled OT Services

Example	Reasons
Mrs. A. is a 69-year-old client who sustained a humeral fracture. She is qualified for services under Medicare Part A. The COTA sees the client 3 times/week for ADL training. Twice weekly a restorative aide provides passive range-of-motion (PROM) therapy.	A skilled level of care is not needed on a daily basis.
Mrs. N. is a 69-year-old client diagnosed with right cerebral vascular accident. Previously, she performed all ADL functions independently. On initial evaluation, client was able to perform ADL functions independently but slowly. Pt status on initial evaluation was independent with ADLs although performance was slow.	Slow performance with ADL functions is not significant enough to require the intervention of a skilled practitioner. The client will likely improve on her own over time without treatment intervention.
Mrs. K. is a 75-year-old client diagnosed with rheumatoid arthritis. OT was ordered to provide an adapted pencil gripper to assist with writing. The COTA provided the gripper.	Treatment does not require the skilled expertise of the COTA. Anyone could provide an adapted pencil gripper.
Mr. O. is a 74-year-old client diagnosed with Alzheimer's disease. He is dependent in feeding. The COTA monitors feeding 3 times/week for 2 weeks.	The client's condition is chronic and has not shown significant improvement. Treatment is routine, therefore not requiring the skilled expertise of the COTA.

TABLE **6-3**

<center>**Justification For Professional Therapy Service**</center>	
Example	**Reasons**
Mrs. B. was admitted into an SNF to recuperate from hip replacement surgery. In addition, she was to learn to ambulate with a walker and independently perform ADL functions, particularly her own dressing. Once Mrs. B. learns these skills, she may return to her retirement home apartment and receive home health care to ensure her continued progress and safety.	The immediate or short term potential for progress toward a less intensive or lesser skilled service area exists.
Mrs. B. was depressed and the COTA primarily treated her for depression rather than the total hip replacement. However, intervention may be considered skilled if the COTA could demonstrate that the treatment was directly related to motivating the client to safely perform ADL functions.	The philosophy and plan of treatment must realistically focus on achievement of outcomes for the specific phase of rehabilitation, such as being an inpatient in a skilled facility.
The COTA focuses Mrs. B.'s treatment on going home with safety considerations.	Treatment must also focus on the plan for the next expected phase such as outpatient or home care.
During treatment, the COTA should address short-term deficits in safely performing ADL functions. The OT treatment should also take into account the performance component of the client's difficulty with problem solving.	Treatment is expected to address the type and degree of deficits and effects of other problems in relation to the short-term or interim goals.
The COTA would thoroughly document changes in Mrs. B.'s status and her motivational level.	The therapist must emphasize variances in the client's response to treatment and new developments.

Allowable Costs for Services Supplied by Outside Providers

OT practitioners who contract their services to an SNF are currently reimbursed per service rendered. In the near future, OT practitioners' contracted services may be reimbursed by salary equivalency, which is a specific dollar amount designated for services rendered in a nursing facility by a therapist under contract. The Health Care Financing Administration (HCFA), which is the government agency that runs the Medicare program, is currently reviewing therapy service reimbursement policies and procedures and developing forthcoming directives.

Billing Procedures for Home Health Care

Although home health care is reimbursable under both Medicare Part A and Part B, most home health agencies choose to bill under Part A. Medicare will reimburse 100% under Part A but only 80% under Part B. Prior hospitalization is not required to receive home health benefits under either Part A or Part B. The number of home health visits allowed depends on the client's progress, although intermediary insurance companies may establish some guidelines for frequency and duration of visits (Steinhauer, 1995). The HCFA designates intermediaries to determine whether payment should be made for Medicare services and to distribute those funds. The OT practitioner should maintain communication with employees of local intermediaries because they may serve as resources for documentation and billing questions.

MEDICAID
Eligibility

Medicare and Medicaid are two separate programs with different eligibility requirements. Medicare is a federally funded program available for individuals who have worked (or whose spouses have worked) for at least 10 years in Medicare-covered employment and are 65 years old or have had a disability for more than 2 years. In contrast, Medicaid is funded by a combination of finances from the state and federal governments. It is designed to benefit low-income individuals and families and anyone whose health and disability status has resulted in low income or high expense. In addition, the Medicaid program does not have an age requirement, although the elder population often receives a larger portion of funds than other age groups. Eligibility is mandated for all beneficiaries of Aid to Families with Dependent Children (AFDC), most Supplemental Security Income beneficiaries, and indigent children and pregnant women. Individual states may also choose to cover people who are above poverty level but need institutional services.

Benefits

States must provide basic health services, including inpatient and outpatient hospital services, laboratory and x-ray examinations, nursing facility services, physician and nurse practitioner services, and family planning services. State administrations may choose to cover any of 30 or more specific services, including OT. States have also been required to ensure that descriptions of their services meet federal guidelines and that all Medicaid recipients are treated equally (Sommers, Browne, Carter, 1996).

In most states, Medicaid provides home health care coverage to Medicaid beneficiaries who are also eligible for care in an SNF. Under this coverage, OT is considered an optional service. Unlike Medicare, the requirement for one of the qualifying services such as nursing, physical therapy, or speech and language pathology as a prerequisite for OT services does not exist. In some states the client does not have to be homebound to qualify for these home healthcare benefits.

Medicaid reimbursement is considered lower than Medicare and in some states requires prior approval. In some states the Medicaid program has become a managed care plan, and more states will likely choose this option. Medicaid pays a high percentage of nursing care expenditures in the nursing home industry. Because of funding restrictions, Medicaid places an emphasis on institutional care rather than other options that might permit elders to remain in their communities. However, the degree of emphasis varies among states because some have waiver programs and demonstration projects that involve broader funding.

FUTURE CHANGES IN HEALTH CARE COSTS

Prediction of the effects of governmental changes on Medicaid and Medicare laws and funding and thereby coverage of OT is difficult. With the "graying of America," costs for programs that service this population will continue to increase, thereby justifying close scrutiny. The trend to encourage Medicare recipients to obtain Medicare managed care plans is a result of cost-containment efforts. Another way to contain costs and prevent abuse of Medicare and Medicaid is to place "salary caps" on OT and other rehabilitation contracted services. That is, a maximum amount is charged to Medicare for OT services, which may ultimately limit salaries. Changes in the Medicaid and Medicare systems toward per diem payments are also possible. With Medicaid the change may be similar to the acute care hospital diagnosis related groups (DRGs) system but based on function rather than diagnosis. The reformed system may be based on the OBRA MDS assessment using a system called *resource related groups (RRGs)*. The RRG system considers many factors, including the client's functional limitations in addition to medical and

functional needs. A Medicare per diem payment may occur in SNFs and with home health care. Changes will be likely to continue for many years. OT practitioners must be strong advocates for their profession by adjusting to change and adapting to new ways to deliver treatment.

SUPPLEMENTARY SECURITY INCOME PROGRAM

The Supplementary Security Income program, which was enacted in 1972, is a federal assistance program that increased the dollars available for the needy elder, blind, and disabled individuals who did not quality for Social Security benefits. This amendment to the Social Security Act established a minimum income program fully funded by the federal government. Unlike Social Security, Supplementary Security Income is not a retirement program (Rich, Baum, 1984). Elders who did not work long enough to receive reasonable Social Security benefits are the primary recipients.

States supplement the federal assistance with their own benefits, which accounts for the differences in monthly payments among states. Despite increases in public programs, some elders remain below the poverty level. In 35 states the criteria for receiving Supplementary Security Income determines Medicaid eligibility. The recipient is eligible for food stamps. The states must permit the individual to deduct medical expenses in determining income, and to establish Medicaid eligibility by "spending down." Spending down implies reducing one's financial assets to meet the eligibility standards in effect since 1972. Over 1 million eligible people do not participate in the program, possibly because they associate the program with welfare.

Many individuals who quality for Supplementary Security Income have the same types of problems as institutionalized elders. Their needs for therapy often go unidentified because they live in social environments rather than medical environments such as an SNF. These social environments may be substandard and provide no case management unless individuals are involved with community-based health programs. These individuals often do not have access to Medicare Part B services because they may not have the resources to buy into the voluntary program. The need for OTR and COTA collaboration and development of services for these individuals is clear, but practitioners need to find creative ways to fund programs and advocate for the needed care. Appropriate services from OT practitioners may reduce the need for institutionalization.

OLDER AMERICANS ACT

In 1965 the Older Americans Act (OAA) was enacted to provide services for elders. The premise of OAA was that services provided to elders at least 60 years of age would enable them to remain in their homes and communities. Funding was established for nutrition programs, senior centers, transportation, housing, and ombudsman and legal services. Differences in these programs exist among states because administration is at the state level. In addition, more opportunity for OT exists in some regions than in others. The OAA was designed to foster independence, but rehabilitative services were not included. The act established the Administration on Aging, an agency specifically responsible for developing new social services for elders.

OAA was reauthorized in 1992 and additional funding was added for resource centers to promote links among acute care, rehabilitative services, and long-term care systems. Some limited references to preventive health services include home injury control services, programs relating to chronic disabling conditions, and provision of information concerning diagnoses. Other limited resources include prevention, treatment, and rehabilitation of age-related diseases and chronic disabling conditions. Resources such as homemakers, chore workers, home-delivered meals, and community-based programs provide respite for caretakers of dependent relatives and friends. Goals to establish OAA-coordinated programs for elders were not reached.

BOX 6-2

Ways for COTAs to Become Involved with Public Policy

- Be able and ready to articulate a clear definition of OT for the public; be visible.
- Serve on OT task forces and committees.
- Volunteer for community committees that advocate for elders, such as an Alzheimer's Association.
- Read public and OT literature as much as possible to keep up on trends.
- Write and submit articles to professional and consumer publications about OT practice.
- Find a mentor who understands public policy.
- Write letters to important people such as legislators, managed care and corporate executives, third-party payers, and case managers.
- Learn the legislative process in your state and testify for relevant issues at public hearings.
- If questions or concerns cannot be answered or addressed on a local level, network with the legislative division of AOTA.

ADVOCACY

Health care is in a state of flux that will directly affect OT practice. Involvement of COTAs in **advocacy** for elders and the OT profession can make a difference. A quotation from Eleanor Roosevelt states "Every person owes a portion of his time and talent to the upbuilding of a profession to which he/she belongs" (Scott, Acquaviva, 1985). Every COTA and OTR must encourage the benefits of OT and establish the role of the profession within society. COTAs must stay informed about all government decisions regarding health care (Box 6-2).

▌ CHAPTER REVIEW QUESTIONS

1 What is SSI and who can benefit from it?
2 Can a COTA complete the MDS?
3 What areas does OBRA address in which occupational therapy can be involved?
4 What is an RAP?
5 What qualifies a person for Medicare Part A OT coverage in an SNF?
6 What is required for OT services in home health care?
7 What makes a person eligible for Medicaid?
8 How can COTAs be advocates for the OT profession?

REFERENCES

Binstock RH: Changing criteria in old-age programs: the introduction of economic status and need for services, *Gerontologist* (34):6, 726, 1994.

Health Care Financing Administration: *Coverage of services, Medicare regulations,* Baltimore, Md, 1987, The Administration.

Lubarsky JM et al: *Medicare resource manual: a guide through the critical steps,* Hindsale, Ill, 1995, Life Services Network of Illinois.

MacClain J: Personal communication, 1996.

Morris JN, Murphy K, Nonemaker S: *Resident assessment instrument (RAI) user's manual,* Baltimore, Md, 1995, Health Care Financing Administration.

Omnibus Budget Reconciliation Act (OBRA), Baltimore, Md, 1995, Health Care Financing Administration: Administration.

Rich BM, Baum M: *The aging: a guide to public policy,* Pittsburgh, 1984, University of Pittsburgh.

Scott SJ, Acquaviva JD: *Lobbying for healthcare,* Rockville, Md, 1985, Government and Legal Affairs Division, American Occupational Therapy Association.

Sommers FP, Browne S, Carter ME: *Medicaid: current law and issues in reform proposals,* Bethesda, Md, 1996, American Occupational Therapy Association.

Steinhauer MJ, editor: *Guidelines for occupational therapy practice in home health,* Rockville, Md, 1995, American Occupational Therapy Association.

OCCUPATIONAL THERAPY INTERVENTION WITH ELDERS

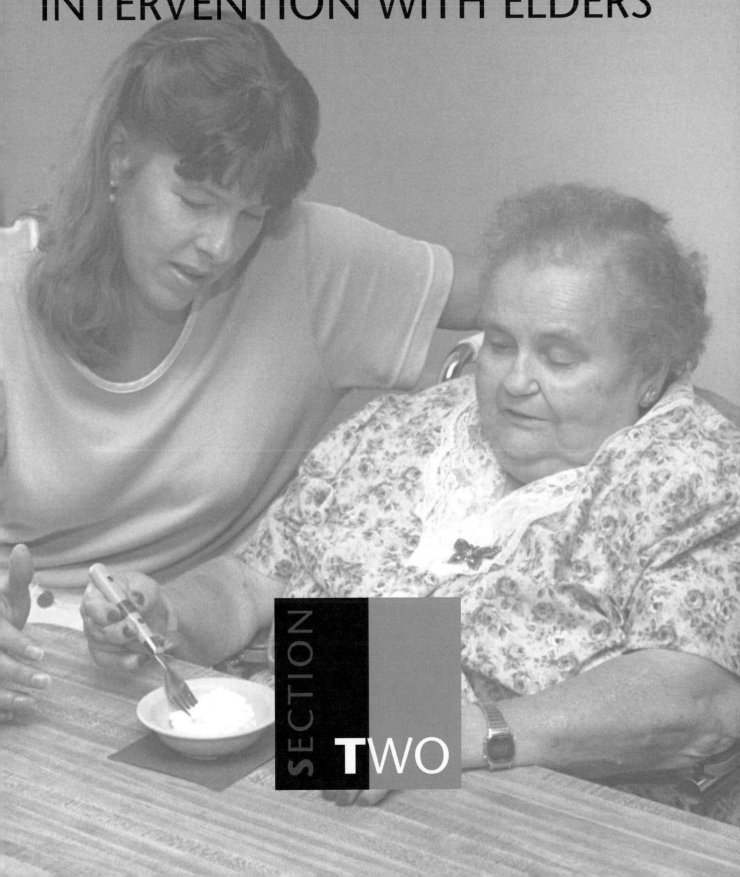

SECTION TWO

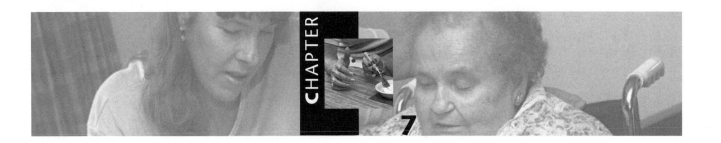

Application of Occupational Therapy Theories With Elders

RENÉ PADILLA

KEY TERMS

clinical practice models, values, dysfunction, skills, occupation, function, assessment,
task, roles, performance, culture, environment, self-care, work, play and leisure,
treatment, context, cognition, maturation, motor action, subsystem, habits

CHAPTER OBJECTIVES

1. Explain the importance and use of practice models in occupational therapy intervention with elders.
2. Briefly summarize principles of four occupational therapy practice models as they relate to aging, including Occupational Performance, Facilitating Growth and Development, Cognitive Disabilities, and the Model of Human Occupation.
3. Demonstrate the ways COTAs can incorporate theoretical principles into practice with elders.

Rose is a recent graduate and a new COTA employee at an acute care hospital in a Midwestern city of 300,000 people. Rose came from a small farming town of German ancestry and has never been out of the state. At the hospital, she is asked to continue OT treatment for Mr. Zia, an 82-year-old Pakistani gentleman who suffered a stroke 5 days previously. The OTR who performed the evaluation told Rose that Mr. Zia has lived in 20 cities throughout the world before coming to this city, where he is an executive in a large company. Rose is to continue working with Mr. Zia on sitting balance and midline alignment using an activity that is meaningful for the client. Given the different backgrounds of client and

practitioner, what process should Rose use to select a meaningful activity?

Mike has worked as a COTA in a 30-bed skilled nursing facility for over a year. The majority of clients admitted have temporary orthopedic impairments in addition to chronic conditions. Mr. Cole, who was recently admitted to the nursing facility, is a 75-year-old gentleman who underwent radiation and chemotherapy for prostate cancer. The treatment was ineffective and the cancer metastasized. Mr. Cole is still fairly mobile and alert and wishes to go home to his wife while he is still able. How should Mike go about prioritizing Mr. Cole's treatment?

Sarah is a COTA working at an adult day-care center in the downtown area of a large city. Sarah has worked at the center for 2 years. The majority of her clients are Hispanic and from rural Mexico. Sarah and the supervising OTR want to develop a group activity program for the clients who have mild Alzheimer's dementia. What techniques should Sarah use to implement an appropriate activity program based on the shared needs of these clients?

Pete has been a COTA at an outpatient rehabilitation center for 10 years. Pete traveled to West Africa 2 years ago to trace several hundred years of his family roots. This was a very significant experience for Pete, whose great grandfather was a slave on a Southern plantation. On Pete's schedule is Mara, a 60-year-old female client with repetitive motion injury of the upper extremities. Mara, a native of the West Indies, has been working at a food packing plant for over 30 years. Her husband died in a car accident 2 months previously. To what extent can Pete rely on his knowledge of the history of Blacks in America to plan Mara's OT treatment?

The previous scenarios are examples of the diversity of people and their needs that the COTA deals with daily. Rose must find a way to treat her client, whose background is so different from her own. Mike must help Mr. Cole prepare for his final stage of life. Sarah must choose one activity that addresses the needs of each client in her group. Pete must make sure he does not impose his own values on Mara. Each COTA is providing OT services. Should their programs look similar?

These COTAs need a common tool that addresses all these situations consistently and according to basic OT philosophic and theoretic principles. Although the programs must maintain a common thread that identifies them as OT treatments, they should be flexible enough to provide individual meaning for each client. OT **clinical practice models** are intended to connect professional philosophy and theory with daily practice.

OVERVIEW OF A PRACTICE MODEL

This chapter reviews four practice models: Occupational Performance (American Occupational Therapy Association [AOTA], 1974; Pedretti, 1995), Facilitating Growth and Development (Llorens, 1976), Cognitive Disabilities (Allen, 1985), and the Model of Human Occupation (Kielhofner, 1995). These models have either specific or inferred applications with the elder population. Several other practice models may also be useful to OT practice with elders (Dutton, Levy, Simon, 1993; Kielhofner, 1992).

The common link between all forms of OT intervention cannot be overemphasized. The philosophy of OT practice includes **values,** beliefs, truths, and principles that should guide the general practice of the profession. One tenet of this philosophy is that the human being is inherently active and can influence self-development, health, and environment with purposeful activity. Thus the human is able to adapt to life's demands and become self-actualized. **Dysfunction** occurs when the human being's ability to adapt is impaired in some way. OT intervention seeks to prevent and remediate dysfunction and facilitate maximal adaptation through the use of purposeful activities (AOTA, 1995). The use of purposeful activity, or occupation, is the common thread for every OT intervention.

Since the OT profession began, the term *occupation* has described the individual's active participation in self-care, work, and leisure (AOTA, 1993), which constitute the ordinary, familiar things people do every day (AOTA, 1995). The person must use combinations of sensorimotor, cognitive, psychologic, and psychosocial **skills** to perform these occupations (AOTA, 1994). Specific environments and different stages of life influence these occupations. Kielhofner (1995) defines *occupation* as "doing culturally meaningful work, play or living tasks in the stream of time and in the contexts of one's physical and social world."

To understand the concepts of **occupations** and use them to facilitate **function** and adaptation, COTAs must have broad knowledge of the biological, social, and medical sciences in addition to OT theoretical premises. OT practice models provide organized frameworks for that knowledge, which allows the therapist to apply pertinent information to a specific client's problem. Thus practice models guide the therapist in creating individual treatment programs that are culturally meaningful and age related and that facilitate development of sensorimotor, cognitive, psychological, and psychosocial skills. By using a practice model for guidance, the four COTAs discussed in the scenarios can ensure professional treatment programs that are tailored to meet the needs of each client.

OT practice models do not offer concrete plans for improvement of function. Instead these models suggest use of various graded occupations that demand development of performance abilities, thereby improving function. COTAs may use the information in the practice models to formulate questions to assess the client's needs, interests, and meanings; select **assessment** tools; and accordingly design a unique intervention strategy. COTAs should be familiar with several practice models because each model usually has a specific focus and does not address all dimensions of occupational functioning.

Occupational Performance

The Occupational Performance Model is concerned with the individual's ability to perform **tasks** that permit satisfaction in the **roles** the individual occupies in society. Successful **performance** requires that the task be appropriate for the individual's developmental stage, **culture,** and physical **environment.** The suggested tasks are organized in three broad categories, or performance areas: **self-care, work,** and **play and leisure** (Figure 7-1). These performance areas influence and are influenced by the individual's life space (that is, the cultural, social, and physical environment). The person must be able to use combinations of skills, or performance components learned through experience. Health is a result of the balance of occupational performance. Thus the Occupational Performance Model is concerned with remediation or compensation of deficits that may occur in the performance areas or performance components. These deficits, which threaten the balance needed for good health, may result from illness, developmental, biological, social, and environmental limitations. The OT practitioner helps the client engage in purposeful activity that establishes or restores optimal balance in occupational performance and roles.

Before applying this model, the COTA must obtain information about the client's performance in the self-care, work, and play and leisure areas. Information may be obtained through interviews and observation. The COTA and supervising OTR should determine the methods and depth of evaluation. Once a deficit in one performance area is identified, the COTA must investigate life space factors that may contribute to the deficit and not assume that the client, family members, and acquaintances recognize the deficit.

The next step is to investigate the client's deficits in performance components that inhibit optimal performance of the self-care, work, and leisure tasks (see Figure 7-1). Performance component skills may be evaluated in a variety of ways ranging from use of specific standardized tests to informal observations of specific components during task completion. For example, joint range of motion is measured using a calibrated goniometer that quantifies the arc of movement at any particular joint. Joint range of motion may also be observed while a client performs a functional activity such as reaching to the back of the head to comb hair or putting an arm into a jacket sleeve. Muscle strength is most often assessed with a manual muscle test, and endurance is determined by the length of time a person can sustain or repeat an action. Cognitive function can be assessed by using standardized tests or by observing the way the client plans and executes a task. Social skills are best assessed by observing the client in a social situation. All possible methods to assess each performance area and component cannot be listed within this chapter. However, the OTR and COTA team

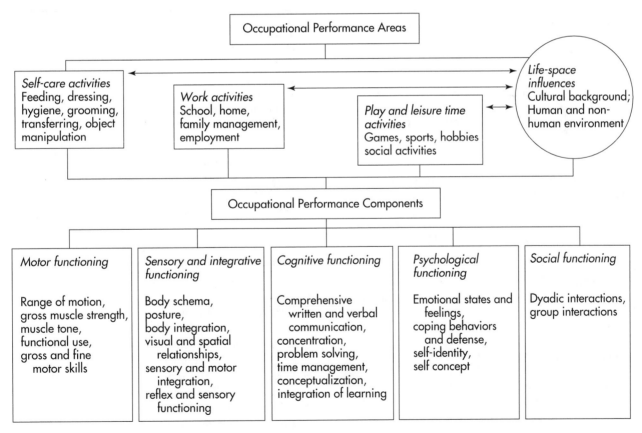

FIGURE 7-1 Occupational performance areas and components. (From American Occupational Therapy Association: *A curriculum guide for occupational therapy educators,* Rockville, Md, 1974, The Association.)

must have a complete picture of the client's functional ability in all performance components to construct a pertinent **treatment** plan for the client. The COTA should be familiar with the evaluation methods because the same method should be used to measure the client's progress.

Once the OTR and COTA have an overview of the client's limitations and environmental **context,** they can prioritize OT needs. Intervention strategies may be selected from a continuum of adjunctive methods, which are procedures that prepare the client for OT but are preliminary to purposeful activity; enabling activities, which stimulate involvement in purposeful activities but are not directly purposeful; purposeful activities, which have an inherent or autonomous goal and are meaningful to the client; and occupational performance and roles, which are activities the client performs daily (Table 7-1). Intervention strategies should address each deficit in both performance components and areas (Figure 7-2). In addition, the client's physical environment may be modified or redesigned to support optimal functioning.

TABLE 7-1

Continuum of Therapeutic Activities	
Activity classification	**Activity examples**
Adjunctive	
Procedures that prepare the client for occupational performance and are preliminary to purposeful activity	Exercise, facilitation/inhibition techniques, positioning, sensory stimulation, splints, braces, physical agent modalities
Enabling	
Activities that stimulate purposeful activities to train specific sensorimotor, perceptual, and cognitive functions needed for self-care, work, and leisure	Driving simulators, skate boards, sanding boards, work simulations
Purposeful	
Activities that have a meaningful goal for the person	Cooking, painting, dressing, reading, writing
Occupational performance and occupational roles	
Groups of activities that form a role in the person's living environment and community	School performance, job performance, home maintenance, leisure involvement

Data from Pedretti L: *Occupational therapy: practice skills for physical dysfunction,* St Louis, 1995, Mosby.

Adjunctive and enabling activities should not form the exclusive method of treatment. Rather, these types of activities should prepare the client to engage in purposeful tasks. Purposeful activity characterizes OT treatment and distinguishes it from other services. OT treatment is discontinued when the client can effectively perform and sustain a balance of occupational roles (Pedretti, 1995).

CASE STUDY

The Occupational Performance Model can help Rose, the COTA discussed earlier, organize information to select a meaningful activity for her client, Mr. Zia. The OTR already identified specific motor and sensory performance component deficits. Rose must interview Mr. Zia and his family to determine his daily self-care, work, and leisure routines before the stroke. She must also ask about the environment in which Mr. Zia will live and acceptable behaviors in which he will engage from the perspective of his Pakistani culture. This information will give Rose insight to Mr. Zia's competence in the three performance areas and the expectations. In addition, interviewing the client and his family will give Rose some information about the **cognitive,** psychological, and social skills Mr. Zia needs to continue finding life meaningful. She may find out that Mr. Zia is a devout Muslim and consequently finds observance of Muslim traditions central in structuring his life. Mr. Zia may react with resistance or anger to expectations to participate in a therapeutic program on Friday, the Sabbath. An interview with the client and his family may reveal that religious rules cause Mr. Zia to feel uncomfortable being touched by a woman. Rose can recruit one of Mr. Zia's male relatives to assist him with some personal care and other activities that require close physical contact because this is most likely the arrangement Mr. Zia will have when discharged home. Finally, Rose might discover that Mr. Zia, like most Pakistani businessmen, often drank tea with his associates. Consequently, Rose may choose tea preparation as an activity to help Mr. Zia develop better trunk control and midline alignment and to instruct his male relative about correct procedures when assisting Mr. Zia with movement. This activity is meaningful for Mr. Zia from the perspectives of both performance areas (particularly work, leisure, and cultural contexts) and components (for example, sitting up, aligning the trunk, sequencing the familiar tea-making activity, and interacting with others while pouring and drinking tea).

Facilitating Growth and Development

The Facilitating Growth and Development Model views the OT practitioner's role as one "concerned with facilitating or promoting optimal growth and development in all ages of man" (Llorens, 1976). An individual's growth and development may be threatened by disease, injury, disability, or trauma. The OT practitioner may be required to assist the individual in coping with illness, trauma, or disability or to help with rehabilitation. The OT practitioner may also seek to prevent maladaptation and promote health maintenance.

This model requires the OT practitioner to understand the developmental tasks and adaptive skills that are usually mastered at different ages. The model describes the belief that the human being "develops simultaneously in the areas of neurophysiological, physical, psychosocial and psychodynamic growth, and in the development of social language, daily living, socio-cultural, and intellectual skills during the life span" (Llorens, 1976). The way the individual integrates and organizes these areas of development to perform in work, education, play, self-care, and leisure activities during each stage of life is of primary concern to OT. In addition to understanding the individual's development, the OT practitioner must understand the ways illness, disease, trauma, and disability may threaten that development. Finally, OT addresses the environmental variables necessary to support the development and maintenance of the important adaptive skills cited by Llorens (1976).

The Facilitating Growth and Development Model synthesizes the work of numerous authors that have contributed to the understanding of human **maturation** (Llorens, 1976). The model includes descriptions of the adaptive skills mentioned during each life stage, including infancy to age 2 years, ages 2 to 3 years, ages 3 to 6 years, ages 6 to 11 years, adolescence, young adulthood, adulthood, and maturity. Each stage is built on the

foundation of the stages the person has completed (Box 7-1). This text, however, focuses on the last stage.

During the OT process the OTR and COTA assess the client's development and determine potential disruptions in each adaptive skill area. The OTR and COTA analyze this information to determine the effects on age-appropriate occupational performance in the areas of work, education, self-care, and play and leisure. The OTR and COTA may then devise intervention strategies that facilitate development of a specific skill needed for successful occupational performance (Box 7-2). Matching the client's needs with the right therapeutic activities requires careful analysis of inherent requirements of each activity.

Depending on the client's needs, selected activities may include sensory, developmental, symbolic, and daily life tasks. These activities are combined with the social interaction that is most beneficial for the client. Sensory activities are those that primarily influence the senses through human action, such as touching, rocking, running, and listening to sounds. Developmental activities involve the use of objects such as crafts and puzzles in play, learning, and skill development situations. The client develops specific performance skills by engaging

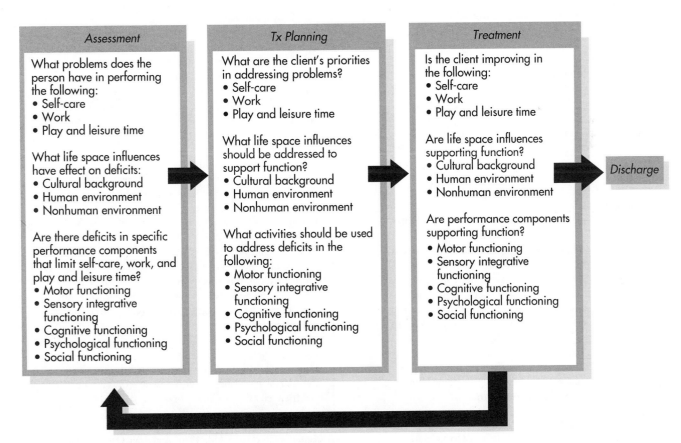

FIGURE 7-2 Steps in the occupational therapy process using the occupational performance model.

BOX 7-1

Characteristics of Maturity

Neurophysiological and physical development
Possible alterations in sensory functions (visual, auditory, tactile, kinesthetic, gustatory, and olfactory), motor behavior (coordination of extremities), information processing (higher level integration, including conceptualization and memory), and physical endurance

Psychosocial—ego integrity and maturity
Acceptance of life experiences and the life cycle

Psychodynamic
Coping with continued growth after middle age, decision making regarding growth or death (giving up on life), dealing with insincerity of friends and acquaintances, inner life trends toward survival, possible decrease in efforts to maintain false pride, often a reduction in defenses, more suspiciousness, and necessity of dealing with psychological deterioration

Sociocultural
Group affiliation: family, social, interest, civic,

Social language development
Predominantly verbal use, some use of nonverbal behavior to communicate

Activities of daily living and developmental tasks
Adjustment to decreasing physical strength and health, adjustment to retirement and reduced income, adjustment to death of spouse, adjustment to one's own impending death, establishment of affiliations with own age group, and meeting of social obligations

Ego-adaptive skills
Ability to function independently; ability to control drives and select appropriate objects; ability to organize stimuli, plan and execute purposeful motion; ability to obtain, organize, and use knowledge; ability to participate in primary group; ability to participate in a variety of relationships; ability to experience self as a holistic, acceptable object; ability to participate in mutually satisfying heterosexual relationships oriented to sexual needs

Intellectual development
Possible neurophysiological and physical development alteration and return of egocentrism

(Data from Llorens LA: *Application of a developmental theory for health and rehabilitation*, Rockville, Md, 1976, American Occupational Therapy Association.)

BOX 7-2

Activity Analysis

Sensory aspects
How much touch and movement does the activity require? To what extent are visual-perception skills used in the activity? Does the activity require auditory perception and discrimination? Are perception and discrimination of smells and taste involved in the activity?

Physical aspects
How much does the activity require bilateral movements of arms and legs? Does the activity require the use of both hands at the same time? Can the activity be completed with one hand? How much muscle strength and joint range of motion does the activity require? How much sitting, standing, and variability in position is necessary to complete the activity? Does the physical performance require much thought organization? Which fine and gross motor movements does the activity require? How much eye-hand coordination is needed for the activity? How much time and what equipment is needed for the activity?

Psychodynamic aspects
Does the activity permit expression of feelings, thoughts, original ideas, and creativity? Is there opportunity for the constructive expression of hostility, aggression, expansiveness, organization, control, narcissism, expiation of guilt, dependence, and independence? How does the activity permit or require sex role identification?

Social aspects
How much contact and guidance from others is required to complete the activity? How much does the activity require the person to work alone or with others? How much socialization does the activity permit?

Attention and skill aspects
How much initiative and self-reliance does the activity require? Does the activity require technical skills? Are manipulative and creative abilities needed? Does the activity require persistence to complete? How much repeated motion is needed?

Practical aspects
How much noise and dirt are created during the activity? What materials and equipment are used and what are their costs? Can waste or scrap material be used?

(Data from Llorens LA: *Application of a developmental theory for health and rehabilitation*, Rockville, Md, 1976, American Occupational Therapy Association.)

in these types of activities. Symbolic activities are designed to help the client satisfy needs and elicit and cope with emotional responses. Examples include gouging wood and kneading clay, which may release muscle tension and help process anger. Another example of a symbolic activity is leading a group in a task. This activity may satisfy the client's need to be heard and feel competent. The emotional response from leading a group may be improved self-esteem. Daily life tasks, also called *activities of daily living*, include tasks such as brushing teeth, getting dressed, cooking, and cleaning. Finally, social interaction includes participation in dyads with the therapist or another person and groups. These activities encourage development of sociocultural competence and language and intellectual skills (Figure 7-3).

According to the Facilitating Growth and Development Model, OT intervention should continue until the client reaches sufficient competence in performing the skills and activities described as developmentally appropriate. The OTR and COTA continually monitor and reevaluate the client's progress in improving, maintaining, or restoring areas of occupational performance and therefore clearly know when the client no longer requires specialized OT services.

CASE STUDY

Mike, the COTA at a skilled nursing facility, may use the Facilitating Growth and Development Model to prepare his client, Mr. Cole, for the final stage of life. Mr. Cole is a 75-year-old gentleman with metastatic prostate cancer who wishes to go home to his wife while he is still able. Although Mr. Cole's physical abilities have deteriorated as a result of his medical condition, Mike must continue to address the physical deficits because this area directly supports Mr. Cole's desire to go home. Mr. Cole's statement that he wants to go home while he is "still able" indicates that he

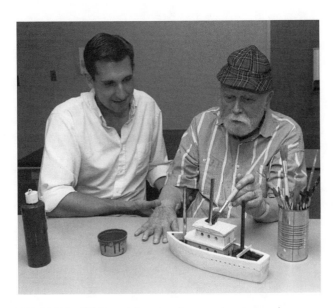

FIGURE 7-3 This activity permits creative expression.

has acknowledged his deterioration, has accepted his life cycle, and is seeking to adjust to the idea of impending death. Mike must focus the OT treatment on helping Mr. Cole prioritize activities to conserve his energy and thereby enable him to actively function in his primary group (wife and family). Accordingly, Mike will select adaptive and durable medical equipment such as a reacher to avoid bending and a raised toilet seat to avoid standing from a low surface. In addition, Mike can teach Mr. Cole methods of carrying objects and sequencing tasks that decrease the amount of effort required. The treatment focus should be on maintenance of social interaction and learning skills rather than on complete independence with ADL functions and work. Consequently, Mike may also work with Mr. Cole on identifying communication skills that help Mr. Cole request assistance and express his appreciation of other people.

Cognitive Disabilities

As its name indicates, the Cognitive Disabilities Model is concerned with OT services that are designed for clients with cognitive impairments. These impairments may be the result of psychiatric illness, medical diseases, brain traumas, or developmental disorders. Psychiatric illnesses such as depression and schizophrenia have associated cognitive impairments. Alzheimer's dementia and cerebrovascular accidents are examples of medical conditions that result in cognitive impairments, and closed head injuries are an example of trauma to the brain that can also result in a brain disorder. Brain dysfunction may also result from use of prescribed medications or other drugs. The cognitive impairment that results from these conditions may be short term or long lasting.

Assertions of the Cognitive Disabilities Model are based on information from neuroscience, biology, psychology, and traditional OT theory. According to this model, *occupation* is synonymous with *voluntary motor action*. Observing voluntary **motor actions** such as dressing, completing a craft, or preparing a simple meal is of primary interest to the OT practitioner because of the inferences that can be made about brain function. Voluntary motor actions are "behavioral responses to a sensory cue that are guided by the mind" (Allen, 1985). That is, voluntary motor actions occur as a consequence of the relationship among the external physical environment of matter, which provides sensory cues; the internal mind, which provides purpose; and the body, which produces behavior in the form of motor activity. Observing a person's voluntary motor action gives the OT practitioner insight to the relationship among these three domains. Each domain is further described by subclassifications.

Based on extensive research, the Cognitive Disabilities Model proposes a categorization of six cognitive levels that describe the way an individual relates matter, behavior, and mind as demonstrated in performance of voluntary motor actions (Allen, 1985) (Table 7-2). Level 1 represents the highest degree of impairment, and level

TABLE 7-2

Allen Cognitive Levels

	Level 1 Automatic actions	Level 2 Postural actions	Level 3 Manual actions	Level 4 Goal-directed actions	Level 5 Exploratory actions	Level 6 Planned actions
Matter						
Sensory cues	Awareness is at threshold of consciousness	Responds to proprioceptive cues	Responds to tactile cues	Follows visible cues	Follows related cues	Follows symbolic cues
Perceptibility	Attends to cues that penetrate subliminal state	Aware of own body and objects that come into contact with it	Aware of immediate external surfaces	Aware of concepts of color and shape of objects	Aware of concepts of space and depth	Aware of intangible concepts
Setting	Mainly internal	Within range of motion	Within arm's reach	Within visual field	Restricted to task environment	Expanded to potential task environments
Sample	Responds to alerting stimuli	Copies demonstrated body action	Identifies material objects	Makes exact match of sample	Conceives tangible possibilities of variations	Conceives hypothetic ideas
Behavior						
Motor actions	Actions are habitual and automatic and have little thought	Spontaneous actions are postural (bending and stretching)	Hands are used to manipulate material objects repetitively	Actions are goal directed but restricted to tangible environment	Possibilities are explored through motor action that causes a visible effect	Actions are preceded by pause to think and plan
Tool use	Needs stimulation to use body parts in habitual tasks	Uses body parts spontaneously	Uses found objects by chance, success is accidental	Uses hand tools as a means to a concrete end	Uses hand tools to vary means and end	Creates tools, uses power tools
Number	Completes one action at a time	Completes one action at a time	Completes one action at a time	Completes one step of task at a time	Completes several steps at a time	Completes indefinite steps

People	Attends to those who shout or touch	Attends to those who move	Attends to the object manipulation of others	Shares goals with others	Shares exploration with others	Shares plans and recognizes autonomy
Directions	Understands single verbs, physical contact is needed for action	Understands pronouns and names of body parts, gross motor, and guided movements	Understands names of material objects and actions on an object	Understands adjectives and adverbs, must see each step in a series	Understands prepositions and explanations, each step and potential errors must be demonstrated	Understands conjunction and conjectures, demonstration is not necessary
Mind						
Attention	Attention is focused on subliminal cues, external attention is very transient	Attends to proprioceptive cues, to own body, and to movement	Attends to tactile cues, focuses attention on the immediate effects of own actions	Attends to clearly visible cues, focuses attention to complete a task, end product sustains attention	Attends to related visual cues; may seek novelty through variation, but must see effects first	Attends to symbolic cues, thinks before testing results
Goal attainment	Is awake, completes very habitual behaviors (eating and drinking)	Chance body movement creates interesting result that may be repeated	Chance movement causes visible results that are repeated many times	Uses several movement schemes to achieve an end goal	Becomes aware of problems when they become visible, uses trial and error approach	Problems are solved covertly, images are used to test solutions
Time	Attention is maintained for seconds at a time	Attention is directed for minutes at a time	Attention is directed for half an hour at a time	Attention is maintained for an hour at a time	Attention is maintained and goals are remembered for weeks at a time	Sense of past, present, and future is maintained

Data from Allen C: *Occupational therapy for psychiatric diseases: measurement and management of psychiatric diseases,* Boston, Mass, 1985, Little, Brown.

6 represents normal performance. As this model has evolved, each cognitive level has been expanded to include several subcategories. Only the global characteristics of each level are described in this text. This practice model may be used to describe client performance and guide selection of activities or tasks that permit the client to function consistently at the highest possible level. (Other chapters in this text describe conditions associated with elders for whom application of the cognitive disabilities model may be appropriate, including side effects of medication in Chapter 15; malnutrition and dehydration in Chapter 20; strokes in Chapter 21; Alzheimer's dementia in Chapter 22; depression, schizophrenia, and drug addiction in Chapter 23; and brain tumors in Chapter 27.)

Observing clients perform activities and tasks that are part of their daily routines is ideal during assessment because these activities are usually important to the client and caregivers. These activities also allow the OTR and COTA team to separate issues related to learning a new activity, which might not accurately convey the client's current cognitive performance. Consequently, task assessment should be preceded by information obtained from the client and caregivers regarding the client's most familiar tasks. After observing the client, the OTR and COTA team can compare the performance with the characteristic behaviors for each cognitive level. The OTR and COTA must remember that a client may function at a variety of levels depending on familiarity with the task and the time of day. Knowledge of the client's optimal functional level helps the OTR and COTA team design intervention strategies that maximize the client's abilities.

Several standardized tests may be used to determine cognitive level, including the Expanded Routine Task Inventory (RTI) (Allen, 1985), and the Allen Cognitive Levels Test (ACL). The RTI evaluates the individual's ability at each of the six levels to complete a variety of routine tasks along a physical scale, such as grooming, dressing, bathing, walking, and exercising, feeding, toileting, taking medication, and using adaptive equipment; a community scale, such as housekeeping, obtaining and preparing food, spending money, doing laundry, traveling, shopping, telephoning, and taking care of a child; a communication scale, such as listening, talking, reading, and writing; and an employment scale, such as maintaining pace and schedule, following instructions, performing simple and complex tasks, getting along with co-workers, following safety precautions and responding to emergencies, and supervising and planning work. The ACL test helps determine cognitive level by assessing response to verbal instructions and problem-solving techniques when a client is presented with a leather lacing project. (Allen, 1985). The large ACL was developed to compensate for visual loss in the elder population, and the Cognitive

Performance Test was developed to provide a standardized, ADL-based instrument for the assessment of functional level in Alzheimer's dementia (Figure 7-4).

Once the client's cognitive level has been determined, the OT intervention goals must be considered. Allen (1985) states that participation in an occupation does not necessarily mean the client will improve. This assumption fails to recognize other possible reasons for recovery, including the fact that the client may recover spontaneously without any treatment. Consequently, the purpose of OT intervention should be to document alterations and improvements in functional abilities, sustain current performance, and reduce pain and distress associated with the symptoms. Goals are not intended to improve cognitive level but to ensure consistency of performance at the safest and least restrictive level. The case of Ray illustrates this point. Ray, who is 70 years old, has Alzheimer's dementia. An OTR and COTA team determined that he is currently functioning at cognitive level 4. This means that Ray can spontaneously complete tasks when cues are clearly visible. A goal for Ray to live independently would not be appropriate because he does not deal with cues that are not within his field of vision and consequently can easily place himself in danger. Appropriate OT goals for Ray according to this model may include consistent initiation of daily self-care routines, initiation of laundry washing, consistent monitoring of Ray in unfamiliar environments, and provision by his caregivers of appropriate cues to maximize his performance.

Once the client's goals have been determined, the COTA may select a variety of activities that match the characteristics of the matter, mind, and behavior domains appropriate to the client's cognitive level. The COTA

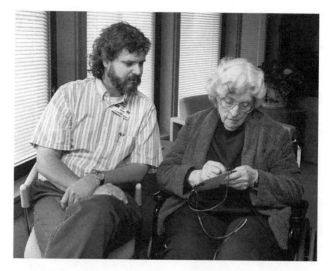

FIGURE 7-4 The large ACL was developed to compensate for visual loss.

must be adept at analyzing a task to know precisely the way it requires matter, mind, and behavior to interact for the client to *successfully* perform a voluntary motor action. Tasks are selected by the degree of demand on the client to perform consistently at a particular cognitive level. The OTR and COTA team evaluated Ray and determined he was at cognitive level 4. Consequently, he can understand basic goals of activities, can purposefully use objects placed within his field of vision, and is able to match examples of tasks demonstrated to him. To reinforce his ability to maintain a sense of accomplishment, the COTA may select a simple woodworking project for Ray. The COTA can place all materials for this project on a table in front of Ray and instruct him to sand the wooden pieces. Telling him to pick up the sandpaper, hold it so the grain comes in contact with the wood, and rub it against the wood is unnecessary. These steps would be obvious to Ray because the materials are in his field of vision. Once Ray completes the sanding, the COTA may instruct him in a similar way to glue the pieces together as shown in the sample, stain the stool, and varnish it. Ray lacks the foresight to plan for potential problems; consequently, the COTA should demonstrate the amount of glue, stain, and varnish needed in addition to the application procedures.

Once the client is performing at a level that most consistently demonstrates remaining task abilities and the environment has been structured to compensate for the client's limitations, skilled OT services should be discontinued. Discharge considerations are made from the beginning of OT intervention. The cognitive disabilities model specifically focuses on preparing the client for discharge to the least restrictive environment. Therefore the COTA must observe voluntary motor actions to understand the way each client interacts with the environment. The COTA and OTR should recommend that the client be discharged to the setting that best supports the client's task abilities.

CASE STUDY

Sarah, the COTA working at an adult day-care center, was asked to develop a group activity program for the clients with mild Alzheimer's dementia. This diagnosis assumes the presence of cognitive deficit, so the Cognitive Disabilities Model is an ideal tool to guide Sarah in her endeavor. The first task for Sarah and the OTR is to determine the cognitive level of each potential group member. Sarah and the OTR may select the Allen Cognitive Test (leather lacing activity) as a tool to evaluate potential members. Most clients at the day program are from rural Mexico, so Sarah and the OTR must first verify that the task is culturally appropriate. Once this has been verified, Sarah and the OTR can administer the leather lacing test and obtain a general impression of overall cognitive level. This information may be used in several ways. Sarah and the OTR may wish to run a group program for each cognitive level. This would facilitate task selection and leadership style for each group.

Sarah would select activities for group members performing at cognitive level 4 that lend themselves to successful outcomes when presented step-by-step. Examples may include simple printing or painting tasks, woodworking kits with few and large pieces, and simple food preparation activities that do not require use of a stove or other potentially dangerous appliance. Sarah could select activities for clients performing at cognitive level 5 that encourage consideration of possible outcomes and that require completion of several steps before needing another set of instructions. Examples may include cooking by following a recipe and decorating a flower pot. If an insufficient number of members is available to form a group for each cognitive level, Sarah will have to organize groups that include the needs of several cognitive levels at once. This approach requires more skill and creativity but may be more realistic given the environment. For this case, Sarah must select activities in which the whole group can simultaneously participate and that permit each member to successfully accomplish something at the individual's own level. By carefully analyzing each activity, Sarah can assign a portion of the tasks involved to each individual, matching the requirements of each portion to the individual's capabilities. Occasionally, Sarah may ask clients who function at higher cognitive levels to assist those at lower levels. Examples of these activities include group murals and more complex cooking projects.

Model of Human Occupation

The Model of Human Occupation was designed for use with any individual experiencing difficulties in performing occupation. This model evolved from earlier research by Reilly (1962) on occupational behavior. Using concepts from General Systems Theory, Open Systems Theory, and Dynamical Systems Theory, this model gives an explanation for the way occupation is motivated, organized, and performed, thereby emphasizing the human system's spontaneous, purposeful, tension-seeking properties and acknowledging its creative properties (Kielhofner, 1995). In addition, this model provides a view of the degree of intimacy between the environment and the performance of occupation.

Human beings maintain constant interaction with the environment and receive many types of input such as olfactory and sensory stimulation and behavior expectations. The individual uses that input in many ways (for example, food becomes energy; sensory stimulation may translate to touch, pain, or temperature; and words are interpreted). This process is known as *throughput*. Part of the result of the process of input and throughput is that a behavior, or output, is produced. Finally, as the person performs the behavior, the experience of doing it and any results from it form the process of feedback, which becomes a new source of input into the system. The Model of Human Occupation explains occupation as the cumulative expression of this process. For example, in meal preparation the cook sees the food items (input), considers what recipe to use (throughput), prepares the food items (output), and feels arm movement as well as sees the result of the preparation (feedback). While seeing that feedback, the cook notices that the food is beginning to turn brown (input), decides it is burning (throughput), removes the pan from the stove (output), and experiences moving the pan until it is off the stove (feedback). To further explain this dynamic interaction between the individual and the environment from which the occupation arises, the Model of Human Occupation describes external and internal environments of the human being as composed of several subsystems.

According to this model, the external environment offers opportunities for certain behaviors while requiring others. For example, the institution of school offers the teacher a room in which to walk around, speak, write on the chalkboard, and sit in a chair. At the same time, the school requires from the teacher the behavior of instruct-

ing the students. The teacher will be fired if those requirements are not met. Providing opportunity and requiring behavior is a complementary relationship. The influence of this relationship comes from several sources in the environment, including the physical realm, such as objects and built or natural structures; the social realm, which includes the tasks deemed appropriate and desirable and the social groups sanctioning the behavior; the settings in which occupation occurs, such as home, neighborhood, school and workplace and gathering, recreation, and resource sites; and the overall culture, such as values, norms, and customs, which affects the individual's life (Figure 7-5).

The earlier example of meal preparation can be used to elaborate on these external environment concepts. To perform this occupation, the cook requires several objects, including food ingredients and seasonings, a knife,

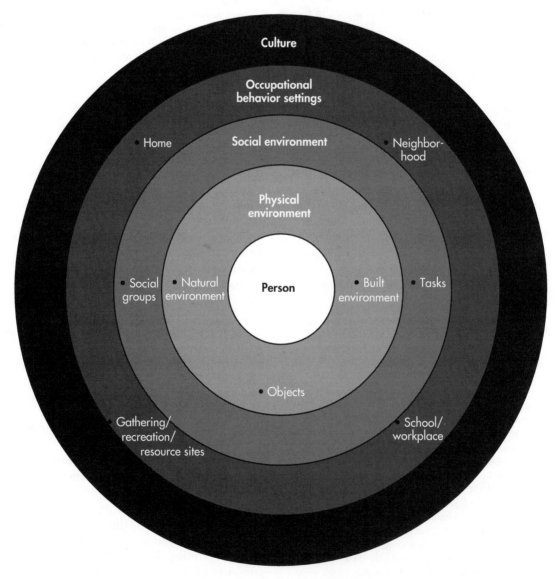

FIGURE 7-5 External environment layers.

some pans, and the stove. The processes of dicing, chopping, stirring, and frying the food are all tasks recognized as cooking. Because of health concerns, the cook may choose to prepare a meal consisting only of vegetables for his family (social group). The setting of the meal is the cook's home, where he can exercise creativity in preparing and seasoning the food and presenting the meal. In addition, the choice of vegetables only may be influenced by a cultural value that an athletic body is preferable to an obese one. If the cook were performing the occupation of cooking as the main task of his job at a restaurant, however, the objects, tasks, social group, setting, and possibly cultural expectations may present completely different opportunities and behavior expectations. There he might use industrial size knives and tools, prepare large amounts of fried fish, be part of a team of cooks, and work in a restaurant that specializes in an ethnic food.

The Model of Human Occupation describes the individual's internal environment as composed of **subsystems** (Figure 7-6). The volition subsystem is responsible for guiding the individual through occupation choices throughout the day. According to this model, occupation choice is influenced by the individual's disposition about expected outcome and by self-knowledge, or awareness of the self as an active participant in this world. Both these influences determine the way the individual anticipates, chooses, and experiences occupation. These concepts are illustrated by George and Pam, an elder couple residing in a senior housing community. Every Saturday night they dress in their best clothes and walk to the common hall to play bridge with other members of their community. They choose to do this because they anticipate the pleasure of friends' company and because they believe they are capable bridge players. Helen, who lives in the same community as George and Pam, chooses not to play bridge. Although she is a champion player, she anticipates feeling out of place because she is a widow and does not have a regular partner.

The volition subsystem is comprised by personal causation, values, and interests. Personal causation refers to the awareness individuals have of their abilities (that is, knowledge of capacity) and to individuals' perceptions that they have control over their behavior (that is, sense of efficacy). An individual is more likely to engage in an occupation he or she feels capable of doing. Values refer to the convictions people have that help them assign significance and standards of performance to the occupations they perform. Each individual has values that form the individual's views of life. These values elicit a sense of obligation to do what one believes is right. Finally, interests refer to the desire to find pleasure, enjoyment, and satisfaction in certain occupations. Interests may also be attractions people feel toward certain occupations and preferences regarding ways occupations are performed.

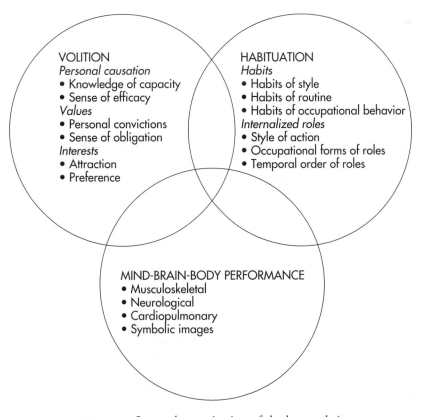

FIGURE 7-6 Internal organization of the human being.

For example, George, Pam, and Helen each have a sense of themselves as good or effective bridge players (personal causation). This sense was developed over time, so that after playing as partners for over 30 years, George and Pam have a specific playing style (preference) and are attracted to the opportunity to play bridge on Saturday nights rather than stay home and watch television. Although Helen may have developed the same interest and personal causation, she believes that playing bridge is most meaningful with your spouse as partner. Because she has no spouse, this value is sufficient to deter her from participating in the Saturday night games at the senior housing community.

In contrast to the volition subsystem, which has to do with conscious choice of occupation, the habituation subsystem has to do with the routine activity of daily life. These routines require very little deliberation because they are built on repetition. The habituation subsystem is comprised of **habits** and internalized roles. Habits have to do with the typical way an individual performs a particular occupation and organizes it within a typical day or week, and the unique style the individual brings to performance. For example, going to the common hall on Saturday night to play bridge is part of George and Pam's weekly routine. While playing bridge, both drink coffee. George typically puts one teaspoon of sugar in his cup before pouring in the coffee, and Pam pours her coffee first and then mixes in the sugar. During the game, George is talkative and Pam is quiet, but both break into song when they win the game.

Internalized roles refer to typical ways in which an individual relates to others. Roles are the identities and behaviors people assume in various social situations. These roles are based on the individual's perceived expectations of others. Thus roles involve obligations and rights of the individual in the various social contexts. According to the Model of Human Occupation, the specific occupational behaviors that encompass a role, the style in which actions in a role occur, and the way an individual's roles are prioritized are of particular interest to the OT practitioner. George, Pam, and Helen each have an image of the role of bridge player. For George and Pam, this role includes the occupations of dressing nicely, walking to the common hall, playing by the rules, and sitting around a table conversing with others. Helen may view the role in a similar way, but has the additional sense that the role of bridge player requires having one's spouse as partner. Because she is a widow, Helen has abandoned the role of bridge player. George and Pam, on the other hand, routinely enter this role on Saturday nights.

The final subsystem of the human being's internal environment is the mind-brain-body performance subsystem. As its name implies, this subsystem represents the complex interplay between the musculoskeletal, neurological, perceptual, and cognitive abilities required to actually perform an occupation or enact a behavior. Interaction with the environment occurs through this subsystem. The individual perceives challenges and opportunities in the environment through the perceptual system and processes this information in the brain. According to the meaning ascribed to the perception, the brain plans an action, which is carried to the muscles, joints, and bones of the limbs that perform the action. Whereas an occupation's meaning is ascribed by the volition subsystem and the social context is determined by the habituation subsystem, the related actions are created by the performance subsystem. George and Pam like to play bridge (volition subsystem) and do so every Saturday night (habituation subsystem). During the bridge game, George and Pam keep in mind the rules and play accordingly. They sit with others around a table and maintain a grasp on the cards (performance subsystem). The complex interplay between mind, brain, and body inherent in the performance of any occupation occurs through specific skills, including motor skills, process skills, and communication-interaction skills (Box 7-3).

A strength of the Model of Human Occupation is the holistic view it provides of any dysfunction. Traditional health practice often focuses on one or two particular traits of a dysfunction rather than on all the contributing factors. All the effects of dysfunction on an individual's life are rarely fully explored (Kielhofner, 1995). This lack of understanding the whole situation may be particularly detrimental to the elder, such as in the case of Calvin, a 78-year-old man recently admitted to the hospital after falling and fracturing his left femur. Upon admission, an x-ray examination was done, Calvin was taken to surgery, and an open reduction of the fracture was performed. A cast was put on Calvin's leg and he was referred to physical and occupational therapy for a brief rehabilitation course. The physical therapist focused rehabilitation on getting in and out of bed and walking with the reduced weight-bearing guidelines recommended by the physician. The OTR evaluated Calvin and identified difficulties in dressing and toileting because of the cast and weight-bearing precautions. The OTR asked the COTA to train Calvin to dress and toilet with adaptive equipment, to which Calvin easily complied. Calvin was discharged to return home in 2 days, at which time the OTR and COTA team documented that Calvin was independent in dressing and toileting with necessary equipment and was aware of home modifications needed to avoid further falls. Unfortunately, nobody on the health team carefully investigated the reason Calvin fell. Although he can care for himself, he finds living alone unbearably lonely. In addition, three of Calvin's lifelong friends died in the past year. Thus Calvin has a deep sense of hopelessness. He occasionally tries to alleviate his feelings of loneliness and despair by drinking alcohol. He fell after one of these drinking episodes. When the admitting health worker at the hospital asked him if he

BOX 7-3

Performance Skills

Motor domains and skills

Posture
Stabilizes
Aligns
Positions

Mobility
Walks
Reaches
Bends

Coordination
Coordinates body parts
Manipulates
Uses fluent movements

Strength and effort
Moves objects
Transports objects
Lifts objects
Calibrates force, speed, and movement

Energy
Endures
Paces work

Communication and interaction domains and skills

Physicality
Gestures
Gazes
Approximates body appropriately
Postures
Contacts

Language
Articulates
Speaks
Focuses speech
Manages
Modulates

Relations
Engages
Relates
Respects
Collaborates

Information exchange
Asks
Expresses
Shares
Asserts

Process domains and skills

Energy
Paces
Attends

Knowledge
Chooses tools and materials
Uses tools and materials appropriately
Handles tools and materials appropriately
Heeds directions
Inquires for directions

Temporal organization
Initiates
Continues
Sequences
Terminates

Organization
Searches and locates
Gathers
Organizes
Restores
Navigates

Adaptation
Notices and responds
Accommodates
Adjusts
Benefits

Social interaction domain and skills

Acknowledging
Turns body or face toward others
Looks at partner
Confirms understanding
Touches others appropriately

Sending
Greets
Answers
Questions
Complies
Encourages
Extends
Clarifies
Sets limits
Thanks

Timing
Times response
Speaks fluently
Takes turns
Times duration
Completes

Coordinating
Approaches
Places self at appropriate distance
Assumes position
Matches language
Disclosure
Expresses emotion

consumed alcohol, Calvin responded truthfully that he did so only occasionally. During his hospital stay Calvin appeared bright and friendly because he received much desired social contact. A more systematic evaluation of Calvin's life would have revealed a deeper problem related to his volition and habituation subsystems. Instead, the OTR and COTA team focused on the obvious performance subsystem problem, which actually was only a symptom of a more complex issue. The team's care should have also addressed Calvin's feelings of hopelessness (volition) and the reduced number of roles he has to help him organize his days (habituation). Furthermore the COTA and OTR should have helped Calvin explore community resources.

According to the Model of Human Occupation, any traditional OT tool is valid for assessment and treatment. Not one single assessment or treatment tool can completely address the complexity of the individual. Some suggested evaluation tools include the Assessment of Communication and Interaction Skills (Salamy, Simon, Kielhofner, 1993), the Assessment of Motor and Process Skills (Fisher, 1994), the Assessment of Occupational Functioning (Watts et al, 1986), the Occupational Case Analysis Interview and Rating Scale (Kaplan, Kielhofner, 1989), and the Occupational Performance History Interview (Kielhofner, Henry, Wakens, 1989). Interest and role checklists, activity configurations, manual muscle tests, range-of-motion tests, and cognitive tests are among the many tools that may be used to evaluate each subsystem. Ultimately, data should be gathered regarding all subsystems of the individual's internal and external environments. Once problems are identified, intervention is prioritized according to the fact that all subsystems are interdependent. In Calvin's case, if the volition and habituation issues had been identified, OT intervention could have focused on helping Calvin find other meaningful activities and resources for continued social contact in addition to addressing his dressing and toileting needs.

CASE STUDY

Pete, the COTA working in an outpatient rehabilitation program, was very aware of his African heritage. He was preparing to treat Mara, a 60-year-old native of the West Indies. However, having the same skin color does not guarantee similar values, the same understanding of responsibilities of various social roles, comparable daily habits, or similar home environments. Pete must understand the environment Mara comes from and currently lives in as well as her sense of self, and the values, roles, and habits that direct her occupational performance. In collaboration with the OTR, Pete conducts the Assessment of Occupational Functioning and a role and interest checklist. In addition, he documents sensation, strength, active and passive range of motion, and gross and fine motor coordination of Mara's upper extremities. From these assessments, Pete discovers that Mara is distressed about her repetitive motion injuries. She is afraid she may lose her job and does not believe she has other

abilities for work. She has performed the same job for 30 years, and this job has been a major source of stability. Mara describes in detail the ways her work tasks must be performed and the objects used in that performance. When Pete attempts to discuss some slight modifications in job performance, Mara states that the foreman might not approve of the changes, even if they do not slow her down or alter the product in any way. She also repeatedly asks Pete if he can "fix" her. Mara's hesitancy to consider modifications and her request that Pete fix her reveal Mara's sense of lack of control over many aspects of her life. In addition, they provide insight to her work values that employees must obey the foreman without question, and there is only one right way to do a job. Further assessment reveals that Mara has very little social contact and support outside of her job. Her husband died recently and her three children all moved to other states to find work. Assessment of Mara's habituation system helps Pete understand that if Mara lost her job, she would lose an important social context that motivates her to continue living. The financial reward from work is obviously not the only benefit she receives from her job. As Pete evaluates Mara's motor functioning, he realizes that she will be unable to sustain the same work load much longer. Even though she would qualify for disability income, Pete must help Mara find daily activities that will provide the regular, predictable social contact she relishes and enable her to feel productive and in control. Pete is able to coordinate Mara's return to part-time work and receipt of some disability compensation with an employment representative and a financial officer. In addition, Pete accompanies Mara to a local seniors' club that combines social outings with volunteer work at a local hospital. The new contacts and opportunities instill in Mara a hope for the future that supports her willingness to explore job modifications. At the same time, Mara's social context broadens, thereby giving Mara a renewed sense of meaning in life.

CONCLUSION

Building on the use of purposeful activity or occupation as a common thread for any OT intervention, each practice model provides a unique way to organize and think about information regarding the individual's function. In addition, each model guides the selection of treatment strategies appropriate for the specific needs of the individual. Finally, the use of practice models assists the COTA in looking beyond the obvious functional deficits, thereby ensuring a more holistic approach to care of complexities of an elder's life.

▮ CHAPTER REVIEW QUESTIONS

1 Explain the meaning of *occupation* and why this concept should be at the core of any OT intervention.
2 Describe at least two ways in which a practice model can help the COTA work with elders.
3 Explain why exclusive use of adjunctive methods and enabling activities as defined in the Occupational Performance Model does not constitute real OT.
4 Considering the definition of intervention strategies proposed in the Occupational Performance Model,

describe at least two purposeful or occupational performance (functional) activities that could be used instead of the following enabling activities:

a. Stacking cones to increase shoulder range of motion

b. Placing pegs in a board to improve fine motor skills

c. Sorting color pegs to improve cognitive skills

d. Squeezing plastic therapeutic putty to increase finger strength

5 You have planned a task group for psychiatric clients during which you plan to carve pumpkins for Halloween. Using the Cognitive Disabilities Model, you conclude that two members of your group are functioning at level 5, two at level 4, and one at level 3. Describe the activity and how you should modify your instructions for each member of your group to have a successful experience.

6 Using the terminology of the Model of Human Occupation, explain how you would prioritize treatment for an elderly Asian-American gentleman who has been admitted to the hospital after a car accident in which his wife and adult son died. He has suffered severe fractures in all his extremities, and there is a possibility of mild head trauma. When you approach this gentleman, he tearfully refuses treatment, stating there is no use or hope for therapy and that he has no other relatives and will be unable to return home.

REFERENCES

Allen C: *Occupational therapy for psychiatric diseases: measurement and management of cognitive disabilities*, Boston, Mass, 1985, Little, Brown, and Company.

Allen C, Earhart C, Blue T: *Occupational therapy treatment goals for the physically and cognitively disabled*, Rockville, Md, 1992, AOTA.

American Occupational Therapy Association: The philosophical base of occupational therapy, *Am J Occup Ther* 49:1026, 1995.

American Occupational Therapy Association: Uniform terminology for occupational therapy- third edition, *Am J Occup Ther* 48, 1047, 1994.

American Occupational Therapy Association: Position paper: purposeful activity, *Am J Occup Ther* 47, 1081, 1993.

American Occupational Therapy Association: *A curriculum guide for occupational therapy educators*, Rockville, Md, 1974, The Association.

Dutton R, Levy L, Simon C: Frames of reference in occupational therapy. In Hopkins H, Smith H, editors: *Willard and Spackman's occupational therapy*, ed 8, Philadelphia, Pa, 1993, JB Lippincott.

Fisher A: *Assessment of motor and process skills (version 8.0)*, unpublished test manual, Ft. Collins, Colo, 1994, Colorado State University.

Kaplan K, Kielhofner G: *Occupational case analysis interview and rating scale*, Thorofare, NJ, 1989, SLACK.

Kielhofner G: *A model of human occupation: theory and application*, ed 2, Baltimore, Md, 1995, Williams & Wilkins.

Kielhofner G: *Conceptual foundations of occupational therapy*, Philadelphia, Pa, 1992, FA Davis.

Kielhofner G, Henry A, Wakens D: *A user's guide to the occupational performance history interview*, Rockville, Md, 1989, American Occupational Therapy Association, Inc.

Llorens L: *Application of a developmental theory for health and rehabilitation*, Rockville, Md, 1976, The American Occupational Therapy Association, Inc.

Pedretti, L: *Occupational therapy: practice skills for physical dysfunction*, St. Louis, 1995, Mosby.

Reilly M: Occupational therapy can be one of the great ideas of 20th century medicine, *Am J Occup Ther* 16:1, 1962.

Salamy M, Simon S, Kielhofner G: *The assessment of communication and interaction skills (research version)*, Chicago, 1993, University of Illinois.

Watts J et al: The assessment of occupational functioning: a screening tool for use in long term care, *Am J Occup Ther* 40:231, 1986.

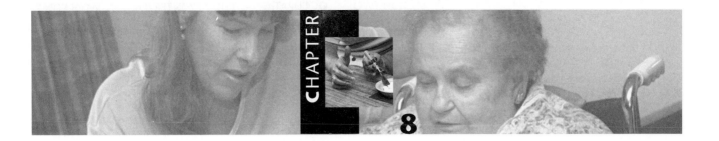

Practice Settings

PAMELA BROWN, HELENE LOHMAN, AND MEG NIEMAN

skilled nursing facility (SNF), subacute unit, adult day care (ADC), inpatient
rehabilitation, outpatient rehabilitation, geropsychiatric units, home health, activity
director, diagnostic related groups

1. Identify key practice locations for COTAs working with elders.
2. Discuss the role of the COTA in each practice setting.
3. Identify future geriatric practice trends.

The majority of COTAs now practice with the elder population. A study done in 1995 by the American Occupational Therapy Association (AOTA) indicates that 62.5% of all COTAs work with clients who are 65 years or older. This percentage has almost doubled since 1990 (Silver-Gleit, 1991; Steib, 1996). One reason for this increase is the current and projected growth of the elder population (American Association of Retired Persons, 1995). Related to this growth is legislation such as the Omnibus Budget Reconciliation Act (OBRA) of 1987 and Medicare. Both the OBRA act and Medicare encourage intervention by rehabilitation professionals to ensure maximal functional levels. In addition, COTAs can provide cost-efficient treatment with function-based outcomes. These factors have been recognized by facilities that hire COTAs and insurers such as managed care organizations.

COTAs are employed to work with elders in many practice settings, including **skilled nursing facilities (SNF), subacute units, adult day care (ADC), inpatient** and **outpatient rehabilitation, geropsychiatric units,** Alzheimer units, **home health,** and group homes. They also work as **activity directors.** This chapter provides an overview of many of these employment areas. COTAs can consider the following guidance questions about each practice setting:

- What is the focus of treatment in the practice setting?
- What trends affect that practice setting?
- What are the COTA's job responsibilities?
- What duties comprise a typical work day?
- Would you consider working in that setting?
- What is the working relationship of the OTR and COTA and other members of the treatment team?

- What level of supervision will be provided by the OTR?

COTA PRACTICE IN SKILLED NURSING FACILITIES

Approximately 39.6% of COTAs consider SNFs their primary employment settings. In fact, SNFs are the main employment settings for COTAs (American Occupational Therapy Association, 1990, 1995). To be classified as an SNF and receive Medicare reimbursement, the institution must have facility or contracted staff and equipment to provide nursing care, rehabilitation, and other health-related services. SNFs have become a primary OT practice setting. COTAs provide cost-efficient, function-based treatment. Currently, some SNFs hire their own OT staff rather than contract from other services. An increase of residents in SNFs because of quick discharge of elders from acute care hospitals is another reason SNFs are primary OT practice settings. This trend reflects changes in the acute care hospital system resulting from the advent of **diagnostic related groups** in the mid 1980s. Diagnostic related groups comprise a billing system set up by Medicare in which elder clients in acute care hospitals are reimbursed by a per diem or set amount for their stay based on diagnoses. With this billing system, financial incentives exist for acute care hospitals to discharge clients quickly. SNFs are often discharge sites of choice. In addition, for clients to be covered under Medicare Part A in an SNF, they currently need to have spent a minimum of 3 days in an acute care hospital. As a result of these factors, COTAs treat more acutely ill clients in SNFs for rehabilitation. After rehabilitation, most elder clients are discharged to their homes or other settings. Others stay in the SNF for long-term care.

COTAs have important roles in assisting the health care team at the SNF to comply with the OBRA law and related Health Care Finance Administration regulations. In this setting, Medicare is often the reimbursement source. Therefore compliance with the Medicare guidelines must be maintained. (Chapter 6 contains specific details about the COTA's role in accordance with these laws.)

COTAs who work at SNFs may be responsible for assisting with assessments, including those required by OBRA regulations, in addition to providing OT treatment. COTAs may gather information for the screening process, implement the treatment plan, provide documentation, and attend interdisciplinary and family team meetings. In addition, COTAs may provide education to staff and consult with other departments such as diet and nutrition, recreation, and nursing (Figure 8-1). COTAs also assist in the daily operation of the OT department.

Terry starts her week by establishing a weekly resident treatment schedule. She sends a copy to the nursing unit and other rehabilitation workers. Before working with clients, she reviews their charts and consults with nursing and other staff as needed.

Terry works with clients who have a variety of diagnoses, including stroke, hip fracture, cancer, chronic obstructive pulmonary disease, and dementia. Because of the diversity in her caseload, she uses a variety of skills to plan treatments. Terry also screens residents in collaboration with the OTR to determine whether the residents require OT services.

Terry educates the nursing staff about a dining program for a resident who suffered a stroke. Earlier she educated the same staff about proper bed and wheelchair positioning. She then instructed a resident who sustained a hip fracture about use of adaptive equipment. She will implement an activities of daily living (ADL) program for this elder. Later Terry will provide education to staff members about ways to increase active participation of residents with dementia. In collaboration with the OTR, Terry also works with an elder who has a humeral fracture to increase the elder's function with an injured arm (Figure 8-2).

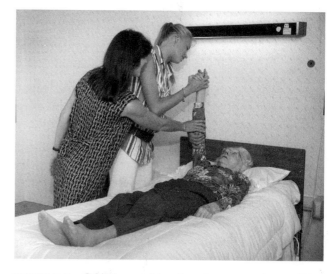

FIGURE **8-1**   COTAs provide education to nursing staff in a variety of areas.

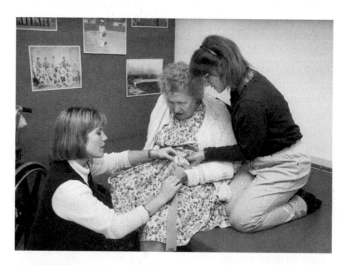

FIGURE **8-2**   COTAs and OTRs collaborate in providing OT treatment.

Terry meets with the OTR to review residents' progress and changes in treatment plans. She then participates in interdisciplinary team meetings to update other staff members on the progress of residents in her caseload. Terry must also make time in her busy day to participate on the Dining Room Committee as the rehabilitation representative. She then completes her daily (or weekly) documentation. Terry feels that her job is satisfying and enjoys working with elders. She enjoys giving other staff members inservices about improved ways to work with the residents and is pleased that staff members follow through with her suggestions. Terry has received excellent reviews from the OTR and SNF administrator about the positive changes with resident care she has implemented. Terry would prefer not to have to stay late on many days to complete her documentation after a busy day. She is also concerned that there is a continuous staff turnover at the SNF. Therefore she must constantly provide feedback regarding various services to maintain good follow through.

COTA PRACTICE ON SUBACUTE UNITS

Subacute units are usually distinct areas that offer ill clients various services, including wound management, respiratory care, cardiac care, orthopedic care, and neurological care. Generally, these units are associated with SNFs. However, they can also be associated with hospitals or be free standing. Subacute units treat clients whose health needs range from acute to long-term care. Subacute units operate from a medical model of delivery (Joint Commission on Accreditation of Health Care Organizations, 1995).

COTAs working on subacute units follow clients of all ages. However, many clients are elders, especially on rehabilitation-focused units. Because much of the client's care is reimbursed by managed care, clients move quickly through the system. COTAs work closely with case managers and the treatment team. Discharge planning is a major focus of OT treatment.

Joe, a newly graduated COTA, works on a subacute unit that specializes in rehabilitation. The majority of the clients on the unit are elders. During his first few weeks on the job, Joe assists the OTR in treating the clients. Joe observes the quick pace of treatment resulting from the influence of managed care. Most clients on the unit follow a "clinical pathway." That is, a structured rehabilitation plan provides for each client's diagnosis. For example, the first day of treatment for a client that has experienced a total hip replacement may involve instructions in safe bed mobility. A set plan is followed with each subsequent day, leading to the ultimate goal of quick discharge through the system.

Once a client referral is received, Joe works closely with the OTR to assess the client and collaborate on the treatment plan. Joe enjoys his new job. He likes the strong interdisciplinary team focus. He also enjoys the quick movement of clients through the system and likes planning treatments for a variety of diagnoses. He is pleased that most of the clients he works with are discharged to their homes. His only frustration is that some clients who do not progress quickly enough are discharged because of reimbursement constraints.

COTA PRACTICE IN ADULT DAY CARE UNITS

Although adult day care (ADC) is not strictly for elder clients, most ADC programs have a majority of elder clientele. The average age of clients is 76 years (Partners in Caregiving, 1995). ADCs are structured programs that provide medical and social support for elders and other clients such as adults with severe physical disabilities or mental illnesses. These programs provide the opportunity for elders to remain at home or in other living situations when independent function decreases. No two ADC programs are exactly alike. Some have a social focus, others have a medical focus, and others are oriented to specific conditions such as Alzheimer's disease. New specialty areas for ADC programs include AIDS and multiple sclerosis care (Moldenhauer, 1996). Many units and centers also offer rehabilitative services to help clients maintain optimal functional levels. Some centers offer respite care as well (Lewis, 1989; Moore, 1988).

COTAs who practice in ADCs may organize therapeutic groups to enhance clients' muscular function and endurance. Other groups may include a cognitive or psychosocial emphasis (Achenbach, 1988). In addition, COTAs may plan specific group activities according to clients' skill levels and special needs. Individual OT treatment may also be offered to work on psychosocial issues and function concerns. COTAs must know the way to make adjustments in each elder's treatment plan after collaborating with the OTR so that all individuals can fully participate in the programs offered. Improving independent living skills to prepare or maintain elders for community living and to increase awareness of community resources is often a focus of treatment (Figure 8-3). Sometimes COTAs are not full-time employees but rather consultants to the program. In that capacity,

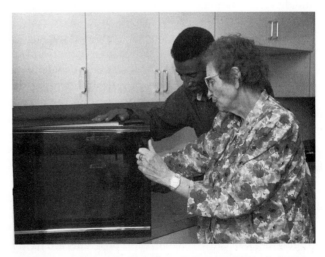

FIGURE 8-3 In Adult Day Care (ADC), COTAs help prepare elders for community living or maintain current living arrangements.

COTAs may consult on individual elder needs or developing groups. COTAs employed full time may observe clientele throughout the day and therefore can recognize and provide intervention when an elder's function appears to be declining. Observation throughout the day may be helpful in cases such as an elder with Alzheimer's disease who functions better at specific times.

> Mary is a COTA employed full time in an ADC program. Mary starts the day by participating in an interdisciplinary team meeting. The attending staff members discuss the status of many ADC clients and make adjustments and changes in treatment plans. After the meeting, Mary leads a group of elders working on range of motion (ROM) and then leads a reminiscent group. In the afternoon, Mary leads a community living group. Next, she works individually with two elders who have experienced strokes. In the late afternoon, Mary meets with an OTR to discuss the ADC clientele. Mary enjoys the ADC setting because of the strong personal relationships she has with many of the elders. She enjoys the creativity of group planning and especially likes the mental health emphasis she provides. She likes helping elders remain in the community. Mary reports that she sometimes is disappointed when she does not see substantial progress in the elders with chronic diagnoses. In addition, Mary must be creative with the limited funds available for program planning.

COTA PRACTICE IN INPATIENT REHABILITATION

In an inpatient rehabilitation program, COTAs treat elders who have various disabilities. The treatment focus in this system is to provide an interdisciplinary approach to maximize functional abilities. As with other practice settings the trend is for shorter lengths of stay (Granger, Ottenbacher, Fiedler, 1995). In addition, a trend for increased specialization in rehabilitation settings with programs such as cardiac units, pain management programs, and driver education programs exists (Punwar, 1994).

Elders covered by Medicare are reimbursed only if they meet certain qualifications ensuring that the needed rehabilitation services require skilled intervention and are of the utmost benefit. These qualifications include being able to endure at least 3 hours of rehabilitation per day and a prognosis that predicts an increase in the client's ability to function on discharge. OT practitioners, particularly COTAs, are vital to the rehabilitation process. The COTA's involvement in this setting has increased over the past 10 years. Currently, 8.7% of COTAs are employed in a rehabilitation hospital (AOTA, 1995; Punwar, 1994). OT treatment includes working with the client in the three performance areas of self-care, work and productivity, and play and leisure (AOTA, 1994) (Figure 8-4). Because rehabilitation programs are tightly structured, OT treatment may involve individual and group treatments. These groups often focus on client discharge to the community or on an increase in the client's independent level of functioning. Examples include range of motion groups, feeding groups, community skills groups, and wheelchair mobility groups (Elmore, Smith, 1993). According to Punwar (1994), groups led by COTAs in inpatient rehabilitation have decreased in some facilities as a result of reimbursement constraints.

> Jeff is a COTA who has worked at a rehabilitation hospital for the past 2 years. Jeff carries a caseload of five to eight clients whom he treats daily. His routine includes a weekly interdisciplinary team meeting. At this meeting, Jeff reports on the progress of his clients and gives input regarding the decisions being made about continued rehabilitation, discontinuation of OT services, and client discharge. Jeff communicates daily on an informal basis with the psychiatrist who supervises the treatment team.
>
> After the weekly meeting, Jeff is responsible for scheduling treatments for each of his clients. Every day he sees three or four clients for morning ADL functions. These activities include bathing, dressing, and functional transfers to and from the bed, toilet, and bathtub. He sees each client for one or two half-hour sessions. Jeff determines which activities are most appropriate for use in treatment according to the elder's long- and short-term goals. He initiates the treatment and keeps a record of each elder's progress. Jeff regularly meets with Mike, an OTR, to collaborate on client progress. During the week, Jeff also attends family meetings and runs a hemiplegia exercise group and a relaxation group for clients with chronic obstructive pulmonary disease. Jeff enjoys the structured days provided in the rehabilitation environment and the close teamwork, which always involves the clients and their families. He likes the accessibility of the psychiatrist to consult. Jeff feels frustrated that the clients are quickly discharged by insurers because they do not make substantial progress.

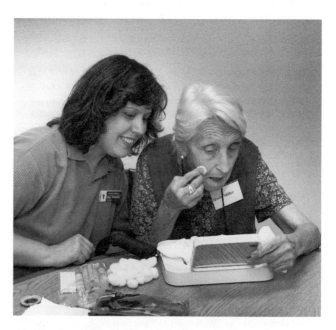

FIGURE 8-4   Self-care is an important performance area for COTAs to address.

COTA PRACTICE IN OUTPATIENT REHABILITATION

For elders who do not need the intense treatment offered in an inpatient setting, outpatient rehabilitation may be a better choice of treatment settings. In addition, with managed care, outpatient treatment is frequently suggested because it is cost effective. The ultimate treatment goal is the same as that of inpatient rehabilitation: to maximize functional abilities.

Elders in outpatient rehabilitation receive OT treatment regularly. COTAs work with clients whose ages and diagnoses vary. Some outpatient clinics may have a specialty such as hand therapy. Emphasis in treatment may be on improving instrumental activities of daily living (IADL) skills, ADL functions, and work, productivity, and leisure skills. All clients should be educated in a home program that supplements the therapy.

Sharon is a COTA who is employed in an outpatient rehabilitation clinic. Once a week, Sharon starts her day by meeting with an OTR to discuss treatment plans and client progress. Sharon collaborates with the OTR and modifies treatment plans as necessary.

Sharon maintains a caseload of six to eight clients. Four of the clients are over 65 years of age. Two elders experienced strokes, one has a Colles wrist fracture, and one had a total hip replacement. A large part of these elders' treatments is provision of caregiver and client education. Sharon collaborates on treatment with the clinic's physical therapy and speech therapy staffs. Sharon also supervises an OTA student regularly. Sharon ends her day by working on documentation. She likes the fast pace of her day, the variety of clients she treats, and the flexibility that is essential because new orders often have to be fit into her schedule. She also enjoys collaborating with other rehabilitation professionals in the clinic. Sharon's only complaint is that her busy day often makes it difficult to complete the documentation. This is especially true when walk-in clients arrive at the clinic.

COTA PRACTICE ON A GEROPSYCHIATRIC UNIT

Working on a geropsychiatric unit provides COTAs with an excellent opportunity to combine their knowledge of physical rehabilitation and mental health. Although clients are primarily admitted for psychiatric reasons, chronic health problems are often encountered. Declining physical abilities such as decreased strength, endurance, mobility, sight, and hearing may contribute to the client's need for admission to the unit. In addition, elders may have experienced losses and subsequent major depression, thereby necessitating admission. The loss of a spouse is one of the greatest adjustments elders face in later years (Cummings, 1993). Elder abuse is another reason for admission to a geropsychiatric unit. Often, admission results in changes in the elder's living accommodations to a safer setting with more supervision after discharge.

In this setting, COTAs provide purposeful activities and treatment to help elders function as independently as possible. Treatment may be individual or in groups. Groups may include assertiveness training, socialization skills, independent living skills, reminiscing skills, remotivation, and discharge planning.

Lynn is a COTA who has been employed in mental health practice for over 10 years, with the last 5 years on a geropsychiatric unit. Lynn starts her day by reviewing charts of newly admitted clients. She then participates in screening interviews of these elders. The interviews consist of questions that, when answered, give some idea of the elder's functional performance level, interests, and roles. Lynn also takes the opportunity to introduce the new clients to OT. Lynn reports the results of the screening interviews to the OTR supervisor. After receiving client orders for OT treatment, Lynn and the OTR co-assess the new clients. Often they use the Allen's Cognitive Level Test to evaluate the client's level of functioning. The results help Lynn plan her treatments.

During the rest of the day, Lynn leads various group sessions. She also provides some individual treatment sessions in which she addresses clients' mental health and physical needs. Lynn completes rounds to report on client progress to the other health professionals on the team. Lynn is actively involved with the discharge planning team. She likes the mental health practice because she provides traditional mental health group approaches and addresses elders' function concerns. She enjoys the creative part of her job, especially group planning. She occasionally feels frustrated when clients have to be discharged to a setting other than their own homes. She also feels troubled when a client is readmitted.

COTA PRACTICE IN HOME HEALTH

According to Rodriguez and Goldberg (1993), most elders prefer to receive therapy in their own homes. Clients function best in their own environments. Currently, home health is a growing practice area as a result of early client discharge from the different treatment settings and because home health is a cost-effective way to provide treatment. Home health agencies have grown from 200 in 1967 to over 10,000 20 years later (Rodriguez, Goldberg, 1993).

Medicare guidelines specifically allow COTAs to treat clients in the home in addition to OTRs. COTAs can be effective therapeutic agents. After the evaluation and establishment of the treatment plan and goals, COTAs may treat clients without the physical presence of an OTR. However, Medicare-certified home health agencies may require extensive supervisory plans. Medicare intermediaries may request to see the supervisory plan that details the types and frequency of supervision the OTR is providing for the COTA (AOTA, 1995). COTAs must have strong clinical and communication skills to work in this setting. Therefore COTAs should have 1 or more years of prior clinical experience before working in home health (Joe, 1994; Thiers, 1994).

COTAs who work in the home setting can directly see problems and therefore may recommend safety adaptations as part of treatment. COTAs may suggest that clutter be removed to prevent falls and that furniture be rearranged to assist with safer transfers. However, COTAs need to be sensitive to the caregiver's feelings about changes in the home. COTAs assume all treatment responsibilities as they would in any setting. Working in the home environment makes therapy more meaningful for the client. In the home setting, COTAs are not only treating the elder but also directly working with family members or other caregivers. COTAs may provide emotional support for the caregivers and assist with caregiver education about realistic goal attainment. Education may also be provided to home health aides. COTAs should arrange their schedules to be at the client's home when the home health aide is present.

Working in this environment presents an advantage to COTAs because activities are based on everyday materials (Figure 8-5). For example, COTA may suggest an elder client make a bed, which would address sequencing, motor planning, balance, and body mechanics.

Interdisciplinary communication must be maintained for coordination of treatment services. This is usually conducted by telephone because all members of the treatment team are not at the client's home at the same time. Visits coordinated with other members of the interdisciplinary team may be helpful for everyone. Documentation in home health care is very thorough and based on functional performance (Joe, 1994). Medicare, managed care organizations, and state, agency, and other standard regulatory systems often control documentation guidelines. Finally, COTAs working in the home health setting need to know and make use of community resources to help clients. (The Appendix contains a list of community resources.)

Mike is a COTA employed by a home health agency. Mike begins his day by driving to the agency headquarters. There he checks in to determine whether any new treatment orders have occurred. Mike travels to clients' homes for the rest of the day. He covers a 30-mile radius serviced by the agency. The clients that he visits live in various parts of the town and surrounding rural area. The socioeconomic status of the clients varies. Some clients are from low-income living situations, and Mike must be creative with limited resources. Other clients come from upper-class backgrounds and have financial resources for any adaptive equipment that might be needed.

In a day, Mike visits four or five clients. Each visit lasts about 1 hour. Mike provides creative OT intervention, often using items at the client's home. For an elderly lady who sustained a wrist fracture, Mike suggests the activity of hanging sheets with clothespins to help strengthen pinch. Mike also spends time at each visit communicating with the client's family members and other caregivers. Mike updates his documentation after each visit. He loves his job for several reasons. He enjoys having different settings throughout the day. He feels the client's home is a more realistic setting than a clinic for OT treatment. He enjoys getting to know the clients and their families as a unit. Mike's main dislikes are the lack of regular on-site OTR supervision and that he must collaborate with numerous OTRs about his caseload. He has learned to compensate by calling them with any questions.

COTA AS AN ACTIVITY DIRECTOR

Activity directors are employed in many settings, including group homes and long-term care facilities for elders, people with mental illness, and people with mental retardation. Activity directors may also be employed in community centers for both well and disabled clients (Ryan, 1993).

Activity directors provide goal-directed, purposeful activities for each client. They must be skilled in assessing a client's strengths and needs and able to analyze and select appropriate activities (Crepeau, 1986). COTA education includes activity analysis and human development throughout the life span. This ideal knowledge allows the COTA to function as an activity director. COTAs have also been educated about physical and

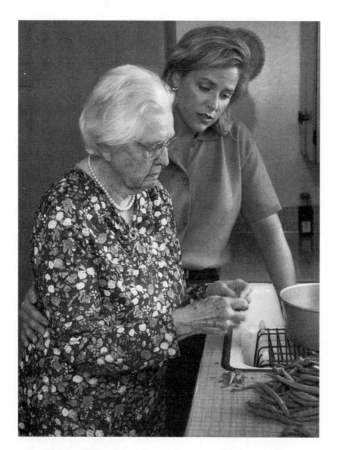

FIGURE 8-5 The home environment presents a myriad of therapeutic activities.

mental disabilities and understand the need for purposeful activities to foster a feeling of well-being (Ryan, 1993). With this knowledge the COTA can work as an activity director with well or ill people of any age (Figure 8-6).

Activity directors must know and follow specific regulations set forth by the Department of Health and Human Services and any other standard-setting agency. In addition, activity directors are responsible for providing proper documentation, program planning and implementation and scheduling. They also assess individual client activity needs, train, and supervise the staff. The activity director's job also includes participating in interdisciplinary team meetings, the care planning process, purchasing of equipment, and preparing of the department budget (Ryan, 1993).

COTAs who function in this role are not providing formal OT services. They do not require OTR supervision, nor do they use the title *COTA*. Qualifying criteria vary according to the geographic region. If OT services are required and the COTA activity director does provide therapy services, an OTR must be involved. In any case, state and any other appropriate standard-setting agency regulations and the Occupational Therapy Standards of Practice must be followed (Ryan, 1993).

Jean is a COTA who is employed as an activity director at a retirement community. Jean has organized a committee of representatives from the retirement community that gives input about activities in which they would like to participate. She also has volunteers who help her provide the ac-

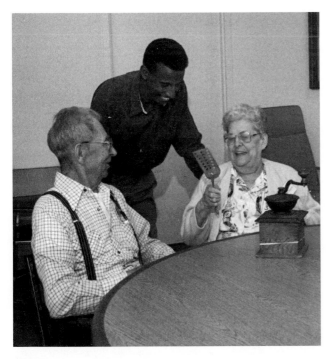

FIGURE 8-6 Activity directors provide purposeful activities to individuals and groups.

tivities. Jean has a very structured schedule of activity groups based on the committee's input for the elders at the retirement community. Some activity groups include craft groups, bridge tournaments, creative writing groups, and current events groups. Jean regularly plans outings to the community to attend various cultural events and visit places of historic interest. Jean enjoys her job, and although she is not functioning in the role of a COTA, she is able to use her OT skills to help plan appropriate activities. She identifies any special needs the residents have and makes appropriate adaptations with activities when necessary. She likes the leadership role she has in managing the activities department. She also enjoys working with well elders. Sometimes she becomes frustrated with the financial planning involved with running an activities department. She has to be creative with limited materials. Sometimes Jean jokes that she feels just like one of the original OTRs, who were reconstruction aides, because of her ability to come up with craft projects using material and paper scraps and other items that would normally be discarded.

CONCLUSION

This chapter has illustrated just some of the practice settings that specialize in elder care and in which the COTA can work. The common thread is that COTAs work with a large proportion of elder clients. However, each setting is different. Some are more fast paced, such as subacute units. In other settings COTAs work with elders over longer periods, such as in adult day care settings. COTAs should consider the following when trying to determine the best place to work:

- Any setting discussed in this chapter involves variety.
- Outpatient rehabilitation or subacute units might be most appropriate if a fast-paced job is desirable.
- Skilled nursing facilities, home health agencies, and outpatient and inpatient rehabilitation settings involve treatment focused on rehabilitation.
- Although COTAs apply a holistic treatment approach in all settings and with all clients, the structure of some settings specifically allows a mental health treatment approach with groups designed to meet mental health needs. These settings include adult day care and geropsychiatric units.
- A position in home health or as an activity director may be a suitable setting for a COTA who has the treatment skills needed to function more independently on the job.

When trying to make a decision about a job, interviewing and observing COTAs at work in a practice area is recommended. The newly graduated COTA must determine the amount of available supervision and any state regulations that apply to the practice setting before making a final decision. Finally, COTAs must remember that no job setting is perfect. The COTA's talent and skills make the job special.

■ CHAPTER REVIEW QUESTIONS

1 Describe the COTA's role in each of the discussed practice settings.

2 Identify the primary employment setting for COTAs and discuss reasons for it being the primary setting.

3 Describe trends affecting outpatient and inpatient rehabilitation practice.

4 What is unique about the COTA's role on a gero-psychiatric unit?

5 Discuss why a more experienced COTA in a home health setting is preferable to a less experienced COTA.

6 Discuss what a COTA can bring to the role of activity director.

REFERENCES

Achenbach C: Occupational therapy in the adult day care center, *Occup Ther For* 111(7):1, 1988.

American Association of Retired Persons: *A profile of older Americans*, Washington, DC, 1995, AARP Fulfillment.

American Occupational Therapy Association: Uniform terminology for occupational therapy, third edition, Am J Occup Ther 48(11):1047, 1994.

Crepeau EL: *Activity programming for the elderly*, Boston, 1986, Little, Brown, and Co.

Cummings G: Basic concepts of human development. In Ryan S, editor: *The certified occupational therapy assistant: principles, concepts and techniques*, Thorofare, NJ, 1993, Slack.

Elmore T, Smith KC: Patients win on the NRH team, *OT Week* 7(21):16, 1993.

Granger CV, Ottenbacher KJ, Fiedler RC: The uniform data system for medical rehabilitation, *Am J Phys Med Rehab* 74:62, 1995.

Joe BE: When in doubt document, *OT Week*, 8(23):16, 1994.

Joint Commission on Accreditation of Healthcare Organizations, *1995 Survey protocol for subacute programs*, Oakbrook Terrace, Ill, 1995, The Commission.

Lewis SC: Occupational therapy and the elderly. *Elder care in occupational therapy*. Thorofare, NJ, 1989, SLACK.

Moldenhauer N: Personal communication, July 1996.

Moore SD: Older adult care. In Davis LJ, Kirkland M, editors: *The role of occupational therapy with the elderly*, Rockville, Md, 1988, American Occupational Therapy Association.

Partners in Caregiving: The Dementia Services Program: Life after diagnosis: adult day services in America, (202)479-6682, Winston Salem, NC, 1995, Partners in Caregiving.

Punwar AJ: *Occupational therapy practice*, Baltimore, 1994, Williams & Wilkins.

Rodriguez GS, Goldbert B: Rehabilitation in the outpatient setting, *Geriatr Rehabil* 9(4), 873, 1993.

Ryan SE, editor: The role of the COTA as an activities director. In *Practice issues in occupational therapy intraprofessional team building*, Thorofare, NJ, 1993, SLACK.

Silver-Gleit I: Member data survey, *OT Week* 5(8):6, 1991.

Steib P: Skilled nursing facilities: top employment settings for COTAs, *OT Week* 47:16, 1996.

Thiers N: The proliferation of home care, *OT Week* 8(23):18, 1994.

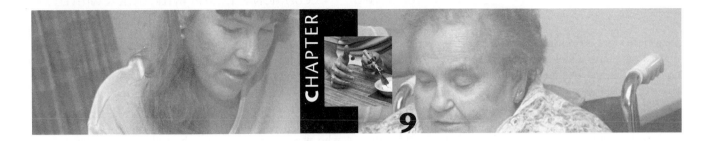

Documentation

SHIRLEY A. BLANCHARD, LORI TAYLOR, RENÉ L. PADILLA, HELENE LOHMAN,
and SUE BYERS-CONNON

KEY TERMS

screening, informed consent, evaluation, assessment, treatment plans,
treatment goals, functional, measurable, progress notes, SOAP notes,
grid system, discharge summary

CHAPTER OBJECTIVES

1. Describe the types of documentation used in occupational therapy practice.
2. Discuss the application of informed consent in occupational therapy practice.
3. List the components of good documentation.

Rhonda, a COTA, received a subpoena to appear at an attorney's office to give a deposition. Mrs. L., an elderly woman that Rhonda worked with 2 years previously at a skilled nursing facility (SNF), recently died. Her death was under investigation. Upon receipt of the subpoena, Rhonda remembered Mrs. L. and wondered what happened to her. Rhonda hoped she had documented thoroughly while caring for Mrs. L.

Rhonda's experience illustrates the importance of clearly and concisely documenting client care. Documentation is the only permanent, legal record of what occurs during treatment. *Documentation* can be defined as written notes or records that describe all information relevant to clients from admission to discharge (Punwar, 1994; Backhaus, 1993).

Effective OT documentation serves many purposes, including facilitating communication among members of the health care team and providing a chronological record detailing the complete course of therapeutic intervention. Documentation reflects the practitioner's reasoning and facilitates continuity of treatment. In addition, written records provide data for research and advancement of the OT profession. These records facilitate training and student education. Documentation can be of assistance in explaining a treatment program to an elder; it also provides a method for ensuring the elder's rights and can be a tool for advocacy. In addition, documentation provides an objective basis from which to evaluate and determine the appropriateness, effectiveness, and medical necessity of intervention. Documentation helps justify continued treatment for utilization reviews and is necessary to ensure payment. Documentation demonstrates compliance with federal and state laws by contributing substantive evidence about the care rendered and whether it met the legal standard of care. Furthermore, documentation is used to obtain facility accreditation from organizations such as the Joint Commission for Accreditation of Health Organizations and the Commission on Accreditation of Rehabilitation Facilities (Jabri, 1996; Scott, 1994). Thus documentation is an important tool to measure the overall quality of elder care.

TYPES OF DOCUMENTATION

Decisions about what to document involve clinical judgement and are based on a collaborative model of care. The OTR and COTA decide what should be documented and how much detail will be included in the reports (Abreu, Lackey, 1994). The content and amount of documentation varies depending on the requirements of the service provider, intermediary requirements, and the type of form used. The American Occupational Therapy Association (AOTA) (1995) identifies various types of documentation, including screening, the initial note to the file, a record of informed consent, results of the initial evaluation, and assessment notes and reports. Also included in the client's file are treatment plans and goals, progress notes, monthly progress reports, 30-day recertification documents, treatment records, discharge summaries, consultation reports, and special reports. Special reports may include referrals to other programs and agencies, legal summaries, notes about home programs, and correspondence. Finally, critical incidence reports or notes are included and functional maintenance programs are identified in the file. Most of these types of documentation are discussed in relation to the OT process in the context of elder care. A medical record must be maintained as a permanent, legal file for each elder referred to OT. The record should be organized, legible, concise, clear, accurate, complete, current, and objective. Correct grammar and spelling should be used (AOTA, 1995).

Screening

A **screening** is a precursor to evaluation to determine whether OT services are warranted. Screenings are brief and not "hands on," because they are done before a physician's formal service order is received. Screenings are not reimbursed by third-party payers. Screenings may serve to identify changes in functional status such as improvements or declines in physical or cognitive abilities, changes in environmental limitations, and safety risks. When performing a screening, the OTR or COTA may use a structured guide to obtain and record a general history about an elder's self-care abilities, social situation, occupational roles, and living environment (AOTA, 1993).

A screening by an OT practitioner may be recommended by any member of an interdisciplinary treatment team. Anyone who comes in contact with an elder may inform OT personnel that a change has occurred in a resident's condition. For example, a member of the housekeeping staff in an SNF may report that a resident who was previously using the toilet independently now urinates on the floor. In such a case a screening by an OTR or COTA would be appropriate to determine if OT services are indicated.

COTAs who work in SNFs will need to be familiar with any regulations that require specific documentation. In an SNF a screening should be performed quarterly or when one or more functional changes have been identified on the resident assessment protocol of the minimum data set (MDS), according to the Omnibus Budget Reconciliation Act of 1987. The MDS, a screening tool coordinated by nursing may include contributions from other disciplines such as OT. (Refer to Chapter 6 for a review of the OBRA regulations.) Each SNF may administer and interpret OBRA guidelines differently, resulting in varied time lines for completion of screenings by the clinician.

Screenings may be done in all COTA practice settings. However, state licensure may vary regarding the COTA's participation in screening. In acute care hospitals, screenings may occur only in certain medical units. The need for OT services may be identified during conferences or rounds when each elder's specific needs are discussed. Screenings may occur in home health and hospice care programs as well.

When appropriate, and on completion of the screening, an order for OT evaluation and possibly treatment is requested from the physician. All recommendations should be documented in the medical record. The initial referral for service may read "Occupational Therapy to evaluate." COTAs should keep in mind that policies and intermediary requirements for ordering OT evaluation and therapy vary greatly among practice areas, facilities, agencies, and physicians.

Informed Consent

Once an order has been received, some facilities require the OTR and COTA team to obtain **informed consent** before evaluating and treating the elder. Informed consent is "the permission obtained from an elder to perform a specific test or procedure" (Anderson, Anderson, Glanze, 1994). The concept of informed consent is largely a result of the consumer rights movement. All health care providers, including OT practitioners, who treat elders have a legal and ethical duty to obtain an elder's informed consent before commencing treatment (Scott, 1994). The need for informed consent is another crucial reason for COTAs and OTRs to work as a team. Both must know clearly what procedures are being performed. No practitioner should obtain consent to perform a procedure that he or she is not legally qualified to do.

Informed consent is recognized as a fundamental right in case law and is utilized in every state. Some cases of medical malpractice involve failure of health care professionals to obtain informed consent. They may not have provided sufficient or pertinent information for the elder to make an informed choice regarding treatment. The process of obtaining informed consent is also recognized by professional practice and accreditation bodies such as the Joint Commission for Accreditation of Health Organizations.

A distinct difference exists between informed consent and consent to pay (Spectra Rehab Alliance Consulting Program, 1994). Consent to pay is obtained during the admission process and covers all expenses related to the current stay in the facility. Neither the COTA nor the OTR is responsible for determining the elder's financial status. Informed consent, on the other hand, is the process of providing the elder with all relevant information at a level that he or she can understand. This information should enable the elder to decide whether to proceed with the treatment program. Consent must be voluntary and given by a competent elder to be legal and ethical. The elder should be informed of the diagnosis or findings of the evaluation and the prognosis if treatment is recommended. The elder must also be informed of the potential complications of the recommended treatment and alternative treatment approaches. The decision not to treat should also be presented as an alternative. Elders have the right to refuse treatment and be informed of the consequences of their actions (Scott, 1994).

Decisions about the way to treat elders should be made on the basis of health-related information, not financial considerations. The AOTA Code of Ethics states that treatment cannot be denied on the basis of ability to pay (AOTA, 1994). An elder who agrees to proceed with treatment has given informed consent.

COTAs should consider the following issues when determining the appropriate person to give consent for treatment:

1. If the treatment team has determined that the elder is competent to give informed consent, then the elder may make the decision.
2. If the treatment team has determined that the elder is not competent to give informed consent, then the person who has durable power of attorney or is the elder's legal guardian may make the decision.
3. If the treatment team has determined that the elder is not competent to give informed consent and that no legal guardian or attorney-in-fact has been appointed to make health care decisions for the elder,

a health care surrogate should give the informed consent. If no health care surrogate has been identified, the facility must refer to state law to determine the way to proceed. In some states an ombudsman may be temporarily assigned as an advocate for the elder. Information regarding state laws is available through the state's Department of Health.

Once permission to treat is received verbally, and preferably in writing, it is documented in the elder's medical record. OT practitioners are now ready to initiate the evaluation process (Scott, 1994).

Evaluation

Once a physician's referral for OT has been obtained, the OTR must acknowledge it in writing in the elder's medical record. COTAs may acknowledge the order as well, but they must make sure that they follow facility procedures for informing the OTR (Thomas, 1996). This procedure may be a simple statement that the order was received and that the evaluation has been scheduled. An OTR must then initiate the evaluation process. The terms **evaluation** and **assessment** must be differentiated. Evaluation refers to " . . . the [whole] process of obtaining and interpreting data necessary for intervention. This includes planning for and documenting the evaluation process results" (AOTA, 1995). Assessment, on the other hand, refers to " . . . specific tools or instruments that are used in the evaluation process" (AOTA, 1995).

Smith (1993) wrote that "in occupational therapy, evaluation is a process of collecting and organizing the relevant information about the elder so that the therapist can plan and implement a meaningful, effective program of treatment." Smith further categorized the steps of evaluation as collection of data, organization of data, setting of treatment objectives, and commitment to continuing evaluation.

The purpose of an evaluation is to establish the baseline information needed to assess an elder's potential for rehabilitation. Evaluation documentation should include a reason for the referral, pertinent medical history, present status, previous functional level, and probable environment upon discharge. This documentation should also reflect assessment findings, treatment plans, and goals (Esposto, 1993). A complete and comprehensive evaluation should answer several questions regarding the client's functional status, including questions regarding the current level of treatment goals, ways to meet the goals, and ways to evaluate progress (AOTA, 1995).

The selection of evaluation tools, the prioritization of problems, and the choice of intervention strategies should be guided by the use of an OT frame of reference or practice model. By using such a framework, the COTA and OTR team can design a meaningful and relevant treatment program for an elder. (Chapter 7 presents a discussion of several OT practice models.) This process also helps establish the medical necessity for OT services. Because Medicare, Medicaid, and other insurers only reimburse for reasonable and medically necessary OT intervention, performing a thorough evaluation and establishing appropriate treatment priorities is imperative. (Chapter 6 explains Medicare requirements for the provision of skilled care.)

The amount of information that is documented during an evaluation and the format in which it is documented mainly depend on the purpose of the evaluation. Other factors that may affect the amount of information documented are the availability of time and space to conduct the evaluation, facility custom, and agency policies (Abreu, Lackey, 1994). Most facilities provide printed forms that are filled out by the practitioner. Evaluation reports typically include the date, the client's medical and social history, physical findings, the status of performance components, and the level at which the client functions in performance areas. In addition, evaluation reports should include an interpretation of findings, a treatment plan, goals, planned interventions or modalities, and the frequency or duration of treatment necessary to achieve the goals.

A thorough evaluation begins with a comprehensive review of the elder's medical record. Such a review will help determine whether any particular precautions must be taken while working with the elder, such as restrictions pertaining to activity level, the amount of weight the elder can bear, and diet. COTAs may assist with data collection or administer standardized tests in cooperation with the OTR after service competency has been established (AOTA, 1993; Backhaus, 1993). A large part of a COTA's role is to interview elders and observe their skill performance while they are engaged in an occupation. Observation skills and objectivity are of utmost importance in this process. Objectivity means that the COTA is able to make a clear distinction between external facts and personal opinion. Important considerations during evaluation and treatment planning also include the elder's personal aspirations and the needs of the family or caregiver, which should always be documented in the record.

COTAs may then summarize and document initial data and reassessment data. Smith (1993) emphasized that data should be "organized into a meaningful, dynamic description of the elder's strengths and limitations, with a focus on those areas in which occupational therapy can be helpful. The elder, the therapist, and others should be able to understand this description readily." Results are also communicated to the OTR, who interprets the results with input from the COTA (Walker, 1995). The OTR and COTA team can then establish priorities and

strategies for intervention. Staying updated on state, facility, and agency regulations is important because they may require OTRs to co-sign all standardized tests and progress notes completed by COTAs during an evaluation.

Once the evaluation has been completed and treatment objectives have been established, the **treatment plan** must be signed by the ordering physician and incorporated in the medical record. This step constitutes a "clarification order." Some facilities or agencies may require OT personnel to complete this step by acknowledging the physician's referral on a physician order form. Once the physician signs the clarification order, the OT practitioner may proceed with OT intervention. Any modifications to the clarification order require written approval by the physician.

TREATMENT PLANS AND GOALS

At the time of evaluation and reassessment, COTAs and OTRs collaboratively develop short-term and long-term **treatment goals.** OT goals should be functional, measurable, and objective and should reflect the elders' needs and desires (AOTA, 1994; Health Care Financing Administration [HCFA], 1990; Jabri, 1996; Trombly, 1995; Smith, 1993). In addition, goals should be related to specific deficits in occupational performance areas and components that have been evaluated (Backhaus, 1993; AOTA, 1993).

For a goal to be considered **functional,** it must include a performance area as described in the Uniform Terminology document (AOTA, 1994). These performance areas include specific activities of daily living, such as grooming or dressing; work or productive activities such as meal preparation, shopping or job performance; and play or leisure activities such as hobby exploration and actual performance.

The **measurable** level at which the elder is expected to perform in these functional areas should be included in the goal (Table 9-1). For example, a goal may state, "Elder will sequence dressing self with moderate assistance in 2 weeks." In cases in which the goal of intervention is to improve a performance component such as joint range of motion or strength, this component must be related to the functional goal (Trombly, 1995). For the previous example, the goal may state, "Elder will independently demonstrate sufficient range of motion in the shoulder to put on a shirt that is buttoned in the front within 3 weeks." In addition, Trombly (1995) writes, "Because all therapy on underlying factors (components) is thus directed toward a specific function, no treatment time is spent on those factors that do not have a functional impact."

As stated earlier, goals should describe the level of function expected after a designated period of treatment intervention. The length of time spent on achieving goals naturally depends on the work setting and elder's

TABLE **9-1**

Measurable Levels of Independence Described by Medicare and Commonly Used by OT Practitioners

Level of assistance	Explanation
Independent	Elder requires no physical or cognitive assistance
Standby	Elder requires supervision by one person to perform procedures safely (often used with elders who have safety concerns)
Minimum	Elder requires 25% physical assistance and occasional cognitive assistance to perform activities safely
Moderate	Elder requires 50% physical assistance and constant cognitive assistance to perform activities safely
Maximum	Elder requires 75% physical and cognitive assistance to perform activities safely
Dependent	Elder requires 100% physical and cognitive assistance

status. Short-term goals represent incremental steps toward reaching long-term goals, and thus these goals must be related.

In 1992 the HCFA created the "HCFA-700" form for documenting the evaluation of outpatients and their plan of care. The HCFA-700 form has never been mandated for use by HCFA, and thus fiscal intermediaries vary regarding when and for which settings this form is required. Some fiscal intermediaries require the HCFA-700 form for Part B Medicare claims for home health. OT practitioners must know what information is required within their own facility and what information is required by the fiscal intermediary that will approve the claims (Thomas, 1996).

The purpose of the HCFA-700 form is to promote a streamlined and consistent national reporting and billing system for the care of elders who receive Medicare benefits (Wyman, 1994). Although anyone, including COTAs, may enter information on this form, OTRs are ultimately responsible for the form's contents. Consequently, it is recommended that OTRs countersign these forms (Walker, 1996). COTAs should become familiar with these forms because many other third-party payers follow similar formats.

Progress Notes

Progress notes are a written form of communication that identify important factors about an elder's progression in treatment, such as specifics regarding times

the elder is seen, the elder's status, the elder's level of cooperation and motivation, and the progress of education and treatment plans. As elders progress or their status of health changes, modifications in treatment plan and modalities may be necessary. COTAs must clearly identify health status or functional changes in the medical record and discuss these changes with the OTR. The elder may need to be reassessed, and the plan of care, including goals, may need to be revised. New goals may also need to be established. The elder's physician should be notified of the recommended changes and the reasons for these changes by written documentation. HCFA designed the "HCFA-701" form for documentation of updated plans of progress, monthly summaries, and discharge information. Verification of receipt of this communication must be stated in writing by the physician. Once approval is received, COTAs may make these modifications in collaboration with the OTR. OTRs may indicate that they agree with these changes by co-signing all the COTA's documentations while reviewing the COTA's progress notes (Backhaus, 1993). In many cases, OTRs may write in the medical record a sentence that confirms the date and change in the plan.

Because of the diversity of documentation requirements mandated by various facilities and fiscal intermediaries, numerous formats exist for documenting progress. Formats include narratives; subjective, objective, assessment, and plan (**SOAP**) **notes;** and **grid systems.** Most practice settings require that each treatment session be documented individually. Other settings may require weekly summaries, monthly summaries, or both, in addition to daily notes. Regardless of format, however, documentation of progress should follow the same standards of objectivity, measurability, and functionality described earlier in this chapter.

SOAP notes. The SOAP note format may be used for initial notes, progress notes, or discharge notes. The acronym *SOAP* represents the four elements in the format of documentation: subjective, objective, assessment, and plan. The subjective section of the note quotes pertinent information contributed by the client, family member, or both while interacting with the therapist. Key words such as "the client . . . states, describes, denies, indicates, and complains about" are used. In this section of the note the person being quoted should always be identified. Because the subjective section is comprised of quotes, the writer should make no interpretations of the meaning behind the words of the client or family member. An example of a subjective section of a SOAP note is as follows: "S: Client complains of difficulty putting on her pants."

The objective section requests concrete facts pertaining to the elder. These facts may include the results of standardized tests evaluating occupational performance components and areas. This section may also list the interventions provided and the results obtained. Education provided to the client or the client's family, caregiver, and other staff members may also be included. An example of an objective section of a SOAP note is as follows: "O: Initial evaluation indicates that client requires maximal assistance in donning pants. Client has difficulty with right/left discrimination and displays poor sitting balance. A daily regimen of dressing training has been initiated. For followup, staff members have been educated about the dressing techniques used."

Assessment data summarize the professional opinion of the COTA or OTR regarding the functional implications associated with the information discussed in the "S" and "O" sections. This section may also inform the reader of any physical, cognitive, or psychosocial precautions relevant to the client's health and safety. The assessment section becomes a reference point for other health care providers, third-party payers, and others who read the medical record and need a quick overview of the client's functional abilities and limitations. An example of the assessment section of the SOAP note is as follows: "A: Client seems to have difficulty with dressing skills because of poor balance and perceptual difficulties. Client attempts all treatment tasks and follows through with them with other staff."

The plan section of the note describes the therapy focus for the upcoming days, treatment goals, modalities and techniques to be used, and possible assessments or discharge plans. An example of the plan section of the SOAP note is as follows: "P: Client will be followed 5× weekly for 1-hour sessions for OT intervention. Plan is to provide daily activities of daily living (ADL) training for the anticipated discharge to home. Treatment goals are as follows: LTG: Client will sequence dressing with minimal assistance by 4 weeks. STG: Client will display improved sitting balance from poor to fair to dress in a seated position by . . . STG: Client will sequence donning and doffing pants with moderate assistance by . . ."

Grid system. Many rehabilitation agencies have adopted a grid system for documenting client progress. The purpose of grids is to provide a quick system for tracking both treatment provided and response to that treatment. A variety of grids exist. In most systems the planned interventions or modalities are listed in a column on one side of the page, and practitioners make check marks in the grid for each corresponding date intervention was provided. Often all clinicians who treat the client must provide their signature, initials, and title, such as *COTA* or *OTR* in another section of the grid. Initials are used to countersign each entry in the grid. If the treatment provided is not consistent with the plan of care, the practitioner must document the reason in narrative form.

Frequently weekly summary narrative notes are written to complement the information in the grid system. Weekly summaries describe the weekly progress and treatment frequency. These summaries should also ex-

plain the reasons that professional skills are needed and address any functional goals the client must reach. Additional progress notes are written when the client demonstrates a change in status, either through improvement or decline. Additional notes may also be written when meetings involving the family have taken place, specific changes in the care plan have been made, or any other relevant information arises.

Discharge Documentation

OTRs are responsible for the actual decision to terminate OT services and for writing the **discharge summary.** COTAs may collaborate with OTRs in writing an informative discharge summary and restorative program (AOTA, 1993). Pertinent information to be included in the discharge summary includes goals achieved, goals not achieved, and an explanation for why goals were not achieved. Discharge summaries must also list treatment modalities used, the elder's response to treatment modalities, and specific instructions and education provided to elders, family members, and caregivers. Discharge recommendations should also be included.

COTAs may develop a restorative or maintenance program at the time of discharge in cooperation with OTRs (AOTA, 1993). The restorative or maintenance program informs the elder, family members, caregivers, and other health care providers of ways in which the elder may maintain or improve current functional status. The maintenance program should be geared to the elder's anticipated discharge setting. For example, if an elder is going home, the maintenance program should include functional activities to be done in the home. OTRs should co-sign these programs before putting them into the permanent record (Box 9-1). Because delineation of practice roles between OTRs and COTAs may differ from state to state, it is important to clarify this duty and others with the appropriate state licensing board.

BOX 9-1

Suggested Restorative or Maintenance Program Checklist

- Detailed, clearly written plan outlining the activities to be performed by the elder, including how often and when the activities are to be performed
- Specific instructions for caregivers
- Treatment precautions
- Family education
- Contact information and reasons to contact OT personnel

Documenting Consultation and Supervision

COTAs have a varied role in the documentation process. This role may be influenced by numerous factors including state supervision requirements, the legal forms being used, and the frequency of treatment. State licensure boards, facilities, rehabilitation agencies, third-party payers, and the AOTA each have documentation guidelines. COTAs must take responsibility for keeping informed and adhering to these regulations.

Delineation of roles and the amount and type of supervision required for COTAs are outlined in the *Occupational Therapy Roles* document published by AOTA (1993). Although specific regulations may vary among states, facilities, and agencies, collaboration between OTRs and COTAs must be demonstrated during the treatment of each elder. One way to demonstrate this collaboration is by keeping a written account of all discussions, reviews, and observations pertaining to treatment of the elder that have occurred between OTRs and COTAs. Some states have specific forms to be used to document information such as the site, type of supervision provided, and time spent. These forms usually require the supervising OTR's name and license number.

If a state does not have a specific form for reporting the amount and type of supervision provided for COTAs, the COTA and OTR team should implement their own system, such as a notebook. Information about each meeting of the COTA and OTR to discuss an elder's status should be recorded. In case the COTA, OTR, facility, or agency is ever audited by the state licensing board, this documentation provides detailed proof about the adequacy of the supervision.

Another way the OTR can document the supervision provided is to write an entry into the permanent record of each elder the OTR and COTA reviewed. For example, the OTR may write the following: "Discussed elder's status with COTA this date. Current plan of care to continue. No changes in modalities or goals at this time. Signed, OTR." Some states may require supervising OTRs to record such entries. If the OTR is not making such entries in the permanent record, the COTA should suggest that this practice be initiated.

DOCUMENTATION ISSUES

Third-party payers encourage outcome-based clinical record reporting with use of standardized tests as a method of determining the effectiveness of intervention. OT intervention with elders is affected by shifting health care reimbursement patterns. The need for high-quality documentation has increased because of changes in health care delivery and in the structure of reimbursement used in managed care systems. The proliferation of SNFs and subacute care rehabilitation units and an increase in rural and home health care practice have also fueled the need for good documentation procedures. Staffing shortages, the effort to reduce cost and maintain quality care, and the increase in cases of fraud and abuse associated with higher utilization of OT services have made objective, accurate, and thorough documentation essential (Schwartz, Ergle-Ramirez, 1996).

The documentation provided by COTAs, whether sparse or detailed, objective or subjective, accurate or inaccurate, or complete or incomplete, crosses many desks. Members of the clinical team, insurance companies, quality assurance representatives, utilization review committees, and Medicare auditors review documentation to justify the cost of therapy services. The content and quality of a document will influence the reader's opinion about the therapist and the capability of the OT profession to provide effective and efficient health care.

Foto et al (1990) describe writing style and editorial intent as a foundation for successful OT reports. Writing style is defined as "the manner by which thoughts are conveyed in writing." Writing style includes grammar, composition, and word use, as well as a format that is logical, coherent, and concise. Editorial intent is determined by the agency requesting the documentation of OT services. One intermediary may request a deficit assessment, whereas a managed care agency may request a functional outcomes report. An employer, on the other hand, may request a functional capacity evaluation. To write effective OT reports, practitioners must know who will be reading the reports and the intent and expectations of the documentation.

COTAs who work well with elders and provide appropriate therapy for their recovery are not wholly effective if insurance companies deny reimbursement because of a lack of adequate documentation. OT consumers may interpret the refusal of Medicare or their insurer to pay as lack of competence of the OT profession (Smith, 1993). OT practitioners must keep in mind that most reviewers of the documentation have no formal training to assist them in understanding what OT is and what constitutes OT expertise (Abeln, 1993). Thus practitioners must take extra care to understand the reimbursement system. Practitioners must also understand documentation requirements, be aware of the audience reading the reports, and know whom to contact in the event that a claim is not approved on the basis of inadequate documentation. Practitioners must also remember that communication through documentation serves as a catalyst for maintaining a referral base with physicians, case managers, other health professionals, and third-party payers. Communication through documentation can also be used in legal situations. Because OT practitioners are legally responsible for documents that they write and sign, their primary concern should be accuracy. Practitioners should consider how their documentation would hold up in a court of law. Indeed, "the burden of proof is on the therapist" (Burghardt et al, 1996).

Rhonda, the COTA mentioned in the beginning of the chapter who received a subpoena to give a deposition regarding the death of an elderly woman with whom she had worked, hoped her documentation was complete. The elderly women's death was being investigated, and Rhonda's documentation was being viewed by many people, including those in the legal system.

When Rhonda arrived at the attorney's office, she met Mark, the OTR with whom she had collaborated for several years. They were allowed to review Mrs. L.'s OT

documentation. As they read the initial evaluation, they recalled that Mrs. L. had suffered a cerebrovascular accident in the left hemisphere. Box 9-2 contains the initial evaluation summary and treatment goals that Mark and Rhonda had collaborated on writing.

Rhonda and Mark noted that the initial evaluation considered performance areas and components and clearly defined Mrs. L.'s status. They also noted that the treatment goals were concise, measurable, and included the performance area of ADL function and the performance components of muscle strength, sequencing, and motor planning. The goals clearly defined a level of assistance. Rhonda and Mark went on to read the first progress note (Box 9-3).

BOX 9-2

Mrs. L's Initial Evaluation

October 9: Mrs. L. is a 78-year-old woman who was evaluated on Oct. 7 by OT. The client sustained a (L) CVA with (R) hemiparesis on Oct. 1. Prior level of function was independent with all home management, activities of daily living, work, and productive tasks. Medical record indicates a past medical history of hypertension. Client was at hospital for 7 days and was transferred to SNF on Oct. 8. Mrs. L. was evaluated while seated in a chair.

Activities of daily living:
At evaluation, Mrs. L. was neatly dressed and groomed. Client requires moderate assistance to motor plan dressing and grooming activities. Feeding requires set-up. Client can take medications after set-up. According to speech therapy evaluation, client displays mild expressive aphasia.

Work/productive activities:
Client is a homemaker and is presently dependent with home management tasks.

Play/leisure
Client enjoys playing bridge.

Sensory motor components:
Client is (R) hand dominant. Client displays impaired 2-point discrimination on involved R side. Stereognosis testing is impaired; client identified three of five objects. Figure ground testing is impaired.
     Lateral trunk strength is poor (2/5). Client requires moderate assistance with bed to chair transfers. R U/E muscle strength is grade 2 + /5. Active assistive ROM for shoulder flexion and abduction is limited to 90 degrees secondary to pain. All other ROM is within functional limits. The McGill-Melzack Pain Questionnaire was used to identify pain level, which was described by Mrs. L. as distressing and rated by the therapists as 2/5. Grasp

strength R U/E is 15 pounds. Grasp strength L U/E is 45 degrees.

Cognitive components:
Client is oriented ×3. Client displayed adequate attention span of 1 hour for evaluation tasks. Client demonstrated difficulty sequencing dressing tasks.

Psychosocial skills:
Client reports "I feel down since I had this stroke. I used to be so independent and enjoyed being a housewife. I will try to work hard in therapy."

Home situation:
According to her social history, Mrs. L. lives with spouse in a one-floor home. Mr. L. is 84 years old and in good health. Mr. L. reports a willingness to participate in Mrs. L.'s care. They have one son who lives out of state.

Long-term goal:
Mrs. L. will independently complete dressing while sitting in a chair within 4 weeks.

Short-term goals:
1. Mrs. L. will increase lateral trunk strength from grade poor (2/5) to grade fair+ (3/5) to dress self with minimal assistance while sitting in a chair located at the edge of the bed within 2 weeks.
2. Mrs. L. will sequence the transfer from supine in bed to sitting in a chair located at the edge of the bed with minimal assistance to dress self within 2 weeks.
3. Mrs. L. will motor plan donning a button-front shirt with minimal assistance within 1 week. OT will follow client 2× daily, 5 days weekly.
M.L. OTR/L and R.W. COTA/L (signed)

Rhonda and Mark critically considered the first progress note and identified several concerns. The note seemed vague and did not provide specific details about the functional status or treatment plan of the client. Mrs. L. current status was not compared to her initial status, and the note did not comment on her level of motivation or cooperation or on her personal goals. In addition, the note did not mention any attempts to educate staff or family members about Mrs. L.'s condition. Rhonda noted that they were specific in defining the exact number of treatment sessions and a reason for a missed session.

Rhonda and Mark continued to carefully review their documentation. They read the progress note written on October 21 (Box 9-4).

Rhonda and Mark breathed a sigh of relief when they read the October 21 note and subsequent documentation. Rhonda noted to Mark that they must have recognized the problems with the first note when writing the next note. Rhonda and Mark were glad that they had been much more specific in the next note and included Mrs. L.'s functional status in the documentation. They also included her previous status as a comparison, and discussed her level of motivation and cooperation and her personal goals. In addition, Rhonda and Mark commented on the family's involvement.

Because of the clear documentation provided by Mark and Rhonda in the remainder of the chart, Rhonda's story had a positive ending. Mark and Rhonda were able to give a thorough testimony to the attorney, and their documentation held up in the court of law.

CONCLUSION

Many issues related to the COTA's role in the documentation process have been discussed. Documentation is a way to communicate information about a client to others. Other people need this information for many reasons, including coordination of care, proving medical necessity, and substantiating the need for reimbursement of services. By understanding who will be reading the documentation that they provide, COTAs can target the documentation to their audience to help guarantee that elders receive the treatment they need. COTAs should keep the following considerations in mind while preparing documentation:

1. Documentation should be completed in a timely manner and must follow the guidelines provided by the AOTA, state, employer, and third-party payers.
2. Entries in a medical record should be in chronological order. If a late entry must be made, documentation should reflect the reason the entry is late, and the entry must be dated and signed.
3. COTAs should use correct grammar and spelling. Writing must be legible.

BOX **9-3**

Mrs. L.'s First Progress Note

October 14
Mrs. L. has been followed by OT 2× daily, 5 days weekly since Oct. 7 for a diagnosis of Left CVA. Mrs. L. missed one session because of an episode of the flu. OT is working on improving sitting balance for dressing skills.

OT will continue to follow.
M.R. OTR/L and R.W. COTA/L (signed)

BOX **9-4**

Mrs. L.'s Second Progress Note

October 21
Mrs. L. continues to be followed by OT 2× daily, 5× weekly since Oct. 14. This week, treatment continued to focus on improving balance and dressing skills. On Oct. 14 resident required moderate assistance with UE dressing. Resident had a poor (2/5) grade of lateral trunk strength that was interfering with sitting balance. Mrs. L. required moderate assistance to sequence transferring from supine to sitting in the chair to do the dressing task and moderate assistance to motor plan donning a shirt.

This week, Mrs. L. displays a fair+ (3/5) lateral trunk strength. Mrs. L. now requires minimal assistance to sequence transferring from being supine to sitting in the chair to do the dressing task. Mrs. L. still requires moderate assistance to motor plan donning a shirt.

On Oct. 12, Mr. and Mrs. L. and the treatment team participated in a family conference in which each discipline team member discussed functional status and possible discharge plans. The plan is for Mrs. L. to be discharged home. Mrs. L. appears motivated and is cooperative in participating in treatment activities. The plan is to also include Mr. L. in therapy sessions. Mrs. L. stated "I want to get better so that I can get home. That is why I am working so hard."

The plan is to initiate LE dressing next week with the STG that resident will motor plan dressing LE with moderate assistance. (Current status with LE dressing is requiring maximal assistance to motor plan the activity). In addition, plan is to work on sequencing transfers from wheelchair to commode and tub bench and to continue to practice UE dressing with the STG for resident to motor plan donning shirt with minimal assistance by the following week.

Occupational therapy will continue to follow 2× daily, 5× weekly.
M.L. OTR/L and R.W. COTA/L (signed)

4. Notes should be written in black ink only. If the pen runs out of ink, COTAs should write "(pen out of ink)" in parentheses, using a second pen.

5. Discharge summaries, home health care, and follow-up instructions provided to the elder, the elder's family, nurses, physicians, and significant others should be documented thoroughly.

6. Documentation should not include unauthorized abbreviations.

7. Another professional should not be blamed for a problem in an elder's permanent record.

8. Subjective information should be documented as such. COTAs should not assume that all the information provided by an elder is factual. For example, if an elder with a stroke reports that he dressed himself independently that morning, the COTA should check with the nurse or caregiver to verify the elder's report and document statements made by all parties.

9. The elder's participation and nonparticipation should be documented.

10. Possible negligence by the elder, the elder's family, or other caregiver should be documented carefully. For example, if the family is not assisting the elder with ADL functions as established by the treatment plan, the COTA could state in the record, "Caregivers verbally refused to follow the treatment plan for assisting with ADL."

11. Information should never be added or changed in a note after this information has been provided to an elder, payer source, or elder's attorney. If changes need to be made, the revision along with an explanation of reasons for changes should be provided to all these people.

12. Writing data in a medical chart and then removing that information for any reason is illegal. If incorrect information was written, a single line should be drawn through the incorrect information. COTAs should sign and write the date above the line. COTAs may then write the correct information following the error. COTAs should not attempt to erase, scratch out, write over, or cover errors with correction fluid.

13. A straight line should be drawn from the end of the entry to the end of the line or margin of the paper. This practice discourages anyone from adding information at a later time.

▌▌ CHAPTER REVIEW QUESTIONS

READ THE FOLLOWING NARRATIVE PROGRESS NOTE AND ANSWER THE QUESTIONS BELOW.

Weekly Progress Note: Nov. 15. Client has been followed by OT 5× weekly for 45-minute to 1-hour sessions since Nov. 7 for a diagnosis of (R) total hip replacement. This week cli-

ent's husband was educated about the hip safety precautions. OT intervention involved applying the hip safety precautions to the self-care skills of bathing and dressing, as well as the home management skills of cleaning and meal preparation. The client required maximal assistance with self-care skills and now requires moderate assistance. The client was dependent with the home management skills and now requires moderate assistance. The client is depressed. The client states, "I want to go home soon but I am scared about being alone." The client has become tearful in two sessions when discussing the possibility of going home. The client had to be corrected 2× this week for not following the hip safety precautions when picking up items from the floor. The plan is to continue to work with the client 5× weekly for 45-minute to 1-hour sessions. OT will continue to work on self-care and home management skills, with the goal for client to be functioning with minimal assistance by 1 week.

1 Critically review the progress note and identify the strengths and weaknesses of this document.

2 The COTA and OTR collaborated to make the following treatment goal: "Client will be more independent with self-care and home management skills." Discuss what is wrong with this goal.

3 Develop one long-term goal and two short-term goals for the client described in this progress note.

4 Convert this narrative progress note into the SOAP format.

REFERENCES

Abeln S: Importance of documentation to patient care reimbursement. In Stewart D, Abelns, editors: *Documenting functional outcomes in physical therapy*, St. Louis, 1993, Mosby.

Abreu B, Lackey P: Documentation and additional considerations. In Royeen C, editor: *AOTA self study series: cognitive rehabilitation*, Rockville, Md, 1994, American Occupational Therapy Association.

American Occupational Therapy Association: Elements of clinical documentation—revision, *Am J Occup Ther* 49(10):1032, 1995.

American Occupational Therapy Association: Uniform terminology for occupational therapy—third edition, *Am J Occup Ther* 48(11): 1055, 1994.

American Occupational Therapy Association: Occupational therapy roles, *Am J Occup Ther* 47(12):1087, 1993.

Anderson K, Anderson L, Glanze W, editors: *Mosby's medical, nursing, and allied health dictionary*, ed 4, St. Louis, 1994, Mosby.

Backhaus H: Documentation. In Ryan S, editor: *Practice issues in occupational therapy: intraprofessional team building*, Thorofare, NJ, 1993, SLACK.

Burghardt R, et al: *Rehabilitation and the law: liability and the occupational therapy practitioner*, Bethesda, Md, 1996, The American Occupational Therapy Association.

Commission on Practice, American Occupational Therapy Association: Clarification of the use of the terms assessment and evaluation, *Am J Occup Ther* 49(10):1072, 1995.

Esposto L: Applying functional outcome assessment to Medicare documentation. In Stewart D, Abeln S, editors: *Documenting functional outcomes in physical therapy*, St. Louis, 1993, Mosby.

Foto M. et al: Reports that work. In Royeen C, editor:*AOTA self study series: assessing function (lesson 9)*, Rockville, Md, 1990, American Occupational Therapy Association.

Health Care Financing Administration: *Medicare intermediary review manual, Pub No 1303*, Washington, DC, 1990, US Department of Health and Human Services.

Jabri J: Documentation of occupational therapy services. In: Pedretti L, editor: *Occupational therapy: practice skills for physical dysfunction*, ed 4, St. Louis, 1996, Mosby.

Punwar AJ: *Occupational therapy: principles and practice*, Baltimore, 1994, Williams & Wilkins.

Scott R: *Legal aspects of documenting patient care*, Gaithersburg, Md, 1994, Aspen.

Schwartz K, Engle-Ramirez J: Occupational therapy and health care reform. In Pedretti L, editor: *Occupational therapy: practice skills for physical dysfunction*, ed 4, St. Louis, 1996, Mosby.

Smith H: Assessment and evaluation: an overview. In Smith H, Hopkins H, editors: *Willard and Spackman's occupational therapy*, ed 8, Philadelphia, Pa, 1993, JB Lippincott.

Spectra Rehab Alliance Consulting Program: *Informed consent/consent to pay guidelines*, Chicago, 1994, Beverly Enterprises.

Thomas J: Personal communication, Oct 1996.

Trombly C, editor: Planning, guiding and documenting therapy. In Trombly C, editor: *Occupational therapy for physical dysfunction*, ed 4, Baltimore, 1995, Williams & Wilkins.

Walker V: COTA focus, *OT Week* May 16, 7, 1996.

Walker V: COTA and the evaluation process, *OT Week* September 14, 13, 1995.

Wyman J: 700/701 forms not perfect, but better: consistency in rehab documentation, *Adv Occup Ther*, 10:5, 1994.

CHAPTER 10

Cultural Diversity of the Aging Population

RENÉ L. PADILLA

KEY TERMS

diversity, culture, values, beliefs, race, gender, age, ethnicity, sexual orientation, religion, ethnocentrism, assimilation, performance context, melting pot, conformity, bias, prejudice, discrimination, minority, homosexual, cognitive style, associative, abstractive, truth, equality

CHAPTER OBJECTIVES

1. Explain the meaning of "diversity" and related terms.
2. Explore personal experiences, beliefs, values, and attitudes regarding diversity.
3. Discuss the need to accept the uniqueness of each individual and the importance of being sensitive to issues of diversity in the practice of occupational therapy with elders.
4. Present strategies to facilitate interaction with elders of diverse backgrounds.

Today is Susan's first day at her first job as a COTA. She has been hired to work as a member of the rehabilitation team in a small nursing home in the town where she grew up. Susan is excited because this job will permit her to stay close to her family and work with elders. When she arrives at the nursing home she and the OTR discuss the cases of the elders who are participating in the rehabilitation program. Susan is told about Mr. Chu, a Chinese gentleman who experienced a stroke and often refuses to get out of bed, and Mrs. Pardo, a Filipino woman who is constantly surrounded by family and consequently cannot get anything accomplished. The OTR also tells Susan about Mr. Cooper, an elderly man dying from acquired immunodeficiency disorder (AIDS); Mrs. Blanche, a retired university professor who is a quadriplegic; and Mr. Perez, who was a migrant farm worker until the accidental amputation of his left arm 4 weeks previously. Susan notes the distinct qualities of each of these elders.

OVERVIEW OF CULTURAL DIVERSITY

The cultural **diversity** of clients adds an exciting and challenging element to the practice of OT. Each client comes from a **culture** with a unique blend of **values** and **beliefs.** This uniqueness affects all aspects of the client's life, including the occupational dimension. The ways in which a person chooses to do a task, interact with family members, move about in a community, look to the future, and view health are in many ways the result of past experiences as well as the expectations of the people with whom that person comes in contact. Consequently,

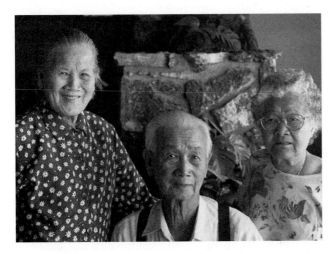

FIGURE **10-1** Cultural diversity makes OT practice exciting and challenging.

COTAs have to deal with many issues that arise from interactions with persons unlike themselves in terms of **race, gender, age, ethnicity, sexual orientation,** family situation, place of birth, **religion,** and level of education, among other factors (Figure 10-1).

Culture, **ethnocentrism, assimilation,** and diversity are discussed to provide a framework for working with elders in a sensitive manner. After this discussion are general guidelines for assessment and treatment. The challenge for COTAs is to create a therapeutic environment in which diversity and difference are valued and in which each elder can work to the fullest potential.

WHAT IS CULTURE?

The concept of culture has long been considered important in the practice of OT. The official definition for licensure of occupational therapy adopted in 1981 by the American Occupational Therapy Association (AOTA) representative assembly states, "Occupational therapy is the use of purposeful activity with individuals who are limited by physical injury or illness, psychosocial dysfunction, developmental or learning disabilities, poverty and cultural differences, or the aging process in order to maximize independence, prevent disability and maintain health" (AOTA, 1981). However, the term *culture* has not been clearly defined in OT professional literature, nor has it been consistently considered in the assessment and treatment process (Krefting, Krefting, 1991). Part of the reason for this lapse may be the breadth of complex concepts encompassed by this one term. For example, AOTA's Uniform Terminology For Occupational Therapy, third edition (1994) lists culture among the **performance contexts** in which occupation generally occurs, with performance contexts defined as " . . . situations or factors that influence an individual's engagement in desired and/or required performance [of occupation]." Performance contexts might be temporal, such as chrono-

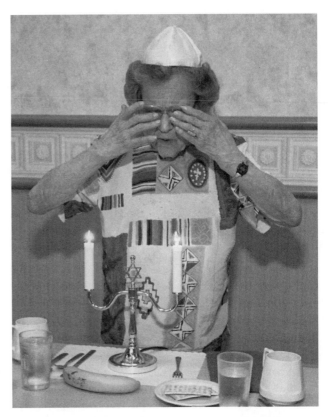

FIGURE **10-2** This Jewish elder practices a religious observance passed down from generation to generation.

logical age, developmental age, place in the life cycle, and health status, or environmental, such as physical, social, and cultural settings. This document defines culture as "customs, beliefs, activity patterns, behavior standards, and expectations accepted by the society of which the individual is a member. Includes political aspects, such as laws that affect access to resources and affirm personal rights. Also includes opportunities for education, employment, and economic support" (AOTA, 1994). Kielhofner (1995) states, "Culture consists of the beliefs and perceptions, values and norms, customs and behaviors that are shared by a group or society, and are passed from one generation to the next through both formal and informal education" (Figure 10-2).

This broad and consequently vague definition of culture is not unique to the OT profession. Entire books in other fields are devoted to describing culture, and authors have been unable to agree on a single definition. Some of the commonalities in those definitions, including that culture is learned and shared with others, may be used as a basis for an understanding of culture. (Benedict, 1989; Krefting, Krefting, 1991).

Culture is learned, or acquired, through socialization (Figure 10-3). Culture is not carried in a person's genetic make-up; rather, it is learned over the course of a lifetime. Obviously, then, the environment in which each person

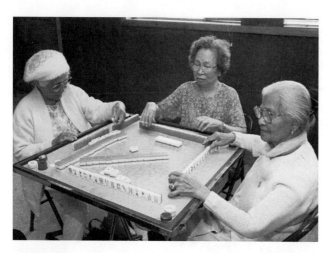

FIGURE **10-3**   This group of elders enjoys a culturally shared game.

lives is central to his or her culture. A person's environment may demand or offer opportunities for some types of behaviors and restrict opportunities for other types. For example, individuals in the United States are offered the opportunity to choose the color of their clothing, but generally wearing of dresses is culturally restricted to females. In the United States, persons are expected to drive on the right side of the street, pay taxes, and go to work according to schedule. Through interaction with the environment, individuals learn a variety of values and beliefs and eventually internalize them. Internalized values direct the interactions among people and with the environment. As a result, people expect that others have internalized the same values and beliefs and consequently behave in the same ways (Hall, 1981). However, culture is the result of each person's unique experiences with the environment and thus is an ongoing learning process.

Another commonality in the various definitions of culture is that, because it is learned from others, it is also shared. What is shared as culture, however, is very dynamic. Because culture is learned throughout one's lifetime, each person learns it at a different point. On the basis of each person's status in learning culture, the person expects something from others and contributes to others' cultural educations. In this way, each person learns and teaches something about culture that is unique. Over time, shared beliefs and values change. These changes in cultural beliefs and values may not be easily observed because the actual behaviors that express them seem to remain the same. However, over time, a periodic recommitment to the dynamic transmittal of beliefs and values has occurred. For example, the attire of women in some regions of the Arabian peninsula has changed very little in the past 200 years. Originally the black gowns, robes, and veils were probably intended to guard the woman's modesty. Many women who wear these garments today, in addition to guarding modesty, do so as a symbol of

resistance to westernization, a concern that was probably not prevalent 200 years ago (Harris, 1989).

Finally, culture is often subconscious (Krefting, Krefting, 1991; Harris, 1989; Peacock, 1986; Hall, 1984). Because learning of culture occurs formally and informally, a person is not usually aware, particularly at a younger age, of learning it. Instead the person simply complies with the demands and restrictions of behavior set in particular environments and chooses behaviors from among those that are permitted. For example, when a child is not permitted to touch a frog found by a pond during a family outing, that child is being formally taught that frogs are dirty and therefore should not be touched, a value the child might internalize and then generalize to other animals. This value is informally reinforced when the child sees other people wince and make gestures of repulsion when they see certain types of animals. When the child sees a younger sibling attempting to touch a frog, the child might tell the sibling not to do so because touching it is "bad." In effect, the child internalized a value received from the culture of his or her family and passed it on to a sibling with the slight reinterpretation that it is "bad" to do the particular behavior. In a similar way all persons continue to learn culture from each physical and social environment in which they participate. When elders enter a nursing home for a short-term or long-term stay, for example, some of the facility's rules of behavior are formally explained, including meal times (and consequently when elders *must* eat), visiting hours (and consequently when elders *must* and *must not* socialize), and lights out time (and consequently when elders *must* sleep). However, elders also informally learn an entirely different set of rules. As they experience the daily routine in the nursing home they learn whether it is acceptable to question the professionals who work there, to decline to participate in scheduled group activities, and even to express their thoughts, feelings, and concerns. Staff members have likely not formally stated, "You are not permitted to state your feelings here." However, this value may be communicated informally by staff members if they cut off conversation when an elder begins to explain feelings or simply never take time to invite an expression of the elder's feelings. In this way values and beliefs become sets of unspoken, implicit, and underlying assumptions that guide interactions with others and the environment.

Culture is a set of beliefs and values that a particular group of people share and re-create constantly through interaction with each other and their environments. These beliefs and values may be conscious or unconscious, and they direct the opportunities, demands, and behavior restrictions that exist for members of a particular group. Essentially every belief and value that humans acquire as members of society can be included in their culture, thus explaining the broadness of the concept of culture.

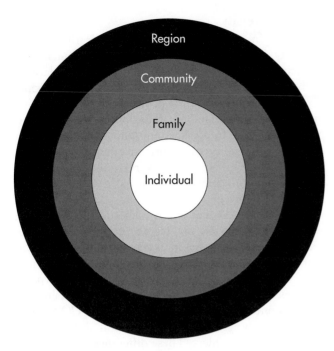

FIGURE 10-4 Levels of culture.

LEVELS OF CULTURE

Various levels exist at which values and beliefs are shared. Krefting and Krefting (1991) propose that a multidimensional view of culture be adopted. In this view, culture can be defined in terms of the individual, the family, the community, and the region (Figure 10-4). At the individual level are the relational, one-to-one interactions through which people learn and express their unique representations of culture. Examples of this level of culture are each person's use of humor, definition of personal space, coping style, and role choices. Included at the level of the family are beliefs and values that are shared within a primary social group—the group in which most of the person's early socialization takes place. This level includes issues such as gender roles, family structure, and style of worship. Each family can be seen as a variation of the culture that is shared at the level of a community or neighborhood, in which economic factors, ethnicity, housing, and other factors may be considered. Communities may be seen as variations in the culture that is shared with a larger region, such as language, geography, and industry. Krefting and Krefting (1991) also note that variation exists at each level and within each group.

Adopting a more relational framework helps overcome some of the difficulties inherent in viewing culture as synonymous with ethnicity. Ethnicity is the part of a person's identity that is derived from membership in a racial, religious, national, or linguistic group (Hartog, Hartog, 1983). The viewing of culture as synonymous with ethnicity relies on generalizations about the people who belong to a particular group and can lead to mistaken assump-

tions about an individual's personality and beliefs. For example, the assumption that all persons of Hispanic ethnicity have brown skin and black hair is not true, because Hispanics of all racial backgrounds exist. Equally, people cannot assume that all whites are educated, that all Jews observe kosher practices, or that everyone who speaks English attaches the same meaning to the word *napkin*.

Equating ethnicity with culture can lead to many misinterpretations. In addition, this practice is often used to justify superiority of one group over another. The term *ethnocentricity* describes the belief held by members of a particular ethnic group that their expression of beliefs and values is better than that of others and consequently that all other groups should aspire to adopt their beliefs and values. In extreme cases of ethnocentricity, a particular ethnic group has attempted to destroy other ethnic groups, as in (Nazi) Germany, Bosnia, and Sudan. Ethnocentrism can be and often is an underlying, subconscious belief that powerfully guides a person's behavior. An unexamined ethnocentric attitude may lead COTAs to place particular emphasis on certain areas of rehabilitation and disregard others that elders may consider essential for their recovery. OT itself can be viewed as a subculture with beliefs and values that guide practitioners toward productivity, leisure, and purposeful activity. This bias may sometimes lead practitioners to ignore the client's wishes and impose their own values in the belief that they are more important and worthwhile.

THE ISSUE OF DIVERSITY

The variety of clients that Susan, the COTA introduced at the beginning of this chapter, will work with underscores a well-known fact about the United States: it is a country of immigrants, a conglomeration of diverse peoples. How is it possible that all these groups live together? The metaphor of the "melting pot" has been used to describe the way in which distinct cultural groups in the United States "melt down" and how differences between groups that were once separate entities disappear. This process is the result of the continuous exposure of groups to one another (Barresi, 1990). Fry (1990) describes a process of **conformity** in which an individual or a cultural group forsakes values, beliefs, and customs to eliminate differences with another culture. In the United States, conformity may be demonstrated by people who Americanize their names, speak only English, abandon religious practices or social rituals, shed their ethnic dress, attend night school, and work hard to become part of the "American dream." Both conformity and the melting pot metaphor imply that new ethnic groups entering the United States will be judged by the degree to which their differences with the values and beliefs of the established American culture disappear. This expectation can easily create **bias, prejudice,** and **discrimination** toward many individuals. The term **minority** is an outgrowth of these

Valuing Diversity

People in the United States are clearly diverse. Diversity is demonstrated through race, gender, age, ethnicity, sexual orientation, family situation, place of birth, religion, and level of education; in addition, people also differ from each other in physical ability or disability, intelligence, socioeconomic class, physical beauty, and personality type. In essence, any dimension of life can create identity groups or cohorts that may or may not be visible. Most people find that several of these dimensions have particular meaning for them.

Ironically, diversity becomes an inclusive concept when we view it as that which makes us different from each other. This view of diversity embraces everyone, because each person is in some way different from everyone else. At the same time, however, each person in some way is also similar to someone else. This viewpoint provides a framework for approaching the diversity that one encounters when working with elders: COTAs can recognize the ways in which they are both different from and similar to the elders. These differences and similarities can be used during therapy to enrich the elder's life. A welcome side effect of this approach is that the COTA's life will often be enriched as well.

Diversity of the Aged Population

A summary of statistical reports on the elder population was presented in Chapter 1. Each of these reports is an example of diversity. The following facts should also be taken into account when considering diversity among the rapidly growing elder population.

Persons over the age of 65 years represent 12.7% of the U.S. population, or 33.2 million people. In 1990, 13% of elders belonged to minority populations, and this number is expected to grow to 25% by the year 2030. The number of elders in minority groups is expected to grow by 328% between 1990 and 2030. A growth of 93% is expected in the white non-Hispanic elder population in that same period. The growth among Asian and Pacific Islander elders is projected to be the largest (693%), followed by Hispanic elders (555%), non-Hispanic black elders (160%), and American Indian, Eskimo, and Aleuts elders (231%) (American Association of Retired Persons [AARP], 1995). A breakdown of the U.S. racial and ethnic population is provided in Figure 10-6. Importantly, these figures represent only the numbers of elders who belong to broad categories, not cultural distinctiveness. Each of the categories listed may include numerous cultures and subcultures. These numbers are used here simply to emphasize that the population served by OT practitioners will increasingly include elders from diverse backgrounds.

No reliable figures are available regarding the sexual preference of persons in the United States who are age 65 years or older. Janus and Janus (1993) estimate that 4% of men and 2% of women in the general population are exclusively **homosexual**. The figures are higher when

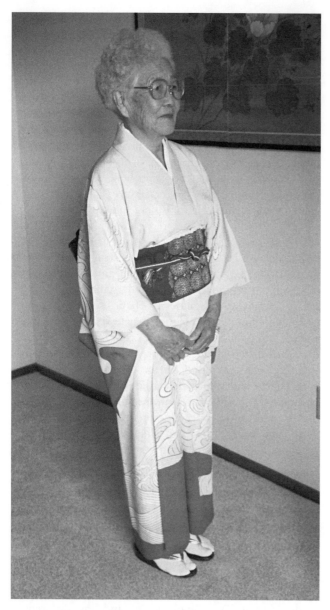

FIGURE 10-5 Maintaining one's cultural dress may be important for some elders.

views. This term is used not only to designate groups that are fewer in number but also groups that have less power and representation within an established culture despite their size.

The realization that some differences such as age, race, gender, and sexual orientation can never be eliminated, even with effort or night school, has led many people to discern that they should also value the other characteristics that make them unique, such as their cultural heritage and their religious practices (Figure 10-5). Cultural pluralism is a value system that recognizes this desire and focuses not on assimilation but on accepting and celebrating the differences that exist among people. Persons who value cultural pluralism believe that these differences add richness to a society rather than detract from it.

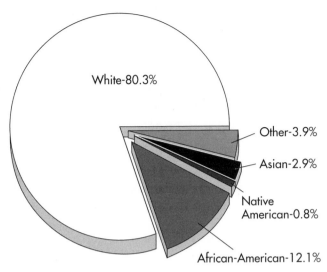

FIGURE **10-6** Breakdown of General Population by Race and Ethnic Origin. (From U.S. Bureau of the Census, 1995.)

bisexual orientation and frequency of homosexual experience are considered. Combining these figures provides the more accurate estimate that 9% of men and 5% of women may be considered homosexual (Janus, Janus, 1993). Studies suggest that these figures are consistent for elders over the age of 65 years (Dorfman et al, 1995; Quam, Whitford, 1992). If this is true, approximately 2.6 million elders are homosexual (Figure 10-7).

The United States is one of the most diverse countries in the world in terms of the religious affiliation of its people. Approximately 89% of persons in the United States say that they have a definite religious preference (U.S. Bureau of Labor Statistics, 1995). The trend toward increased religious diversity is fueled both by conversion and immigration. Since 1957 the Christian population (i.e., Catholics and Protestants) in the United States has dropped from 92% to 81% of all persons, whereas the number of practitioners of other religions, including Buddhism, Hinduism, and Islam, has increased from 1% to 6%. Information on the distribution of faiths of the general U.S. population is provided in Figure 10-8.

In 1992, 13.5% of all persons in the United States lived below the poverty line. This number looks quite different when minority groups are considered individually. For example, 31.9% of African-Americans, 28.1% of Hispanics, and 28.2% of American Indians are impoverished. Only about 41% of those in the United States who live beneath the poverty line receive Medicaid (AARP, 1995) (Figure 10-9).

Sensitivity to Culture and Diversity in Treatment

To be culturally sensitive, persons must acknowledge their own prejudices and biases. COTAs should realize that prejudices are learned behaviors and can be unlearned through increased contact with and understand-

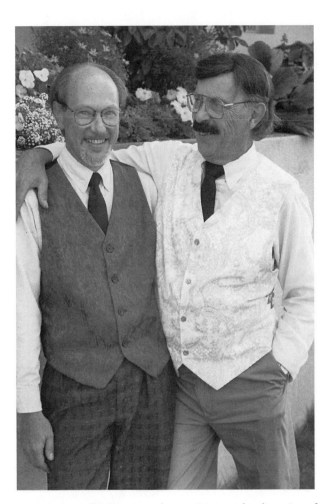

FIGURE **10-7** COTAs must be sensitive to the diversity of gender and age of life partners.

ing of people of diverse cultural groups. Furthermore, communication always takes place between individuals, not cultures. Gropper (1996) suggests that in the clinical encounter the cultures of both the client and the clinician play important roles in successful outcomes. Cooper writes that misunderstandings and miscommunication between clients and clinicians usually result from cultural differences, and that the clinician's responsibility is to adapt to the client's culture rather than demanding that the client adapt to the clinician's culture to receive service. Kohls and Knight (1994) proposed that in addition to the cultures of the client and the clinician, the culture of the institution in which the interaction takes place in many ways directs interaction between the client and clinician. In health care, institutional culture has strongly valued the biomedical approach to treatment, which places the control of health care with the physician rather than with the client. In addition, the U.S. medical system has placed little emphasis on the development of specific programs to address the needs of elders from culturally diverse groups.

Culture and diversity are extremely broad and complex concepts. Attempts to make generalizations about various

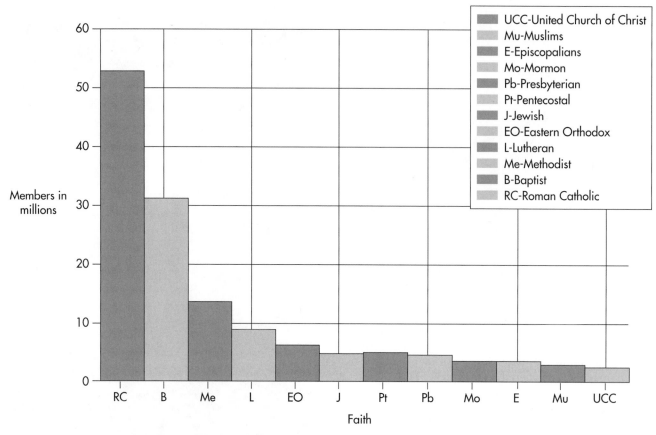

Legend:
- UCC-United Church of Christ
- Mu-Muslims
- E-Episcopalians
- Mo-Mormon
- Pb-Presbyterian
- Pt-Pentecostal
- J-Jewish
- EO-Eastern Orthodox
- L-Lutheran
- Me-Methodist
- B-Baptist
- RC-Roman Catholic

FIGURE **10-8**   Distribution of the 12 largest faiths in the general population. (From *Health Sciences Library Desk Reference*, Omaha, 1996, Creighton University.)

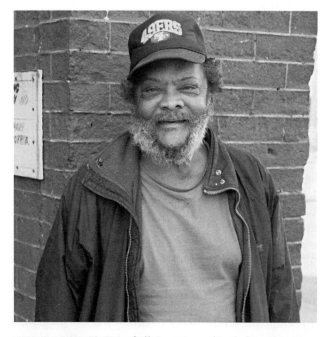

FIGURE **10-9**   13.5% of all Americans live below the poverty level. This 72-year-old man has been in and out of homeless shelters for the past 15 years.

groups would be useless because COTAs are certain to come across elders who do not fit the expected behavior. Few persons are perfect representations of their culture. Generalizations may also limit the COTA's ability to see each client as a unique individual. Consequently, COTAs should be cognizant of general issues about culture that should be assessed and remembered at every step of the OT program. COTAs must realize that cultural sensitivity is an ongoing process. In addition, COTAs should not assume that by following the guidelines presented in the following sections, they have done everything necessary to provide culturally appropriate OT services. The COTA's responsibility is to develop ongoing strategies that allow the client to maintain personal integrity and be treated with respect as an individual.

The two most important strategies COTAs can employ are asking questions and observing behavior carefully. The values and beliefs that encompass "culture" direct elders in their particular way of performing ADL functions and work and leisure occupations. Consequently, COTAs must be oriented to the elder's culture to provide relevant and meaningful treatment. This cultural orientation should include an understanding of (1) the cognitive style of the elder, (2) what he or she accepts as evidence, and (3) the value system that forms the basis of the elder's behavior. A fourth and final area of understanding has to do with communication style. If elders are unable to answer questions regarding these areas for themselves, COTAs should attempt to obtain this information from the elder's family or friends. If this is not an option, the COTA should obtain information about the elder's culture from other sources such as a co-worker who is of the same national origin as the elder and library materials. However, COTAs should remember that the more removed the information source is from the elder, the less likely that the information may apply to that particular elder.

Let us return briefly to Susan, the COTA starting a new job who was introduced at the beginning of this chapter. One of the elders with whom Susan would be working was Mr. Chu, a Chinese gentleman who refused to get out of bed. The OTR informed Susan that soon after Mr. Chu's admission, several of the elders who had Alzheimer's disease and were disoriented had become agitated in Mr. Chu's presence because they associated him with World War II experiences. The nursing home staff did not want Mr. Chu to be offended by this behavior, so they moved him to a private room. When Susan entered Mr. Chu's room, she said, "Hello! I'm from occupational therapy and I'm here to help you get out of bed and do your ADLs." As anticipated, he signaled his refusal to cooperate by turning his head and closing his eyes. He remained silent whenever Susan spoke to him. When she attempted to put her hand behind his shoulder to help him sit up, he grabbed her wrist and pushed her arm away. Susan was perplexed. She called Jon, a therapist of Japanese descent whom she had met at an orientation session a week earlier, and asked him to provide any insight into Mr. Chu's behavior. Jon told Susan that in general Asians are very circumspect, preferring to be with members of their own group, and that Mr. Chu was probably reacting to the fact that Susan was not Asian. Jon suggested that a family member be called in to enlist Mr. Chu's cooperation. Susan contacted Mr. Chu's son, Edwin, who met her later that afternoon at Mr. Chu's bedside. After some discussion with his father, Edwin informed Susan that Mr. Chu refused to get out of bed because he believed he had been placed in a private room to isolate him because he was Chinese. He viewed being informed about OT intervention plans as further evidence that he was being treated differently. Susan explained the staff's concern that Mr. Chu would be offended by the comments and behavior of the other elders. Mr. Chu said he understood that such behavior was part of an illness. Susan facilitated Mr. Chu's move to a room with three other elders, and he began to participate daily in the OT program. Susan was careful to ask Mr. Chu what he wanted to accomplish in each session. Jon's report

about Asians wanting to be with members of their own group was only partially true. Mr. Chu wished to be with other elders, not specifically other Chinese people. Susan was able to discover this only with the help of someone very familiar with Mr. Chu.

Cognitive Style

COTAs need to understand how elders organize information. This process does not refer to an assessment of cognitive functions that indicate the presence or absence of brain dysfunction (Allen, 1985; Allen, Earhart, Blue, 1992). Rather, cognitive style refers to the types of information a person ignores and accepts in everyday life. Because cognitive style is the result of habits, it tends to be automatic or subconscious. Studies of cognitive style suggest that people are either open-minded or closed-minded and that cultural patterns are reflected in these styles (Morrison, Conaway, Borden, 1994). Open-minded persons seek out additional information before making decisions and tend to admit that they do not have all the answers and need to learn more before reaching proper conclusions. Open-minded persons usually ask many questions, want to hear about alternatives, and often ask COTAs to make personal recommendations regarding alternatives. Closed-minded individuals, on the other hand, see only a narrow range of data and ignore additional information. These persons usually take this approach because they function under strict sets of rules about behavior. For example, a devout Hindu elder would likely be appalled at being served beef at a meal and would not be willing to consider the potential nutritional benefits of this meal. Similarly, the dietitian who offers this meal to a Hindu elder may do so on the basis of a closed-minded cognitive style, assuming that beef is the ideal and only source of the particular nutrients the elder needs. Both persons are functioning under rules of behavior, with the Hindu elder's rules dictated by religious practice and the dietician's rules dictated by professional training. Other examples of a closed-minded cognitive style include the female elder who refuses to work with a male COTA during dressing training because she believes this is not proper, and the explosive retired executive who bellows that he does not wish to walk with a cane despite safety concerns. Both these people have attended to only part of the data available; that is, the data contrary to the rules of behavior under which they function. Their cognitive styles have limited their abilities to consider the benefits of the alternatives. Studies show that most cultures produce closed-minded citizens (Morrison, Conaway, Borden, 1994).

Another aspect of cognitive style is the way in which people process information, which can be divided into **associative** and **abstractive** processing styles. Persons who think associatively filter new data through the screen of personal experience. In other words, these persons tend to understand new information only in terms of similar past experiences. On the other hand, abstractive thinkers deal with new information through imagination or by considering hypothetical situations. An example of an associative thinker is an elder who has had a stroke and wants the COTA to provide him with a set of weights because using weights was how he increased upper extremity strength when he was younger. An example of an abstractive thinker is an elderly woman who asks the COTA to write down the principles of joint protection and is able to apply that information to all situations in which she may find herself. When approaching an associative thinker with a new task, COTAs should point out the ways in which it is similar to other tasks the elder has accomplished. Often elders who are associative thinkers need one or more demonstrations of the task and do best with small incremental increases in task complexity. Alternately, when approaching an abstractive thinker with a new task, COTAs should emphasize the desired outcome and permit the elder to think of ways in which to reach the goal. For example, when teaching an elder who thinks associatively to transfer to the toilet, COTAs should point out the ways in which this transfer are similar to the transfer of getting to the wheelchair from the bed. When teaching the elder who thinks abstractly to transfer to the toilet, COTAs should point out that the goal is to maintain alignment when standing, pivot on both legs, and sit by bending the knees.

What is Accepted as Truth

When COTAs engage person in therapy, they assume the persons will act in their own best interest. Based on this assumption, COTAs can ask the question, How do clients decide if it is in their best interest to learn the task presented to them? Or, in a broader sense, what is the truth? Persons from different cultures arrive at truth in different ways. These methods of arriving at truth can be boiled down to faith, fact, and feeling. The process of evaluating truth tends to be more conscious in contrast to the automatic cognitive style discussed previously.

The person who acts on the basis of faith uses a belief system such as that derived from a religion or political ideology to determine what is good or bad. For example, many people believe in self-sufficiency and may decline to use a wheelchair or other adaptive equipment that would clearly help them reduce fatigue. Their belief in self-sufficiency operates independently of the fact that they are too fatigued to stay awake for more than an hour. Other examples of persons who act on the basis of faith include the elder who refuses a blood transfusion because this procedure is explicitly prohibited by her religion, and the elder who calls on a priest, rabbi, or pastor before making a decision about care. Before OT treatment is

initiated, COTAs should always ask if the elder wishes to observe any particular rules and consider the elder's response when selecting therapeutic occupations.

Obviously, people who act on the basis of fact want to see evidence to support the COTA's recommendation or prioritization of a certain intervention. These people often want to know the benefits a certain intervention has proved to give in the past. To make plans for their future, these people often wish to know the length and cost of required OT services. People who act on the basis of fact may stop participating in a particular activity if they do not see the exact results they anticipated. COTAs may find it helpful to have these elders participate in some form of group treatment that allows them to directly observe results of OT intervention with other elders. In addition, written information about their conditions and about resources can be useful for these elders.

Most common are people who arrive at truth on the basis of feelings (Morrison, Conaway, Borden, 1994). Such people are those who "go with their gut instincts." When faced with a difficult decision they often choose the option that "feels right" over the one that seems most logical if this option makes them too uncomfortable. People who function on the basis of feelings often need to establish a comfortable rapport with the COTA before committing themselves wholeheartedly to working with the COTA. Building a relationship with these persons may take a long time. However, once the relationship is established it is very strong. People who function on the basis of feeling will probably want the COTA to continue treating them after they are discharged from a facility if further services are needed; they place less importance on cost considerations than on continuing the relationship. As with any client, COTAs should consistently and periodically ask elders how they are feeling about their situations and permit them time to process feelings as needed.

Value Systems

Each culture has a system for separating right from wrong or good from evil. A person's cognitive style and the way in which the person evaluates truth provide general clues about the values of that person's culture. However, more specific value systems exist that form the basis for behavior. Althen (1988) identified eight values and assumptions that characterize dominant American culture, including the importance of individualism and privacy, the belief in the **equality** of all persons, and informality in interactions with others. In addition, this author described emphasis on the future, change, progress, punctuality, materialism, and achievement as salient American values. In this chapter the locus of decision making, sources of anxiety reduction, issues of equality and inequality, and use of time are discussed. Numerous other value systems also direct behavior, but these four systems will be covered here because they are more related than other systems to the concerns of OT.

Locus of decision making. Locus of decision making is related to the extent to which a culture prizes individualism as opposed to collectivism. Individualism refers to the degree to which a person considers only him or herself when making a decision. Collectivism refers to the degree to which a person must abide with the consensus of the collective group. Pure individualism and collectivism are rare. In most countries, people consider others when making a decision but are not bound by the desires of the group. Returning to the concept of "levels of culture" discussed previously in this chapter may be helpful at this point. Locus of decision making may be considered as a series of concentric circles (see Figure 10-4). In the center is the smallest circle, the individual. At this level the individual considers mainly himself or herself when making a decision. The next circle, slightly larger, is usually the family. Many cultures expect the individual to consider what is best for the family when making a decision. The next circle represents a larger group, the community. This community could be an ethnic group, a religion, or even the individual's country. Some cultures expect people to consider the best interests of the entire, expansive group.

Examples of the ways people use these different levels of consideration when making a decision are easy to come by in OT practice. An individualistic elder is one who makes decisions about when and how he will be discharged home without consulting his spouse or family. This elder might believe that his spouse or family has a responsibility to care for him—a value that they may not necessarily share. Another elder who considers her family when making a decision may refuse to be discharged home out of consideration to her grown children because they would have to adjust their lifestyles to accommodate her needs. Another elder may decide to attempt to continue living independently to defy society's stereotype of dependence of elders.

Another way of thinking about individualism versus collectivism is to consider the degree of privacy a person seeks. Elders from cultures that highly value privacy may be quite perplexed by the number of health care professionals who seem to know about their issues. On the other hand, elders from other cultures that do not have rigid standards of privacy may feel isolated if they are not permitted to have constant contact with family or friends. The OT culture values independence, privacy, and individualism, but these values may be in conflict with an elder's needs if not carefully considered. One of the paradoxes of medical care in the United States is that, at the same time that we defend privacy rights in documentation, we assume that the individual will be completely comfortable undressing or toileting in our presence, and we do not give thought to the

possibility that the elder may feel embarrassed by these experiences.

Sources of anxiety reduction. Every human being is subject to stress. How do individuals handle stress and reduce anxiety? Most people turn to four basic sources of security and stability: interpersonal relationships, religion, technology, and the law (Morrison, Conaway, Borden, 1994; Harris, 1989; Hall, 1981). A person who must make a decision about an important health-related issue or adapt to a traumatic event is under stress. COTAs will find it helpful to know where or to whom elders turn for help and advice. If an elder is going to ask his or her spouse or family for advice, the COTA should include that spouse or family in therapy from the beginning of intervention so they clearly understand the issues at hand.

Elders who rely on religion as a source of anxiety reduction often need COTAs to help them obtain special considerations regarding religious practices. Understanding every nuance in the elder's religion is not as important as acknowledging the importance and appreciating the comfort that the elder finds in religious observances.

Reliance on technology as a source of anxiety reduction can be manifested when elders seek yet another medical test to confirm or refute a diagnosis. These clients may rely on medication as the solution to their problems or may collect a myriad of adaptive equipment or "gadgets." OT practitioners often have a bias toward relieving anxiety by prescribing the use of adaptive equipment without considering fully the extent to which the elder truly needs it.

Issues of equality/inequality. An important characteristic of all cultures is the division of power. Who controls the financial resources, and who controls decision making within the family? A sacred tenet in the United States is that "All men are created equal." Despite this tenet, prejudice against many groups still exists. All cultures have disadvantaged groups. Unequal status may be defined by economic situation, race, or gender, for example. Members of socially and economically advantaged classes may project a sense of entitlement to health care services and may treat COTAs and other health care workers as servants. On the other hand, members of a poverty-stricken underclass may eye COTAs with suspicion or defer to any recommendation out of fear of retaliation through withdrawal of needed services.

COTAs should also analyze issues of male and female equality. Female COTAs, in particular, may find it useful to know the way women are regarded in the elder's culture. In most cultures men are more likely to be obeyed and trusted when they occupy positions of authority, but this is not always the case for women (Bateson, 1989). COTAs must understand who will be best suited to act as a caregiver on the basis of the elder's cultural values regarding gender roles. A COTA who is of the opposite gender of the elder may wish to initiate OT treatment around issues less likely to bring up conflicts regarding privacy or authority until more rapport is built and the elder is able to appreciate the COTA's genuine concern for his or her welfare.

Use of time. Time is consciously and unconsciously formulated and used in each culture. Time is often treated as a language, a way of handling priorities, and a way of revealing how people feel about each other. Cultures can be divided into those that prefer a monochronic use of time and those that prefer a polychronic use of time (Hall, 1984). Elders from monochronic cultures will probably prefer to organize their life with a "one thing at a time" and "time is money" mentality. For these elders, adherence to schedules is highly important. They are likely to be offended if they are kept waiting for an appointment or if they perceive that the COTA is attending to too many issues at once. People from a monochronic culture prefer having the COTA's undivided attention and expect time to be used efficiently. These people are not necessarily unfriendly but prefer social "chit-chat" to be kept to a minimum if they are paying for a particular technical service. In contrast, elders from a polychronic culture organize their lives around social relationships. For them the time spent with someone is directly correlated to their personal value. Often these elders feel rushed by schedules. They may be late for an appointment because they encountered an acquaintance whom they did not want to offend by rushing off to a therapy appointment. With these elders, COTAs may find that sessions are most effective when a lot of conversation takes place. People from polychronic cultures may also wish to know many details about the COTA's life as a way of showing that they value the professional. When elders of a polychronic culture arrive late for an appointment, they may be offended if the COTA refuses to squeeze them into the schedule.

Communication Style

The meaning people give to the information they obtain through interaction with others largely depends on the way that information is transmitted. Cultures differ in the amount of information that is transmitted through verbal and nonverbal language. Cultures also differ in regard to the amount of information that is transmitted through the context of the situation (Lynch, 1992). Context includes the relationship to the individual with whom one is communicating. For example, after living together for more than 50 years, an elder couple does not always have to spell things out for each to know the other's feelings. Each partner may know the other's feelings simply by the way they move and the tone of their voices. Their shared experiences over 50 years have given

them high context, so that meaning is not lost when words are not spoken.

Hall (1984) has noted that high-context cultures rely less on verbal communication than on understanding through shared experience and history. In high-context cultures, fewer words are spoken and more emphasis is placed on nonverbal cues and messages. High-context cultures tend to be formal, reliant on hierarchy, and rooted in the past, and thus they change more slowly and tend to provide more stability for their members (Hecht, Anderson, Ribeau, 1989). When words are used in high-context cultures, communication is more indirect. People in these cultures usually express themselves through stories that imply their opinions (Bateson, 1989).

In contrast, persons from low-context cultures typically focus on precise, direct, and logical verbal communication. These persons may not process the gestures, environmental clues, and unarticulated moods that are central to communication in high-context cultures. Low-context cultures may be more responsive to and comfortable with change but often lack a sense of continuity and connection with the past (Hecht, Anderson, Ribeau, 1989).

Misunderstanding may easily arise when COTAs and elders, family members, or caregivers use a different level of context in their communication. Persons from high-context cultures may consider detailed verbal instructions insensitive and mechanistic; they may feel they are being "talked down to." Persons from low-context cultures may be uncomfortable with long pauses and may also feel impatient with indirect communication such as storytelling. The COTA's responsibility is to become aware of the style of communication of the elder, family, member, or caregiver and adapt to that style. COTAs must note that nonverbal communication such as facial expressions, eye contact, and touching may have completely different meanings in different cultures. COTAs can learn these things by listening carefully, observing how the family interacts, and adapting OT practice style as new discoveries are made about the elder's culture.

CASE STUDY

Mrs. Pardo is a 70-year-old Filipino woman who was admitted to a skilled nursing facility (SNF) after an infection developed in her right hip. She had a total hip replacement 3 weeks before being transferred to the SNF. Because of the infection Mrs. Pardo had not received much therapy. A week ago the OTR was finally able to complete an OT evaluation. Susan, a newly hired COTA, will continue the OT program. When discussing the case with Susan, the OTR stated that although Mrs. Pardo has been trained in getting from a supine position to a sitting position at the edge of the bed and in dressing, her family routinely provides this care. The OTR has not discussed with Mrs. Pardo or her family the need for these activities to be done independently. Part of

Susan's responsibility, according to the OTR, is to "convince them to not fuss over her so much."

Susan reviewed Mrs. Pardo's medical record before meeting her. It appeared that Mrs. Pardo's condition was stable and the infection was under control. Several professionals had documented that she was quite weak and deconditioned, presumably because of prolonged bed rest. Susan reviewed the OT evaluation results and treatment goals, which seemed quite straightforward. The general objective was for Mrs. Pardo to become independent in ADL functions and transfer while observing specific hip precautions for at least 6 more weeks. These precautions included touch-toe weightbearing on the right leg, as well as avoiding right leg internal rotation and right hip flexion grater than 60 degrees. Susan also noted that Mrs. Pardo was a widow who lived with one of her five adult daughters.

One of Mrs. Pardo's daughters and two of her adolescent grandchildren were present when Susan met Mrs. Pardo. When Susan introduced herself, Mrs. Pardo smiled and introduced her relatives. She also told Susan she reminded her of someone she had met years ago while working as a sales representative for an American firm. Once Mrs. Pardo found out where Susan was from she asked if Susan knew the relatives of an acquaintance of hers, who was from Susan's town. Finally, Susan stated she was there to work on transfers and dressing. Because Susan wanted to see how Mrs. Pardo performed these activities independently, she asked the relatives to leave the room for a few minutes. Once they left, Susan sensed a change in Mrs. Pardo. Although she followed all of Susan's directions quickly, she seemed to be avoiding eye contact. When Susan asked her if everything was all right, Mrs. Pardo responded affirmatively. Susan observed that Mrs. Pardo required minimal assistance to get out of the hospital bed, sit in a commode chair, and dress herself with a gown while observing all hip precautions. Noting that Mrs. Pardo appeared fatigued, Susan said she would return at 3 o'clock that afternoon to work on Mrs. Pardo's self-bathing ability. Susan asked if Mrs. Pardo was aware of any scheduling conflicts, to which Mrs. Pardo responded, "No." When Susan left the room, she asked Mrs. Pardo's daughter if she would be available to observe the bath that afternoon. The daughter said she would be there without fail.

Later that afternoon Susan entered Mrs. Pardo's room at the same moment a different daughter was helping Mrs. Pardo get into bed. Alarmed that hip precautions were not being followed, Susan immediately asked the daughter to let her take over and demonstrate the appropriate method of transferring to the bed. The daughter angrily stated that Mrs. Pardo was too tired for therapy and proceeded to complete the task without Susan's assistance. Susan was taken aback and told Mrs. Pardo she would return in the morning for the bath.

That evening Susan could not stop thinking about the afternoon's events. She was aware that she had somehow offended Mrs. Pardo's daughter, and she wondered why Mrs. Pardo had gone back to bed knowing that Susan would be coming to work with her at 3:00 p.m. Susan decided to carefully analyze what had happened. She remembered how friendly and talkative Mrs. Pardo had been at the beginning of the session, which was perhaps a sign that she valued relationships highly and wanted Susan to know she was appreciated. Susan thought about the change in Mrs. Pardo

when her family left and wondered if she felt alone without family to support her. Why had Mrs. Pardo said that everything was all right but then avoided eye contact? Was this her way of letting Susan know that she did not want to do the task without directly opposing the plan for the session? Susan thought about the tasks they had accomplished and wondered if Mrs. Pardo had ever before been required to get out of a hospital bed, sit on a commode in front of another person, and dress in a hospital gown? Did these tasks have anything to do with her real life? Finally, Susan remembered how she had entered the room while Mrs. Pardo's daughter was helping her get into bed. Susan realized that she had blurted out orders without even introducing herself. Had she caused the daughter to feel embarrassed and incompetent? Was the daughter's anger a way of regaining control?

After evaluating the situation, Susan concluded that Mrs. Pardo probably could not relate to the artificial ADL tasks presented to her. She also suspected that Mrs. Pardo relied on family members for support in making decisions and reducing anxiety. Mrs. Pardo also seemed to value the feelings of other people and avoided direct confrontation. The daughter might have been angry because Susan confronted her directly. Susan decided that the next day she would approach the treatment session with Mrs. Pardo differently. First, she would schedule the session when a family member could be present. She also planned to spend some time simply conversing with Mrs. Pardo and her family members, and she planned to spend more time chit-chatting during the session. Susan decided to take Mrs. Pardo to the simulated apartment in the rehabilitation department, where they could work in a more realistic home setting with a real bed and chair and Mrs. Pardo could also work on dressing with her own clothes.

The next day, Susan carried out her plan with great success. Susan had realized that Mrs. Pardo was an associative thinker who needed new tasks to be associated with more familiar routines. Susan had also realized that Mrs. Pardo valued family ties and social relationships greatly and consequently would not risk offending others with a direct refusal. In addition, Susan realized that Mrs. Pardo relied on family as a source of anxiety reduction. Finally, Susan had recognized that Mrs. Pardo was from a polychronic culture that valued a more social than prescriptive approach to rehabilitation.

CONCLUSION

This chapter provides a framework that COTAs can use to approach elders from diverse backgrounds. Concepts of culture and diversity were discussed, with special attention given to the ways these differences can contribute to the elder's ability to obtain meaning in therapy. Emphasis was also placed on the fact that both culture and diversity are very broad and complex terms. Consequently, a cultural model was presented to aid COTAs in designing individualized OT services for each elder. COTAs may use this information as guide for culturally sensitive practice and remain open to new experiences they encounter with each elder. Before attempting to treat elders from other backgrounds, COTAs must become

BOX 10-1

Attitude Self-Analysis

Do I believe it is important to consider culture when treating elders?

Am I willing to lower my defenses and take risks?

Am I willing to practice behaviors that may feel unfamiliar and uncomfortable to benefit the elder with whom I am working?

Am I willing to set aside some of my own cherished beliefs to make room for others whose values are unknown?

Am I willing to change the ways I think and behave?

Am I sufficiently familiar with my own heritage, including place of family origin, time, and reasons for immigration, and language(s) spoken?

What values, beliefs, and customs are identified with my own cultural heritage?

In what ways do my beliefs, values, and customs interfere with my ability to understand those of others?

Do I view elders as a resource in understanding their cultural beliefs, family dynamics, and views of health?

Do I encourage elders to use resources from within their cultures that they see as important?

aware of and analyze their own prejudices and biases about the dimensions of life that create diversity (Box 10-1).

▎ **C**HAPTER **R**EVIEW **Q**UESTIONS

1 Explain why it is difficult to define the term *culture*.

2 Give examples of ways in which you have learned and shared a particular value.

3 Give examples of values and beliefs that connect individuals with the various other levels of culture, including family, community, and country.

4 Explain how appreciating diversity can affect OT intervention with elders.

5 Describe your own cognitive style and explain how you base your actions on faith, fact, or feelings. Also describe how you arrive at decisions about your own health behaviors and what you rely on to reduce anxiety in difficult times.

6 Describe at least three ways in which issues of equality and inequality may affect OT intervention with elders.

7 Explain ways in which you tend to behave on a monochronic and polychronic basis. Describe how this tendency may interfere with your ability to provide treatment to elders.

8 Describe at least three other strategies Susan can use with Mrs. Pardo that would take into consideration Mrs. Pardo's cultural context.

REFERENCES

Allen C, Earhart C, Blue T: *Occupational therapy goals for the physically and cognitively disabled*, Rockville, Md, 1992, American Occupational Therapy Association.

Allen C: *Occupational therapy for psychiatric diseases: measurement and management of cognitive disabilities*, Boston, 1985, Little, Brown.

Althen G: *American ways*, Yarmouth, Me, 1988, Intercultural Press.

American Association of Retired Persons: *A profile of older Americans*, Washington, DC, 1995, The Association.

American Occupational Therapy Association: Uniform terminology for occupational therapy, ed 3, *Am J Occup Ther* 48(11): 1047, 1994.

American Occupational Therapy Association Representative Assembly: Official definition for licensure, *Am J Occup Ther* 35(6): 789, 1981.

Barresi C: Ethnogerontology: social aging in national, racial, and cultural groups. In Ferraro K, editor: *Gerontology: perspectives and issues*, New York, 1990, Springer.

Bateson MC: Foreword. In Benedict R, editor: *Patterns of culture*, Boston, 1989, Houghton Mifflin.

Benedict R: *Patterns of culture*, Boston, 1989, Houghton Mifflin.

Dorfman R et al: Old, sad, and alone: the myth of the aging homosexual, *Gerontol Soc Work*, 24, 29, 1995.

Fry C: Cross-cultural comparisons of aging. In Ferraro K, editor: *Gerontology: perspectives and issues*, New York, 1990, Springer.

Gropper R: *Culture and the clinical encounter: an intercultural sensitizer for the health professions*, Yarmouth, Me, 1996, Intercultural Press.

Hall E: *The dance of life: the other dimensions of time*, New York, 1984, Anchor Books.

Hall E: *Beyond culture*, New York, 1981, Anchor Books.

Harris M: *Cows, pigs, wars, and witches: the riddles of culture*, New York, 1989, Vintage Books.

Hartog J, Hartog E: Cultural aspects of health and illness behaviors in hospital, *West J Med* 139:910, 1983.

Hecht M, Andersen P, Ribeau S: The cultural dimensions of nonverbal communication. In Asante M, Gudykunst W, editors: *Handbook for international and intercultural communication*, Newbury Park, Calif, 1989, Sage.

Janus S, Janus C: *The Janus report on sexual behavior*, New York, 1993, John Wiley & Sons.

Kielhofner G: *A model of human occupation: theory and application*, ed 2, Baltimore, 1995, Williams & Wilkins.

Kohls R, Knight J: *Developing intercultural awareness: a cross-cultural training handbook*, ed 2, Yarmouth, Me, 1994, Intercultural Press.

Krefting L, Krefting D: Cultural influences on performance. In Christiansen C, Baum C, editors: *Occupational therapy: overcoming human performance deficits*, Thorofare, NJ, 1991, SLACK.

Lynch E: Developing cross-cultural competence. In Lynch E, Hanson M, editors: *Developing cross-cultural competence: a guide for working with young children and their families*, Baltimore, 1992, Paul H. Brookes.

Morrison T, Conaway W, Borden G: *Kiss, bow, or shake hands: how to do business in sixty countries*, Holbrook, Mass, 1994, Bob Adams.

Peacock J: *The anthropological lens: harsh light, soft focus*, London, 1986, Cambridge University Press.

Quam J, Whitford G: Adaptation and age-related expectations of older gay and lesbian adults, *Gerontologist* 32:367, 1992.

U.S. Bureau of Labor Statistics: Personal communication, December 12, 1995.

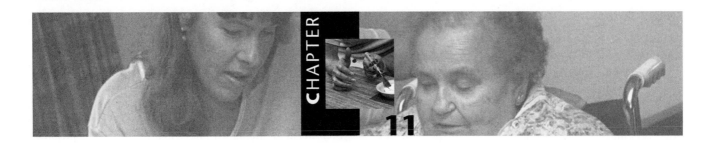

Ethical Aspects in the Work With Elders

KATE H. BROWN AND CAROL J. SCHWOPE

KEY TERMS

client autonomy, informed consent, ethical dilemma, ethical distress, distributive justice, least restrictive environment, benefits, burdens, Institutional Ethics Committee, confidentiality, empathy, whistle-blowing, American Occupational Therapy Association (AOTA) Standards and Ethics Commission (SEC), National Board for Certification in Occupational Therapy (NBCOT), State Regulatory Boards

CHAPTER OBJECTIVES

1. Discuss steps for ethical consideration.
2. Become familiar with the language of ethics.
3. Refine and explain personal and professional ethical commitments.

Sheila, Maryann, and Chris are three friends who graduated from the same OTA program a few years ago. They have gathered to discuss a problem Sheila has been having at the psychiatric hospital where she works. Maryann works in a long-term care facility. Chris is employed in a rehabilitation clinic. Recently his employer expanded to home care, so Chris has begun seeing clients in their homes as well as in the clinic.

In this chapter the three COTAs mentioned above discuss a variety of ethical questions arising from the complexities of their job demands. These discussions include a series of steps for ethical consideration, which students and clinicians can use in responding to ethical challenges in their practices. Some of the language of ethics is reflected in the American Occupational Therapy Association Code of Ethics (AOTA, 1994a). Other ethics commentaries that guide professional practice are intro-

duced as well. The authors hope that COTAs will take the opportunity to refine and explain the ethical commitments that shape their personal integrity when working with elders.

AN OVERVIEW: ETHICS AND ELDER CARE

The health care environment is in the midst of great change. In recent years, OT practice has been especially influenced by the pressures of new technologies and cost controls. On one hand, these pressures have contributed positively to OT practice. For example, technologies such as hip replacements, pacemakers, and organ transplants have increased the practitioner's capacity to respond more effectively to clients' needs. Increased attention to the way health care dollars are spent has also made us focus on which treatments to use and why.

On the other hand, some technologies—especially those capable of sustaining life—sometimes pose complex questions that clients, clinicians, and society are ill-prepared to answer. The ethics of continuing to artificially feed a person in a permanent vegetative state is one example. Another question concerns the ethics involved with providing access for all persons to expensive new technologies.

Cost-control strategies can also create ethical challenges for practitioners. Traditionally, health care professionals have served their clients' best interests before their own. Increasingly, however, financial constraints force practitioners to decide the best way to uphold this commitment. For instance, cost controls on health care expenditures are sometimes linked to salary incentives in managed care organizations, which can tempt practitioners away from their professional responsibilities. Other ethically problematic cost-driven practices include "creative" documentation for reimbursement and accepting referrals for marginally necessary or needless treatments. Creative documentation refers to the practice of exaggerating a problem, altering a diagnosis, or implying better prognosis so that more client visits can be approved. When actual fraud is present, such practices are liable to legal and ethical inquiry and punishment.

Frequently, cost controls can translate into fewer staff for more clients. When these staffing changes contribute to inadequate supervision or require COTAs to use modalities for which they are not sufficiently trained, COTAs are placed in another ethically questionable position in terms of their professional standards of practice.

Regardless of the clinical and financial environment of practice, special ethical concerns are raised for COTAs working with elders. Elders have a wide range of health care needs. Their occupational goals are diverse, and they require personalized treatment plans, which may require the practitioner to develop particular ethical sensitivities.

Consider the example of ethical decision making in health care. Generally in the United States, most people believe that adults should be the primary decision makers about their own health care because **client autonomy** is important. Client autonomy refers to the idea that adults have the right to determine what happens to them in a health care setting.

The value of client autonomy is expressed in many ways. For instance, because of client autonomy, health care providers are careful to get **informed consent** from clients before doing a procedure, especially if the procedure is risky. Before consenting, clients need to know the risks and benefits of the procedure, whether there are alternatives, and the way their health will be affected if intervention is refused. Once clients have this information, client autonomy necessitates that they be allowed to accept or refuse the treatment.

How is client autonomy translated into care for elders? Elders vary in their capacities for independent function

and thought, and thus their capacities for autonomous decision making. Some elders are no longer able to make decisions on their own behalf. But often the extent of this inability and its consequences for decision making are unclear. Of course, physical dependency is not always accompanied by mental dependency. COTAs must remember that clients who have lost most of their physical independence may still retain the ability to make independent decisions.

In addition, caregivers need to appreciate that elders' capacities for independent decision making may fluctuate because of their physical or mental conditions. For instance, persons with Alzheimer's disease, Parkinson's disease, or stroke may be more fully alert at certain times of the day than other times.

Elders also vary in their capacities to respond to different kinds of decision-making tasks. In a nursing home, for instance, a resident who is able to walk to a dining hall without assistance at the appropriate time may be unable to choose a balanced diet. Another resident may be mentally competent to decide what to eat but unable to keep reliable bank records. The task, the circumstance, and clients' mental and emotional states will determine their decision-making capacities.

Client decision making is just one area of ethical concern for COTAs. In this chapter, through exploration of the situations presented by the three COTAs, Chris, Sheila, and Maryann, a number of other issues are presented (Figure 11-1). The chapter is organized around

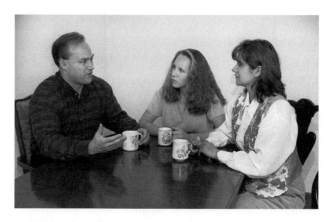

FIGURE **11-1**   Discussions with peers may help clarify ethical dilemmas.

BOX **11-1**

Steps for Ethical Consideration
Awareness—What is going on?   Reflection—What do I think should happen?   Support—With whom do I need to talk?   Action—What will I do?

a four-step method for working through an ethical problem (Box 11-1). Each step is illustrated with specific cases experienced by the three friends.

Awareness: What is Going On?

The first step in approaching an ethical problem is to figure out what is going on. This may seem obvious at first, but actually the situation can be quite complicated, and before COTAs take action, they must consider a number of factors.

What kind of ethical problem is it? COTAs may find it helpful to start by figuring out the kind of problem they are facing. Ethicists differentiate three kinds of problems (Purtilo, 1993). An **ethical dilemma** refers to a situation in which there are two or more ethically correct options for action. However, with each choice, the COTA compromises something of value. **Ethical distress** refers to a situation in which the COTA knows which course of action to take for the client's benefit but is unable to do so without some personal risk. The barrier often is established by someone who has more institutional authority than the COTA. **Distributive justice** problems arise when there is not enough of something that is valued. The COTA must distribute the item or service in a fair way, or in the language of ethics, a "just" way (Box 11-2).

Who is involved? The question of persons involved must be considered when approaching an ethical problem. Usually the COTA is involved, and most likely the COTA's client is involved. But who else has a stake in the ethical problem the COTA faces? It is not enough to know only who is involved; COTAs must also investigate their beliefs and values to anticipate areas of agreement and disagreement about the proposed course of action. The client's family often needs to be involved in medical decision making, but their involvement may result in an ethical dilemma for the COTA.

For example, the family of one of Chris' home care clients asks him for help in placing their relative in a nursing home. The client has begun to wander from his home and has gotten lost several times. Chris knows that his client values his independence and will resist the move to a facility; on the other hand, Chris recognizes that the client might endanger himself. He respects the wishes of both the client and the client's family. What other value, besides the client's autonomy, should Chris consider? In addition to Chris, the family, and the client, who else is likely to be involved?

Which laws and institutional rules apply? Sometimes laws and institutional rules help clarify COTAs' roles in a given ethics problem. Some laws are federal, meaning that they apply in every state, but other laws apply only within a particular state's jurisdiction. COTAs are responsible for knowing which laws apply to their practice. Many institutions have legal counselors who can answer questions about specific legal issues. Supervisors can also help clarify their legal and institutional responsibilities.

Each institution has established guidelines and rules that specify the expectations they have for staff, clients, and administrators.

The influence of law in defining ethical practice is illustrated in a case about the use of restraints that Sheila was asked to help resolve at the psychiatric hospital where she works. Sheila's client is a 68-year-old woman who was admitted to the acute care psychiatry department because of agitation and uncontrollable behavior. The client's charted diagnosis reads, "Axis I schizoaffective bipolar type, axis III hypertension, degenerative joint disease, chronic obstructive pulmonary disease, chronic constipation, head trauma (grade 9; no further details)." Staff

BOX 11-2

Examples of Ethical Problems

Ethical dilemma
Maryann works in a long-term care facility. A client who has had a stroke asks Maryann whether she will regain fine motor control of her hand. If Maryann tells her she probably will not regain all of her fine motor control, the client is likely to fall into a deep depression. If Maryann does not tell her the full extent of her prognosis, she probably will find out anyway, and then her trust in Maryann might diminish.

What are two of the actions Maryann could take?

What values are compromised if either action is taken?

Ethical distress
Sheila works at a psychiatric hospital. She has just learned that her client is to be discharged tomorrow. She knows he lives alone and will most likely not be able to regulate his medications appropriately. Sheila voices her concerns, but her supervisor tells her that the client's insurance coverage has run out, so they have no choice but to discharge him.

Is it ethically wrong to discharge this client? Why?

What barrier(s) does Sheila confront when questioning the discharge plan?

Distributive justice
Chris works at a rehabilitation clinic but has begun seeing clients in their homes as well. One of Chris' clients has been admitted to the rehabilitation program with clear payment guidelines from his insurance company: there will be no reimbursement for equipment of any type. The client needs a wrist support splint, but this item is considered equipment by the insurance company.

Should Chris ignore the need for a splint because of restricted payment guidelines?

Can you name at least three other scarcities in health care that are likely to raise issues of distributive justice for you as a COTA?

---

members do not particularly like this client; they often construe her behavior as violent. She calls other clients, residents, and staff derogatory names; she tells lies about them and accuses them of mistreating her. At times, she claims she is unable to walk and demands use of a wheelchair. She often stages a fall by throwing herself from the wheelchair onto the floor. The staff recommends she be restrained in a chair for her own safety.

When Sheila brought this case to her friends for discussion, Maryann pointed out that given the client's age her case was most likely covered by Medicare. This means that legally, like the staff in her nursing home, the staff in the psychiatric hospital should follow the guidelines for restraints defined by the Omnibus Budget Reconciliation Act (OBRA) of 1987. Maryann explained that this federal legislation requires health care providers to ensure client safety in the **least restrictive environment.** When Chris pointed out that no one wanted to be around this client, Sheila voiced her suspicion that maybe the restraints were being used as punishment, not client safety. If this was the case, she didn't think this was an ethical use of restraints, and the others agreed. The three friends began thinking of ways that OT could help in designing the least restrictive environment for this client. "After all," said Chris, "even unpleasant clients deserve the right to make choices and have some liberty, as long as they are not hurting themselves or others."

What guidance does the AOTA code of ethics provide? "Ethics are the human effort to catch hold of those human events and occasions that are liable to go badly and then turn them to our good as best we can" (Jonsen, 1990). This quote is a good starting point from which to begin exploring the reasons that the American Occupational Therapy Association Code of Ethics (AOTA, 1994a) serves as a guide for OT personnel in the issues they encounter daily. The Code of Ethics has six principles. These principles are similar to a list of desired behaviors for OT personnel. OT personnel must demonstrate concern for the well-being of their clients and respect their clients' rights. OT personnel must be competent, comply with laws and rules that apply to OT personnel, and provide accurate information about services they provide. And finally, OT personnel must be fair and discreet and demonstrate integrity with colleagues and other professionals.

Not only is the Occupational Therapy Code of Ethics a guide for behavior, it is also a regulatory code in that guidelines for conduct are stated and sanctions are provided for failure to follow the code. These sanctions are stated in the enforcement procedures for the Code of Ethics (AOTA, 1994a). Often the principles stated in the Code of Ethics are also found in local, state, and federal laws.

What are my options? OT practitioners need to be aware of the range of options before deciding what action should be taken in a given ethics case. As noted, sometimes COTAs' options are defined by law. Ethical options may also be limited by personal religious prohibitions and beliefs. Often, however, personal and professional duties are not well defined. In such cases, ethicists suggest that health care providers, clients, and families try to estimate the consequences of a given option. These consequences can be weighed against the consequences of other options. The ethically preferable course of action will be that which carries the most chance of a good outcome **(benefits)** and the least amount of damage **(burdens).**

This calculation of consequences is illustrated with a case Chris discussed with Maryann and Sheila. At the rehabilitation hospital where Chris works, the burn unit was considering the best way to treat a comatose 85-year-old man. The team was trying to decide whether to treat the client's severe burns or to provide him with palliative care until he died. To decide which course to take, the burn unit team was considering whether the burdens of treatment, including excruciating pain from grafts and range-of-motion exercises, were ethically warranted given his questionable survival. They also wondered about the quality of his life if he did survive. It was clear he would never return to his home and would need long-term care in a nursing facility for the rest of his life. The client's family felt that this prospect of the future would be demoralizing for their relative because he had always cherished his independence. But some members of the staff argued that, with rehabilitation, the client might learn to adapt to and even enjoy a more social environment. Questions that arise for Chris out of this example include the following: What burdens are created by aggressive treatment in this case? What benefits are created by such treatment? What burdens are created by palliative care? What benefits are created by palliative care?

In accordance with professional values, COTAs should calculate these ratios of benefits and burdens in light of the client's well-being, not in terms of the staff's convenience or the client's relatives' inheritance. This kind of assurance is necessary for maintaining a bond of trust between health professionals and their clients, who expect professionals to work on behalf of their best interests.

Reflection: What Do I Think Should Happen?

After COTAs are aware of all the facts and options in a given case, they must decide what they want to happen and be able to explain their position. First, COTAs must determine what actions seem most wrong or right. This process may begin as a gut feeling that persists. Sensitivity to such feelings is an important component for reflective ethical practice. In addition, COTAs' legally defined roles or religious tenets may affect their ethical inclinations. Ethical reflection involves careful and critical examination of feelings, a rational estimate of benefits and burdens, and a sense of professional duty.

Often this stage of ethical consideration requires some emotional and even physical detachment as COTAs step back from the problem to reflect on their ethical commitments and reasoning. Sometimes the urgency of a situation requires rapid reflection, but nonetheless, ethicists recommend a conscious period of time be taken for serious consideration of preferences and motivations for choosing a given course of action. Each person finds personal methods of reflection that best fit the person's reasoning style.

Some health professionals find it useful to talk through a problem with a group of trusted advisors, including the OTR team partner. Such a group can be informal—like the group of COTAs highlighted in this chapter—or more formal, as in the case of an **Institutional Ethics Committee.** Typically, Institutional Ethics Committees (sometimes referred to as Hospital Ethics Committees) are composed of staff, administrators, legal counsel, and a community representative. These committees often provide interdisciplinary consideration for a particular problem. Just as with an informal group of peers, these committees can only recommend a resolution; legally or ethically COTAs are not usually bound to comply with their advice.

When choosing to talk over an ethics problem with someone else, COTAs must respect the **confidentiality** of those involved. COTAs should make every effort to see that information about clients, colleagues, or institutions is shared in a way that does not reveal anyone's identity. The client's name should not be used, especially with persons not involved directly with the client's care. Similar care needs to be taken when the behavior of an institution or a peer is discussed.

Freewriting (Goldberg, 1986) is another method used for ethical reflection. Freewriting involves writing whatever comes to mind without worrying about language, spelling, and grammar. Usually the exercise is limited to 10 minutes, during which the writer does not stop writing. The key is to suspend the usual breaks in writing and let uncensored thoughts pour onto the page. The usefulness of this technique is in uncovering deep ethical feelings.

This technique may reveal previously unrealized opinions or persuasive reasons for a stance. The freewriting technique requires only that COTAs trust themselves to be revealed.

Two weeks ago Maryann was placed in a bind with one of her favorite clients, Mrs. Henry. Three months earlier Mrs. Henry had come to the facility after experiencing a stroke. Despite Maryann's best efforts to help Mrs. Henry regain endurance and sitting balance, Maryann's supervising OTR concluded that Mrs. Henry was not likely to improve any further and recommended discontinuing her therapy. Mrs. Henry's family asked Maryann to continue

the treatments anyway. They could tell how much their mother enjoyed the attention. They were worried that Mrs. Henry would lose hope and her health would deteriorate further. Maryann explained that without demonstrable improvement, Medicare was not likely to reimburse the facility for this therapy. In response, the family appealed to Maryann's sense of loyalty to their mother, asking her to be creative about how she documented the effect of the therapy.

Maryann faced an ethical dilemma between loyalty to someone she cared for and the obligation to truthfully document OT intervention. She decided to freewrite for 10 minutes to better determine a response (Box 11-3). To her surprise, she found her response guided by her ethical preference. (This breakthrough appears in boldface at the end of the freewrite.)

Caring professionals are often confronted with the limits of their empathetic relationships with clients. Especially in long-term care environments, professionals

BOX 11-3

Maryann's Free Writing

Let's see. It's 1:48, so that gives me until 1:58. I can't believe I'm writing this. This feels really stupid. OK. OK. The thing is, I don't know what to do for Mrs. H. She's such a sweet old lady. Even though she can't speak, she communicates with her eyes. They shine so gratefully when we are together. I can tell she appreciates my work. But it really bugs me that her family has pressured me to document progress when there isn't any. I can see their point, and in fact I want to do anything at all to help her because I really care about her. I feel really close, maybe because she can't speak, so I have to be with her when we work together. Be there for her eye to eye. That's the trouble though, it would be a lie to say she is improving from the therapy. But I don't want to give up hope. This isn't any more clear than when I started writing. What time is it? Don't stop to look. Keep writing. OK. So. What am I supposed to do? The Code says #1, we are supposed to work for each patient's well-being. But it also says we are supposed to tell the truth. So what help is that? I could get my OTR to fudge a bit on the chart, at least for a couple of weeks. But that's fraud. What is the bottom line? Why is it that caring for Mrs. H seems incompatible with telling the truth? Why not keep seeing Mrs. H., stopping by her room to cheer her up, even though insurance doesn't cover that. I wouldn't be doing therapy. I'd be there as her friend. **I think that's what I'll do. I'll just have to tell the family that the therapy will end, but I won't desert their mother. And maybe I can help teach them how they can work with her so she feels like she is getting attention.** I can't believe it, but I actually feel lighter. And in exactly 10 minutes to the second!

may find that relating to their clients through the rigid shield of professional distance is unrealistic and uncomfortable. On the other hand, clients must be protected from a caregiver's overinvolvement, as in the extreme case of sexual liaisons, and also from a caregiver's subjective biases, as in the case of discrimination. Finding a balance between genuine caring for clients and realistic boundaries for professional involvement is a lifelong goal for all health care professionals that requires on-going ethical introspection.

Useful tools for ethical reflection include prayer, meditation, a walk in nature, and reading a poem or short story, even if the content of the work seems unrelated to the problem at hand. Possibly, the astronomer's wisdom in finding a faint star works equally well for ethics: you can better see the star if you look just to the side of it. These and the aforementioned methods for reflective ethical practice suggest that before responding to an ethical issue, COTAs must step away from the urgency of the problem to gain perspective about their responsibilities.

Support: With Whom Do I Need to Talk?

Although ethical issues admittedly involve conscious reflection, they should not be considered in isolation from others. Ethical commitments are shaped by social influences including upbringing, professional codes, and the circumstances of a given event. Likewise, the outcomes of most ethical decisions have social effects. Before acting according to ethical convictions, COTAs should solicit the support of others who will be affected by the issue at hand. In many instances of ethics in health care, this means communicating with the client, the client's family, and other staff members. Sometimes the Institutional Ethics Committee can also provide institutional support for a COTA's position. Others who are more directly involved in a given issue may have more influence than the COTA when voicing their ethical positions. In addition, others may have more moral authority given the particular circumstances under consideration. The usual practice in the United States is to prioritize the wishes of adult clients above those of others, even when the adult's wishes run counter to expert opinion. Other professionals on the health care team, by virtue of status, training, and tradition, may claim decision-making authority as well.

When COTAs have limited influence, they must express their position and the reasons that support it so that others have the benefit of these insights. Also, by expressing their positions, COTAs can sometimes avoid the experience of ethical distress when asked to participate in an intervention that conflicts with their ethical views. The more rational the COTAs' arguments in support of their position, the more persuasive COTAs will be in defending their objections, even if the course of events cannot be changed.

In cases in which COTAs are asked to do something that is ethically questionable, they have the responsibility to involve those with supervisory jurisdiction over them. COTAs should document such communications, especially if there are legal ramifications or if job security is at risk. Following is an example of this kind of dilemma.

In the last year, since his rehabilitation clinic changed to a managed care model, Chris has observed that he is increasingly asked to do treatments that OTRs previously did. Most of the time Chris appreciates the opportunity for more responsibility and feels comfortable doing what is asked of him. However, recently he was asked by the referring physician to work with a client who needed paraffin baths for her arthritic fingers. After explaining the situation, Chris and his friends discussed the issue.

"Absolutely not! You haven't had any training for this modality, and you might burn the client or something," said Sheila.

"I think it's really unfair that they asked you to do this, Chris. This puts you in a tough position about something that isn't your problem. They are just trying to save money by asking you to do this instead of asking an OTR," added Maryann.

"That may well be," replied Chris, "but I still have to deal with it one way or another."

"What you have here is a perfect example of ethical distress, I'd say. And I don't envy you at all," stated Sheila.

"So what are you going to do?" asked Maryann.

"Well, I like my job and I don't think this is worth quitting over, at least not without first communicating my distress to my supervisor. Like you, Maryann, I worry that I might hurt someone inadvertently, and this goes against my sense of professional duty to do no harm. You know how strongly this is reinforced by the AOTA code. I think there may also be legal liability issues involved, so maybe I need to talk with the risk manager of the clinic. But first I will talk with my supervisor and ask her what she thinks. I will also ask her to negotiate on behalf of the patient to get someone more qualified to do the paraffin baths."

"We're behind you on this one, buddy. The other COTAs at the clinic will be, too. I bet if you called the AOTA national office, their ethics consultant would back you up," suggested Sheila.

"But whatever you do, I think you better document everything that is said and done carefully so there is a clear record of your reasons for refusing and your efforts to negotiate a change in your assignment," cautioned Maryann.

Action: What Will I Do?

Inevitably, even in the most complex ethics cases, COTAs need to take some action. Doing nothing can also be perceived ethically as an action. If the previous steps have been considered in good conscience and the client's best interests have been prioritized, COTAs usually have an ethical basis for action. COTAs may retain a sense of uncertainty, but at least they will have the comfort of knowing that they have given deep thought to their position to articulate the basis for their action. Generally speaking, COTAs will most likely not have to act alone because of the input received from others.

Reporting the unethical behavior of a professional colleague or an institution is one of the most difficult actions to take. Nevertheless, if unethical conduct has been observed, COTAs have an ethical obligation to report this behavior to the authorities. In some states, this obligation is underscored by law. Thus if COTAs know of a wrongdoing and do not report it, the law considers them guilty as well.

Reporting another's unethical behavior is sometimes referred to as **whistle-blowing.** Especially when the COTA's job may be threatened, it can take courage to follow through with such a report. If possible, COTAs should work with the support of others, especially those in a supervisory position. Obviously this is difficult when a supervisor is the person to be reported. Regardless of the circumstance, COTAs should make sure to document their actions so their systematic efforts to address the problem are well established, especially if the COTA is in a less powerful position than the person being reported. Sometimes in a twist of logic, the whistle-blower is scapegoated, or blamed for another's unethical behavior. If COTAs have kept good records of their attempts to correct or resolve the situation, they will be more easily cleared of such an accusation.

Often, co-workers will have also observed the unethical behavior and may feel similarly vulnerable. COTAs can sometimes increase the effectiveness of their responses if they work with others. When sharing information with others to gain support for their actions, COTAs must respect the confidentiality of persons and institutions, providing information fairly and appropriately. If warranted, the authorities will dispense an appropriate punishment for wrongdoing after an investigation.

Who are the relevant authorities? The **American Occupational Therapy Association (AOTA) Standards and Ethics Commission (SEC)** prepared a detailed discussion of where to go to seek guidance about reporting unethical conduct. It names three major bodies with jurisdiction over professional behavior (Hansen, 1992).

COTAs may call or write the AOTA SEC. After discussing the possible violation of the Code of Ethics, COTAs can decide whether to file a formal complaint with the SEC. The SEC is responsible for writing the Code of Ethics and for imposing sanctions against AOTA members who do not follow it. Depending on the seriousness of the unethical behavior, the SEC will suggest "public censure, temporary suspension of mem-

bership, or revocation or permanent loss of membership" (Hansen, 1992).

The **National Board for Certification in Occupational Therapy (NBCOT)** is responsible for certifying OTRs and COTAs. Depending on the significance of the unethical behavior that is reported, and after a thorough and confidential investigation, the NBCOT may take action against the practitioner in question. The most severe punishment available through the NBCOT is permanent denial or revocation of certification.

State Regulatory Boards, created by state legislatures, may also be helpful. These boards have the power to intervene if they determine the public to be at risk because of a practitioner's incompetence, lack of qualifications, or unlawful behavior. State boards can publicly reprimand a practitioner or, if warranted, may even prohibit someone from practicing in that state.

Finally, COTAs should gather copies of their state's licensure laws, the AOTA Code of Ethics (AOTA, 1994a), and other documents from the AOTA that can help clarify ethical issues. Documents such as "Standards of Practice for Occupational Therapy" (AOTA, 1994b), "Guide for Supervision of Occupational Therapy Personnel" (AOTA, 1995), and "Occupational Therapy Roles" (AOTA, 1993) can also give COTAs a basis for their ethical arguments.

CONCLUSION

Working with elders carries special rewards and responsibilities. Clinical and ethical competency is necessary to maximize clients' functional capacities and contribute to the dignity and self-worth required for autonomous decision making. COTAs bring comfort to their clients through skillful treatment and by acting as the client's agent in ensuring ethical care. A healing bond of trust is reinforced each time clients witness COTAs responding with a sense of ethical commitment in the fulfillment of their clients' best interests.

This chapter reviewed ethical challenges in geriatric care settings and presented a step-by-step method for responding in a conscientious, informed manner. The authors hope readers will follow the strategies described when responding to events in their practices.

■ CHAPTER REVIEW QUESTIONS

1 Recall the discussion Sheila, Maryann, and Chris had about one of Sheila's clients at the psychiatric center who was being placed in restraints. At the end of that conversation, Chris stated, "After all, even unpleasant patients deserve the right to make choices and have some liberty, as long as they are not hurting themselves or others." What ethical term did you learn earlier in the chapter that summarizes Chris' statement?

2 Reread the case of Chris, the COTA expected to use paraffin baths with a client.

A. Identify the benefits and burdens to the client if Chris were to administer the paraffin bath.

B. Based on your calculations, is it ethical for Chris to do the procedure?

C. Who, if anyone, would you involve in supporting your decision if you were asked to use a modality for which you had not been trained?

3 Imagine that you are sitting with the three COTAs discussing the case that is described below. Suggest how you would guide their response to the ethical challenges facing Chris.

Chris is concerned about recent changes in his supervision at the rehabilitation clinic, especially in the new home care work he is doing. He never sees his supervising OTR anymore. She does her evaluations in the evenings or on weekends, when he is not at work. She wants him to mail his notes for her to cosign, but he worries about client confidentiality, especially if the notes got lost in the mail. However, Chris is most concerned about some of the treatment being ordered for his older home care clients. He often feels pushed to provide three or four units (15 minutes) of treatment when his older clients seem able to tolerate only one or two units per session. He suspects that the extra treatments are motivated by financial reasons and not by the well-being of his clients.

A. Awareness

(1) What kind of ethical problem(s) is Chris facing?

(2) Who is involved?

(3) What laws and institutional rules apply?

(4) What guidance does the AOTA Code of Ethics give?

(5) What are Chris' options?

B. Reflection

(1) Suggest strategies Chris can use for reflection.

(2) Provide reasons for your preferred response(s) to the problem(s) he faces.

C. Support

Suggest strategies Chris might use for building support.

D. Action

What should Chris do?

REFERENCES

American Occupational Therapy Association: Guide for supervision of occupational therapy personnel, *Am J Occup Ther* 49:1027, 1995.

American Occupational Therapy Association: *Reference guide to the occupational therapy code of ethics*, Bethesda, Md, 1994a, The Association.

American Occupational Therapy Association: Standards of practice for occupational therapy, *Am J Occup Ther* 48:1039, 1994b.

American Occupational Therapy Association: *Occupational therapy roles*, 47:1087, 1993.

Goldberg N: *Writing down the bones: freeing the writer within*, Berkeley, Calif, 1986, Shambhala Press.

Hansen R: Ethical jurisdiction of occupational therapy: the role of AOTA, AOTCB, and State Regulatory Boards, *OT Week* 6(3):6, 1992.

Jonsen AR: *The new medicine and the old ethics*, Cambridge, Mass, 1990, Harvard University.

Purtilo R: *Ethical dimensions in the health professions*, Philadelphia, 1993, WB Saunders.

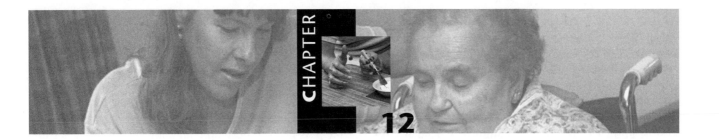

CHAPTER 12

Working With Families and Caregivers of Elders

ADA BOONE AND BARBARA JO RODRIGUES

KEY TERMS

social support system, family, caregivers, education, role changes, stress, community resources, abuse, neglect

CHAPTER OBJECTIVES

1. Define the COTA's role in family and caregiver training.
2. Understand role changes within family systems at the onset of debilitating conditions in elders.
3. Discuss communication strategies that maximize comprehension during elder, family, and caregiver education.
4. Identify stressors that affect quality of care, ability to cope, and emotional responses in the elder/caregiver relationship.
5. Identify techniques to minimize caregiver stress.
6. Define and identify signs of elder abuse and neglect and discuss reporting requirements.

To provide optimal care, COTAs must consider the many factors that influence an elder's functional abilities. When planning treatment, the OTR and COTA team considers not only physical and cognitive skills but also psychosocial factors that affect occupational performance potential. **Social support systems** such as spouse and **family** can significantly affect the outcome of OT intervention (Snow, 1988). COTAs must be able to interact with elders and their social support systems, especially the family, and treat elders and their families as units of care. This chapter addresses interaction between family members and **caregivers.**

COTAs' ROLES

For COTAs to define their roles in facilitating family interaction, they must first understand the family caregiver's role. Family members are not necessarily inherently skilled at caregiving. Frequently this role is unfamiliar and possibly unwanted. Caregivers must keep elders safe and clean and ensure that their daily physical needs are met. They must help elders maintain socialization and a sense of dignity (Peiffer, Crooker, 1990). These tasks can be overwhelming for a family member who has little or no experience with debilitating and chronic illness. Ensuring that caregivers and elders work together effectively is crucial (Rogers, 1988). COTAs should act as facilitators, educators, and resource personnel.

Development of elders' and caregivers' skills is achieved through selected activities with graded successes facilitated by COTAs. Activities that include family members and caregivers should be introduced as early as possible in the OT program to minimize dependence on COTAs. Facilitating interdependence between elders and their families and caregivers will ease the transition from one level of care to the next.

Effective elder, family, and caregiver **education** is a central component of care. Knowledge is empowering and encourages elders, family members, and caregivers to be responsible. Activities selected during the early stages of intervention need not be complex. They may include directions on positioning, simple passive range-of-motion exercises, and communication strategies. More training can follow as discharge planning progresses and the role of the caregiver becomes more clearly defined. Elder, family, and caregiver education is often required for activities of daily living, mobility, upper extremity management, behavioral management, and cognitive intervention strategies (Figure 12-1). COTAs may help elders, family members, and caregivers understand the physician's diagnosis and prognosis of the medical condition and the functional implications of the condition. Insight regarding the specific physical, cognitive, and psychosocial impairments will aid caregivers in providing safe and appropriate assistance. Sometimes understanding the reasons for doing a certain task is more important than

demonstrating proficiency in its performance (Snow, 1988). For example, understanding principles of wrist protection that can be applied to every situation is more important for caregivers than correctly supervising the elder's use of radial wrist deviation to open a door each time. To maximize the effectiveness of the education, COTAs need to develop communication strategies (Box 12-1).

COTAs also act as resources for elders, family members, and caregivers. Depending on facility role delineation, COTAs may provide information about community and support services as well as medical equipment vendors, paid caregivers, and respite programs. In collaboration with OTRs, COTAs may also serve as liaisons with other services. (Some resources are listed in this book's appendix.)

COTAs can learn much about elders', family members' and caregivers' values, desires, and insights through frequent and close interaction. Elders may be unable to express themselves for many reasons. Some limitations

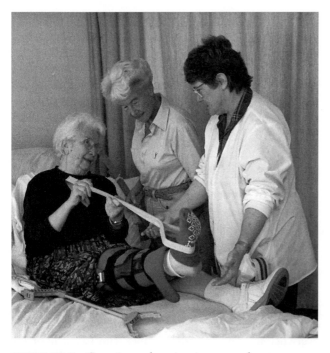

FIGURE 12-1 Caregiver education is a central component of the care COTAs provide.

BOX 12-1

Considerations for Effective Communication

1. Initially, make frequent, brief contacts to develop the relationship. This will familiarize the elder, family members, and caregivers with COTAs and their purpose.
2. Manage the environment in which communication occurs. Minimize distractions and interruptions.
3. Use responsive listening techniques. Maintain good eye contact, intermittently acknowledge statements made, and use body language that allows all parties to listen and respond. Be an active listener.
4. Use common terminology that nonmedical persons understand. If a common term is available, use it. For example, use *shoulder blade* for *scapula*. Otherwise, define and explain concepts in simple terms.
5. Always respect client confidentiality. If able, secure permission from clients before discussing details with others.
6. Use open-ended questions to encourage self-expression. Be comfortable with brief silences.
7. Organize your ideas and avoid skipping between subjects. Focus on one topic at a time and clarify what you don't understand.
8. Provide education that will enable elders and their families to make informed choices. Do not offer advice or your personal opinion. Always acknowledge the right of choice.
9. Communicate with respect and warmth. Be supportive. Respond to feedback when given.
10. Do not promise if you cannot deliver.

may be premorbid, whereas others, such as aphasia, may result from illness. COTAs may act as advocates for elders, helping meet needs that might otherwise go unacknowledged. COTAs may also act as advocates for family members and caregivers.

Like elders, families and caregivers may have needs that become evident only after close and frequent interaction. Because each individual's ability to provide caregiving differs, the OTR and COTA team must consider everyone's abilities when planning for discharge and family training.

All members of the treatment team, including COTAs, must educate elders, family members, and caregivers about the team's treatment recommendations. Recommendations may include plans for discharge, supervision, follow-up treatment, and home programs, and they must be clearly documented. When elders, families, and caregivers choose not to follow the team's recommendation, it is crucial to document all responses and actions to serve as a legal record if anyone is harmed. The more elders, family members, and caregivers are included in the formulation of plans, the more likely they are to comply with home programs and other discharge recommendations (Humphrey, Gonzalez, Taylor, 1993).

ROLE CHANGES IN THE FAMILY

Greater therapeutic outcomes are achieved when intervention does not focus solely on elders but also includes families and caregivers (Snow, 1988). In addition to developing the elder's performance skills, "in the family-centered approach, the emphasis is on enabling that family to maximize function and social interaction of the dependent family member" (Humphrey, Gonzalez, Taylor, 1993). This is especially important when lifestyle changes are required because of functional impairments.

Ideally elders will consult family members when caregiving needs become evident (Figure 12-2). However, many variables affect a family system's abilities to meet the elder's needs. Some of these variables may include the treatment setting itself, cognitive deficits, psychological issues, the prior quality of family relationships, cultural and social influences, geographic distance, scheduling conflicts, financial resources, and advanced directives. COTAs must take all these factors into consideration during collaborative planning.

COTAs must consider role changes that occur for both elders and family during the course of an illness. OT should be designed around elders' and family members' skill levels. From that foundation, COTAs can facilitate adjustment to disability. With the onset of illness or disability, elders may feel a loss of independence, which can mean a major change in their sense of control and their role within the family.

Role changes also occur within the family unit during elders' illnesses. Spouses may feel a deep sense of loss of a partner and may resent being solely responsible for previously shared tasks. In addition to a sense of loss, children must deal with the role reversal of being a parent to their own parent. Elders' disabilities and needs for caregiving may come at a time in children's lives when, for the first time, they find themselves free of family responsibilities and are planning for their own retirement. Family members are usually unprepared for the sudden changes that may occur with acute illnesses.

Roles within the family unit tend to be adjusted and adapted to gradually when elders have chronic or degenerative diseases. However, as the functional impairments accumulate into a major disability with significant activity limitations, modifications in roles are required (Davis, 1988). Not knowing the length of the illness is often a source of added frustration (Peiffer, Crooker, 1990). In addition, chronic conditions may involve long-term adaptations that demand a higher degree of self-care and responsibility on the part of elders and caregivers (Hasselkus, 1988).

Caregiver Stresses

An entire generation is moving into the caregiving role for their aging parents. These caregivers are changing their lives to assist their parents through the illness process. In addition to grieving for their parent, these caregivers may also be experiencing a loss of their own independence, privacy, financial security, safety, and comfort within their own homes. These losses may leave caregivers ultimately feeling guilty about their inadequacies or angry toward the debilitated elder.

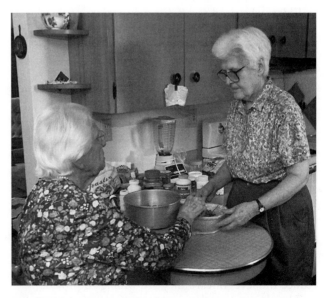

FIGURE 12-2 75% of caregivers are women, 25% of whom are caring for their children as well as their elder parent.

Life changes for caregivers and their families. This changing process may be gradual, beginning with the elder experiencing mild confusion and only requiring assistance with bills. The change may have been sudden and immediate, with the elder surviving a stroke and needing total physical care. The care required may be temporary or permanent with no hope for rehabilitation. No matter what the situation, this change of life is stressful for everyone involved.

Approximately 12 million Americans assist 5 million ill family members or friends who need help to remain at home. Statistics indicate that 75% of caregivers are women, 25% of whom are caring for their children as well as their elder parent. Half of all caregivers also work outside the home (U.S. Department of Health and Human Services, 1996). An estimated 16% to 23% of families across the United States are caring for adults with cognitive impairments, and 70% of the 4 million Americans with Alzheimer's disease are cared for at home (Family Caregiver Alliance, 1996). Financial concerns and home and life management add **stress** to caregivers' lives (Figure 12-2).

Advice from physicians, nurses, and therapists and attempts at self-education about an unfamiliar illness can also add stress. The need to learn the language of health care workers can be stressful, especially for caregivers for whom English is a second language or caregivers who are functionally illiterate.

Stress may also be increased by family members who offer suggestions for caring for elders. When decisions are made by several relatives but one family member or caregiver is responsible for following through with the group's decisions, the caregiver can easily become overwhelmed and feel resentful.

Elders who need caregiving may require various levels of assistance, and their conditions may change frequently. At times little assistance may be needed, but there may be long periods when much more assistance is required. Other family members may not understand the fluctuating assistance levels, and their perceptions of the work required to maintain the elder at home may be mistaken.

Family members may not understand their own emotions or those of the primary caregiver. Family members may deny feelings of guilt, frustration, anger, or grief. They may also be in denial about the level of care required and may not be ready to assist. Family members who are unable to understand their own emotions or the illness and needs of the elder may become angry with the caregiver for not allowing the elder more independence. They may be resentful and suspicious of the caregiver's motives or intentions, which can devastate caregivers and reduce the level of care they are willing to provide.

The demands and constraints of caregiving can become overwhelming. Caregivers may feel isolated and believe that they must be the sole providers of care. They may think they have no time for friends or support

BOX 12-2

Signs of Caregiver Stress

Too much stress can be damaging to both the caregiver and the elder. The following stress indicators, experienced frequently or simultaneously, can lead to more serious health problems.

1. The caregiver may deny the disease and its effect on the person who's been diagnosed. "I know Mom's going to get better."
2. The caregiver may express anger that no effective treatments or cures currently exist for chronic conditions such as Alzheimer's disease* and that people don't understand what's going on. "If he asks me that question one more time, I'll scream."
3. The caregiver may withdraw socially from friends and activities that once brought pleasure. "I don't care about getting together with the neighbors anymore."
4. The caregiver may express anxiety about facing another day and what the future holds. "What happens when he needs more care than I can provide?"
5. The caregiver may experience depression, which eventually breaks the spirit and affects coping ability. "I don't care anymore."
6. The caregiver may be exhausted, which makes it nearly impossible to complete necessary tasks. "I'm too tired for this."
7. The caregiver may experience sleeplessness caused by worrying. "What if she wanders out of the house or falls and hurts herself?"
8. The caregiver may express irritability, which may lead to moodiness and trigger negative responses and reactions. "Leave me alone!"
9. Lack of concentration on the part of the caregiver makes it difficult to perform familiar tasks. "I was so busy, I forgot we had an appointment."
10. The caregiver experiences mental and physical health problems. "I can't remember the last time I felt good."

Adapted from the Alzheimer's Association: *Ten signs of caregiver stress,* Chicago, 1995, The Association (brochure).

*For more information on Alzheimer's disease and services provided by the Alzheimer's Association, call 1-800-272-3900.

systems. Responsibilities can quickly become burdens, and caregivers may feel that if they do not provide the needed assistance, they are letting the elder down. Caregivers may refuse assistance from others because they feel the home is not clean enough for others to visit, or they believe they are the only ones who can properly care for the elder. Caregivers may forget that the level of care they now provide is the result of months of practice and learning through trial and error. COTAs must become adept at identifying signs of caregiver stress to ensure that the elders' needs are being met (Box 12-2).

BOX 12-3

Ways to Reduce Caregiver Stress*

1. Get a diagnosis as early as possible.
Symptoms may appear gradually, and if a person seems physically healthy, it's easy to ignore unusual behavior or attribute it to something else. See a physician when warning signs are present. Some dementia symptoms are treatable. Once you know what you're dealing with, you'll be able to better manage the present and plan for the future.

2. Know what resources are available.
For your own well-being and that of the person for whom you are caring, become familiar with care resources available in your community. Adult day care, in-home assistance, visiting nurses, and Meals-on-Wheels are just some of the community services that can help.

3. Become an educated caregiver.
As the disease progresses, different caregiving skills and capabilities are necessary. Care techniques and suggestions can help you better understand and cope with many of the challenging behaviors and personality changes.

4. Get help.
Trying to do everything by yourself will leave you exhausted. The support of family, friends, and community resources can be an enormous help. If assistance is not offered, ask for it. If you have difficulty asking for assistance, have someone close to you advocate for you. If stress becomes overwhelming, don't be afraid to seek professional help. Support group meetings and help lines are also good sources of comfort and reassurance.

5. Take care of yourself.
Caregivers frequently devote themselves totally to those they care for and, in the process, neglect their own needs. Pay attention to yourself. Watch your diet, exercise, and get plenty of rest. Use respite services to take time off for shopping, a movie, or an uninterrupted visit with a friend. Those close to you, including the one for whom you are caring, want you to take care of yourself.

6. Manage your level of stress.
Stress can cause physical problems (blurred vision, stomach irritation, high blood pressure) and changes in behavior (irritability, lack of concentration, loss of appetite). Note your symptoms. Use relaxation techniques that work for you and consult a physician.

7. Accept changes as they occur.
Elders change, and so do their needs. They often require care beyond what you can provide at home. A thorough investigation of available care options should make transitions easier as will support and assistance from those who care about you and your loved one.

8. Do legal and financial planning.
Consult an attorney and discuss issues related to durable power of attorney, living wills and trusts, future medical care, housing, and other key considerations. Planning now will alleviate stress later. If possible and appropriate, involve the elder and other family members in planning activities and decisions.

9. Be realistic.
The care you provide does make a difference. Neither you nor the elder can control many of the circumstances and behaviors that will occur. Give yourself permission to grieve for the losses you experience, but also focus on the positive moments as they occur and enjoy your good memories.

10. Give yourself credit, not guilt.
You're only human. Occasionally, you may lose patience and at times be unable to provide all of the care the way you'd like. Remember, you're doing the best you can, so give yourself credit. Being a devoted caregiver is not something to feel guilty about. Your loved one needs you, and you are there. That's something to be proud of.

Adapted from the Alzheimer's Association: *Ten signs of caregiver stress*, Chicago, 1995, The Alzheimer's Association (brochure).

*For more information on Alzheimer's disease and services provided by the Alzheimer's Association, call 1-800-272-3900.

Family resources. COTAs should continually assess the familys' needs and resources and offer the best referrals possible, keeping in mind that family members may feel isolated and disconnected or may be reluctant to ask for assistance. It may first be necessary to assist family members in identifying their needs and willingness to accept assistance. The suggestion that they read a book about caregivers or attend a caregiver support group may be met with resistance. However, COTAs must provide support and guidance while family members go through the process of realizing their own needs. When family members are ready to ask for assistance, COTAs must be ready with reliable resources and referrals. Successful experiences encourage families to use available **community resources.** COTAs must help family members and caregivers understand that caring for themselves and accepting help will ultimately help them care for the elder. Caring for themselves and accepting help may also make it possible to offer care at home for a longer period (Box 12-3 and Figure 12-3).

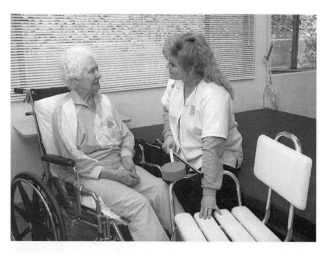

FIGURE 12-3   Careful discharge planning can help elders and caregivers feel less overwhelmed with changes.

Many community and national resources are available for families and caregivers. Support groups, publications, videos, and resources can be found in virtually every large community. In rural areas, organizations may be contacted by phone, in writing, or through computer technology. (An extensive resource and referral list is included in the appendix at the end of this book.)

RECOGNIZING SIGNS AND REPORTING ELDER ABUSE OR NEGLECT

Unfortunately, **abuse** and **neglect** of elders do occur. All professionals working with elders must be informed of their responsibilities and prepare themselves to act on their behalf should abuse or neglect be suspected. Federal definitions of elder abuse have been included in the Older Americans Act since 1987. Each state also has its own definition of elder abuse through legislation on adult protective services. COTAs should contact their state's ombudsman or Adult Protective Services Office for more detailed and specific guidelines. Only general definitions and guidelines are presented here. Elders have a right to direct their own care, refuse care, and be protected from being taken advantage of or hurt by others.

The National Aging Resource Center on Elder Abuse has identified and defined six types of elder abuse (Tatara, 1995). Physical abuse is identified as nonaccidental use of physical force that results in bodily injury, pain, or impairment. Sexual abuse is defined as nonconsensual sexual contact of any kind with an elder. Emotional or psychological abuse is willful infliction of mental or emotional anguish by threat, humiliation, or other verbal or nonverbal abusive conduct. Neglect is the willful or nonwillful failure by the caregiver to fulfill caretaking obligations or duties. Financial or material exploitation is an unauthorized use of an elder's funds, property, or resources. Self-abuse and neglect are abusive or neglectful methods of conduct of elders directed at themselves that threaten their health or safety.

Abuse may occur in the home or community setting as well as in residential care, skilled nursing facilities, or day health programs. In an effort to protect elders, every health care provider must be aware of signs and indicators of abuse. Indicators of abuse have been outlined in many documents available through agencies on aging (Disk, 1992). Physical abuse indicators include the presence of unexplained, inconsistent, and incompatible injuries. These may be bruises or welts, particularly if bilateral, clustered, or in patterns or if in various stages of healing. Other signs are burns, particularly those that appear to be caused by cigarettes, caustic materials, and friction from ties; fractures or sprains; and lacerations or abrasions. Evidence of confinement, such as food dishes or remnants, excretory vessels, and ties on furniture should be evaluated. Behavioral signs of physical abuse include extremes in behavior, fearfulness, nonresponsiveness, agitation, trembling, hesitation to talk openly, implausible stories, anger, depression, withdrawal, contradictory statements not caused by mental dysfunction, and confusion (Disk, 1992). Because many of these indicators are also common symptoms of dementia and other forms of mental illness, careful observation skills are required to confirm or rule out causes of behaviors.

Indicators of neglect include unattended physical or mental problems such as neglected bedsores, untreated injuries, skin disorders and rashes, poor hygiene, and torn or unwashed clothing. Hunger, malnutrition, and dehydration not caused by illness, and pallor, sunken eyes, and sunken cheeks may be potential signs of neglect. Unsanitary conditions in the home, fire hazards, inadequate heating or cooling, and insufficient food and water supply are associated with elder neglect. Neglect may also be indicated by the elder's helplessness, nonresponsiveness, and dependent behavior. Refusal to be helped, desire for social isolation, aggressiveness, agitation, detachment, hopelessness, and low self-esteem may also indicate other types of abuse, such as mental suffering or abandonment (Disk, 1992).

Sexual abuse may go unreported because of the elder's fear, embarrassment, shame, communication difficulties, or concern for the abuser. Sexual abuse may be identified by the presence of sexually transmitted diseases, genital discharge or infection, physical trauma to the anal or genital area, difficulty walking or sitting because of genital or anal pain, and painful urination or defecation. Behavioral indicators of sexual abuse may include changes in customary behavior, eating or sleeping disturbances, fears, phobias, overly compulsive behavior, inability to make eye contact, weeping, and fear of being left alone (Disk, 1992).

Fiduciary abuse indicators include inappropriate activity in bank accounts such as withdrawals from the automatic teller machine when the client is unable to leave home, elder's lack of understanding of having given power of attorney to a care custodian, and another person's unusual interest in the amount of money being spent on care. Refusal to spend money on care, unpaid or overdue bills, and change of title of the home suggest the possibility of fiduciary abuse. Other possible indicators include a recently redrawn will of an elder who is confused, lack of amenities for elders when their estate can afford them, and missing personal belongings. Isolating elders from friends and family, promising lifelong care in return for property, and requesting signatures on checks of incapacitated elders are additional signs of abuse (Disk, 1992).

Many states have enacted mandatory reporting laws that require professionals who regularly work with elders, including health workers such as COTAs and law enforcement and human service personnel, to report abuse. State and local agencies designated to receive and investigate reports and provide referral services to victims, families, and elders at risk for abuse include the Adult Protective Services Agency, long-term care ombudsman programs, law enforcement or local social service agencies, area agencies on aging, aging service providers, and aging advocacy groups. If elder abuse is suspected, these agencies can assist COTAs.

COTAs must report physical abuse if they witness an incident that reasonably appears to be physical abuse; find a physical injury of a suspicious nature, location, or repetition; or listen to an incident related by an elder or dependent adult. An immediate telephone call followed by a written report is often required. This report should include identifying information about the person reporting, the victim, and the caregiver. In addition, the incident and condition of the victim and any other information leading the reporter to suspect abuse must be included. Although many facilities have designated personnel to carry out reporting, it is each individual's duty to report suspected abuse. Failure to report is a punishable misdemeanor in states with mandatory reporting laws.

CASE STUDY

Albert is a 72-year-old man who had a right cerebrovascular accident (CVA) with consequent left hemiplegia. Albert has left glenohumeral subluxation and moderate edema in the hand. He has severe unilateral neglect, is incontinent, often is labile, and has very poor short-term memory. Albert has many difficulties with motor control and task completion. This experience has triggered severe depression and thoughts of suicide. Albert experienced depression before suffering the CVA. In the last 10 years he attempted suicide twice.

Before the CVA Albert was completely independent. He lived with his 69-year-old wife, who has advanced-stage Parkinson's disease. She requires a wheelchair for mobility and a paid caregiver for self-care and home management. She has had an anxiety disorder for many years. Just before experiencing the CVA, Albert named his brother as the primary agent for both his own and his wife's durable power of attorney. The couple has a 40-year-old son who lives in the same

town but is unable to provide much care for his parents because of employment responsibilities.

When Albert was admitted to the hospital for the CVA, he received treatment from various services, including OT. His progress was slow because of poor activity tolerance. Once he was medically stable, Albert was transferred to a skilled nursing facility (SNF) that provides rehabilitation services, including OT. Because the SNF was close to home, it was easier for Albert's wife to visit him.

At the time of the evaluation at the SNF, Albert required maximal assistance for functional self-care and mobility. He was at significant risk for falling because of his unilateral neglect and mobility impairments. With Albert's agreement, his family was encouraged to observe treatment sessions early in his rehabilitation. Initially time was spent answering the family's questions about Albert's functional deficits. They were also instructed on therapy they could do at the SNF during their visits, such as retrograde massage for his arm, left-sided stimulation, and basic positioning. Because of the subluxation problem, the family was not taught to assist with passive range-of-motion exercises. Instead, they were directed to ensure safe positioning of the arm at all times.

Two weeks after Albert's arrival at the SNF, his brother met with the interdisciplinary team and explained that Albert's wife would be visiting less frequently because it upset her too much to see her husband's condition. The brother expressed the family's hope that someday Albert would regain sufficient skills to return home. However, he also stated that he realized this might never happen.

After 10 weeks of therapy, Albert required minimal assistance in most activities and only occasional verbal directions. Albert also was able to use a memory book consistently and took initiative to verbally direct those giving him assistance. He was continent of bowel and bladder. Although he still occasionally spoke of suicide, his energy level had improved and with it, his sense of despair and hopelessness.

Albert's brother visited regularly. His wife came more frequently as Albert's abilities improved, but she often visited for only brief periods. The COTA spent time during each of these visits making sure that Albert could demonstrate his accomplishments. During a team meeting that included Albert and his wife, son, and brother, and OTR and COTA team explained that based on Albert's progress so far, he would likely be able to return home with a minimal level of assistance (about 25%). He would also most likely need to remain in a wheelchair. The COTA recommended a home evaluation to determine needed modifications and equipment.

Although the home was already wheelchair accessible and the wife's caregiver was willing to provide additional assistance for Albert, the wife stated that she would be too nervous to have him in the home for fear he would have another CVA. Albert's brother and son stated that the wife's anxiety would make it too difficult for anyone to provide assistance for both elders at the same time. Albert stated that he did not believe it would be prudent to cause his wife additional worries even if his functional abilities were to improve and an additional caregiver could be found. Tearfully he requested long-term placement.

Considering Albert's story, answer the following questions:

1. Are there strategies the COTA could have implemented earlier to help Albert succeed with his goal to return home?
2. What new strategies do you think the COTA should implement now that Albert has requested placement in long-term care?

CHAPTER REVIEW QUESTIONS

1 While working at an SNF you approach a new elder who says, "My husband just left me here all alone. Oh, please help me, I want to go home." How should you respond?

2 You work in a rehabilitation unit. You recommend a tub transfer bench for an elder with hemiplegia. Medicare will not cover the expense of this bench. The family says, "We'll just rig something up when we get home." How should you respond?

3 You are working on an Alzheimer's disease special unit. An elder comes up to you, grabs your arm and says, "Momma, where have you been? I've been so afraid." As the elder continues to cling to your arm, you notice the elder's family members are watching. The elder's behavior escalates whenever a family member approaches. How should you respond?

4 The grown daughter of an elder approaches you and states, "My father has been an alcoholic all my life. He has been so mean to my mother. His being in the hospital is the first peace she's had in years. Please don't let my father come home." How should you respond?

5 You have worked closely with an elder for 2 weeks. After a week-long vacation you return to learn that the elder has refused treatment most of the week you were absent. The elder had stated, "I don't want anyone new! My family doesn't know how to help me." What steps should you have taken to minimize the elder's dependence on you?

6 On admission of their 87-year-old widowed father to an acute-care hospital, three adult children state that it is their desire to take him home and share the caregiving responsibilities when he is ready for discharge. During the 3-week hospitalization, staff members have seen the children visit only once. They have also not returned repeated phone calls by the social worker. What input should the COTA give to the treatment team in preparation for discharge?

7 The 20-year-old granddaughter of an elder comes in every day to visit her grandmother. The young woman reports that her mother wants to visit but has not been able to get out of bed. She also described depressive symptoms she has noticed in her mother. What do you recommend for the granddaughter? What should you do for the mother?

REFERENCES

Davis L: Coping with illness. In Davis L, Kirkland M, editors: *The role of occupational therapy with the elderly*, Rockville, Md, 1988, American Occupational Therapy Association.

Disk K: *The elderly and dependent adults as crime victims: abuse and neglect of California's elderly*, Sacramento, 1992, State Dept. of Health.

Family Caregiver Alliance: *About brain impairments: quick facts about common brain impairments*, San Francisco, Calif, 1996, The Alliance.

Hasselkus B: Elder education. In Davis L, Kirkland M, editors: *The role of occupational therapy with the elderly*, Rockville, Md, 1988, American Occupational Therapy Association.

Humphrey R, Gonzalez S, Taylor E: Family involvement in practice: issues and attitudes, *Am J Occup Ther* 47(7):587, 1993.

Peiffer M, Crooker B: Our story: two perspectives of family caregiving, *Occup Ther Pract* 2(1):50, 1990.

Rogers J: Roles and functions of occupational therapy in gerontic practice. In Davis L, Kirkland M, editors: *The role of occupational therapy with the elderly*, Rockville, Md, 1988, American Occupational Therapy Association.

Snow T: Working with the family. In Davis L, Kirkland M, editors: *The role of occupational therapy with the elderly*, Rockville, Md, 1988, American Occupational Therapy Association.

Tatara T: *Understanding the nature and extent of elder abuse in domestic settings*, Washington, DC, 1995, National Center on Elder Abuse.

Administration on Aging: *Elder action: action ideas for older persons and their families*, Washington, DC, 1996, US Department of Health and Human Services.

Addressing Sexuality of Elders

HELENE LOHMAN

KEY TERMS

sexuality, values, myths, physiological changes, nursing facilities, PLISSIT model

CHAPTER OBJECTIVES

1. Discuss the ways values can influence attitudes about elder sexuality.
2. Identify primary myths about elder sexuality.
3. Describe normal age related sexual physiological changes.
4. Discuss the treatment team members' roles in addressing elders' sexual concerns.
5. Discuss the ways elders' sexuality is commonly dealt with in nursing facilities.
6. List the components of the PLISSIT model and discuss ways the COTA can apply this model.
7. Identify strategies for elder sexual education.
8. List treatment ideas for addressing sexual concerns of elders who experience strokes, heart disease, and arthritis.
9. Increase personal comfort in discussing elder sexual concerns.

A common treatment goal for elder clients is improving ADL functions. Thirteen categories to address ADL functions, including sexual expression, are listed in *The uniform terminology for occupational therapy—third edition* (American Occupational Therapy Association [AOTA], 1994). Sexual expression is defined as "engaging in desired sexual and intimate activities" (AOTA, 1994). At any age, sexual expression should be considered an important part of a person's life. However, sexual expression may be ignored in clinical treatment for many reasons, including discomfort with one's own sexuality or with an elder or disabled person remaining sexually active. Other reasons may include a lack of understanding of normal sexual changes with aging and a lack of knowledge about sexual function with regard to age and disability. Dealing with

the elder's concerns about sexual function should be part of clinical treatment. This chapter helps the COTA learn about this important but often ignored area of ADL intervention. Furthermore, the chapter will help clarify myths and misconceptions (Figure 13-1).

VALUES ABOUT SEXUALITY

Each generation has certain values reflective of society. In addition, all individuals have their own value systems. The current elder population is from a generation that did not often discuss sexuality. For some it was a necessity for procreation and not a source of enjoyment. These are deeply held values that can influence the elder's comfort level when discussing sexual feelings during clinical treatment. In addition, the COTA may feel uncomfort-

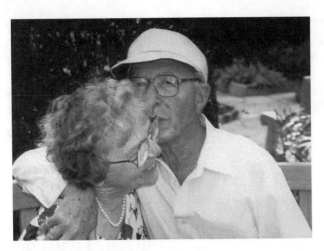

FIGURE 13-1 Sexual expression is an important part of a person's life at any age. (Courtesy Helene Lohman.)

able discussing sexual concerns with the elder, because sexuality is not usually an open topic. Exercises 13-1 and 13-2 should be completed before further reading to explore values regarding elders and sexuality.

EXERCISE 13-1: GENERATIONAL SEXUAL ATTITUDES/VALUES INVENTORY

Answer the following questions while considering your generation and the current elder generation (that is, 65 years and older). Fill in "yes" or "no" for each. Then discuss or contemplate your findings.

Yes = Acceptable
No = Unacceptable

1. It is appropriate to openly discuss sexual needs and concerns.
   Your generation _____
   Current elder generation _____
2. Sexual activity is acceptable in a nonmarriage situation.
   Your generation _____
   Current elder generation _____
3. Sexual activity is appropriate if the purpose is physical pleasure.
   Your generation _____
   Current elder generation _____
4. Sexual activity is only for procreation.
   Your generation _____
   Current elder generation _____
5. The naked body is very private. Nudity is unacceptable.
   Your generation _____
   Current elder generation _____

6. Women should discuss their sexual needs with their partners.
   Your generation _____
   Current elder generation _____
7. It is appropriate for women to initiate sex.
   Your generation _____
   Current elder generation _____
8. Masturbation is a normal sexual act.
   Your generation _____
   Current elder generation _____
9. Sexual activity between people of the same sex is acceptable.
   Your generation _____
   Current elder generation _____
10. Sexual activity between adults of different generations is unacceptable.
    Your generation _____
    Current elder generation _____

(Adapted from Lohman H, Runyon C: An occupational therapy module to increase sensitivity about geriatric sexuality, *Phys Occup Ther Geriatr* 11(2):57, 1993.)

EXERCISE 13-2: PERSONAL VALUES ASSESSMENT

This exercise helps identify personal values and attitudes. Answer the following questions honestly. On completion of this exercise, any uncomfortable feelings may be handled by using this chapter as an educational tool to help dispel myths and misconceptions and clarify normal physiological changes resulting from aging. After reading the chapter, the COTA can retake this personal value assessment to determine whether uncomfortable feelings have decreased.

1. Elders in nursing facilities should not be sexually active.
   Agree _____ Disagree _____
2. My grandparents (or parents) should not be sexually active.
   Agree _____ Disagree _____
3. It is acceptable for elder men to remain sexually active.
   Agree _____ Disagree _____
4. It is acceptable for elder women to remain sexually active.
   Agree _____ Disagree _____
5. It is immoral for elders to engage in recreational sex.
   Agree _____ Disagree _____
6. Sexual education is not necessary for elders.
   Agree _____ Disagree _____
7. Sexual education is not necessary for nursing facility staff.
   Agree _____ Disagree _____

8. Nursing facilities should provide large enough beds for couples to sleep together.

Agree _____ Disagree _____

9. Nursing facilities should provide privacy for residents who desire sexual activity.

Agree _____ Disagree _____

(Adapted from White CB: The aging sexuality attitudes and knowledge scale (ASKAS): a scale for the assessment of attitudes and knowledge regarding sexuality in the aged, *Arch Sex Behav* 11(6):491, 1982.)

MYTHS ABOUT ELDERS AND SEXUAL FUNCTIONING

The media has provided people with misinformation and myths about elder sexual functioning. Television and magazine advertisements encourage people to ignore or cover up the aging process. Greeting cards make fun of aging and suggest that lying about age is acceptable. Some media sources encourage myths about sexuality such as "the dirty old man syndrome." In addition, myths can be perpetuated by family members, peers, or elders themselves. With this inundation of misinformation, many people believe myths instead of truths about the sexual functioning of elders. Exercise 13-3 helps determine personal myths about elders and sexuality.

▮ EXERCISE 13-3: MYTHS ABOUT GERIATRIC SEXUALITY

Answer *T* if the statement reflects a myth, or *F* if the statement does not reflect a myth.

1. T F Elders are no longer interested in sexuality.
2. T F Elders no longer engage in sexual activity
3. T F Elders engage in a wide variety of sexual activity, including intercourse, cuddling, caressing, mutual stimulation, and oral sex.
4. T F Elders in nursing facilities should be segregated according to gender; sexual functioning should be prohibited.
5. T F Elder women are unattractive.
6. T F More elder men remain sexually active than older women.
7. T F Elders are too frail to engage in sexual activity.
8. T F Inability to maintain an erection (impotence) is *not* a natural consequence of aging.

See page 136 for answer key.

(Adapted from Comfort A, Dial L: Sexuality and aging: an overview, *Clin Geriatr Med* 7(1):1, 1991; Goodwin A, Scott L: Sexuality in second half of life. In Doress PB, Siegal DL, editors: *Ourselves growing older*, New York, 1987, Simon and Schuster; Hammond D: Love, sex, and marriage in later years. In Deichman ES, Kociechki R, editors: *Working with the elderly: an introduction*, Buffalo, NY, 1989, Prometheus Books; Morrison-Beedy D, Robbins L: Sexual assessment and the aging female, *Nurse Pract* 14:36, 1989; Pfeiffer E, Verwoerdt A, Wang HS: Sexual behavior in aged men and women, *Arch Gen Psychiatr* 19:753, 1968.)

Discussion of Myths

Studies over many years show that elders are interested in sex and remain sexually active to some degree. Some studies found that as a person ages, a gradual decline in sexual activity occurs, with the population 75 years and older engaging in sex less frequently than younger persons. (Pfeiffer, Verwoerdt, Wang, 1968; Kaplan, 1990; Lohman, Runyon, 1995).

For women, sexual activity often stops because of lack of a partner. Approximately half of older women are widows, and almost five times as many widows as widowers exist (American Association of Retired Persons [AARP], 1995). In addition, some elder women believe the myth that they are unattractive and therefore should remain abstinent. Furthermore, the current elder generation's values are strongly against women being sexually active without a husband. Both older men and older women may experience pressure from their children to remain abstinent. Adult children often find it difficult to think of their parents as having normal sexual desires, especially if the parent is in a nursing facility.

Impotence is by no means a natural consequence of male aging. Men can continue normal sexual activity throughout their lives. Minor physiological changes may have some effect on sexual functioning. For example, a benefit from physiological aging can be delayed ejaculation, which can increase sexual pleasure for the partner (Laflin, 1990).

Most elders, especially the young old (that is, those 65 to 75 years of age), have active lives in which sexuality can remain an important component. Most likely, if a couple has always been sexually active, they will continue to be so as they grow older. As with any age group, communication is important for a positive sexual relationship. Frailty and disability do not automatically necessitate cause for an elder to be abstinent, although that is often the case (Figure 13-2).

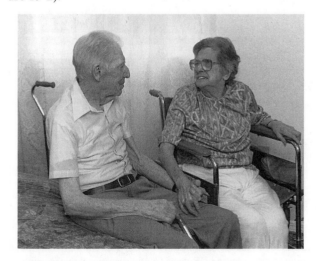

FIGURE 13-2 When elders become frail or disabled, they do not necessarily become asexual.

Society often ignores homosexuality in elders. The percentage of elders who are homosexual is estimated to be the same as that of younger persons (Dorfman et al, 1995). Myths and stereotypes about homosexuality continue to exist as people age. Health care professionals can educate elders about sexual functioning and thereby help dispel these myths.

NORMAL AGE-RELATED PHYSIOLOGICAL CHANGES IN MEN AND WOMEN

With normal aging, physiological changes might affect sexual functioning. Knowledge of these changes may help the COTA counsel the elder (Box 13-1). Not all these

BOX 13-1

Age-Related Physiological Changes and Sexual Responses

Women
1. Decrease in rate and amount of vaginal lubrication may possibly lead to painful intercourse (Thienhaus, 1988).
2. Orgasmic changes include a decrease in the number of involuntary contractions by 50% and an acceleration of postorgasmic decrescendo or clitoral retraction (Thienhaus, 1988)
3. Structural changes or atrophy may occur in the labia or uterus in addition to a reduction in the expansion of the vagina width (Goodwin & Scott, 1987; Thienhaus, 1988; Laflin, 1990).
4. Thinning of the lining of the vagina can result in irritation and painful intercourse (McGracken, 1988).

Men
1. Erection is slower and less full and disappears quickly after orgasm. Erection has a longer refractory period, usually of 12 to 24 hours after ejaculation to achieve erection again (McGracken 1988; Thienhaus, 1988; Laflin, 1990).
2. Decrease in muscle tone occurs (Thienhaus, 1988).
3. Testicles do not achieve full elevation and do not increase in size with erection (Thienhaus, 1988).
4. Decreased volume of sperm occurs. Although fertility level is decreased, men do not become sterile (Laflin, 1990).
5. Ejaculatory control increases, and ejaculation may occur every third sexual episode as a result of less preoccupation with orgasm (Laflin, 1990).
6. Ejaculation is less strong, and orgasm is often less intense (Laflin, 1990).
7. Decrease in ejaculatory testosterone occurs (Laflin, 1990).

Adapted from Lohman H, Runyon C: An occupational therapy module to increase sensitivity about geriatric sexuality, *Phys Occup Ther Geriatr* 11(2):57, 1993.

changes happen to every elder, and the degree varies among individuals (Glass, 1988). In addition, COTAs should be aware of the concept "use it or lose it." Elders who remain sexually active may not experience some of these physiological changes or to the same degree as elders who do not remain sexually active. Furthermore, these physiological changes are just one aspect of sexuality. The psychological aspects of sexual functioning must never be ignored. The ways a person reacts to and perceives these physiological changes ultimately affect sexual functioning. COTAs can apply this knowledge to educate elders. For example, a commercially available lubricant can supplement decreased vaginal secretion and help reduce abrasion from thinning of the vaginal lining. Lubrication may also prevent dyspareunia, or painful intercourse (Lohman, Runyon, 1995).

ROLE OF THE TREATMENT TEAM IN SEXUAL EDUCATION

COTAs and OTRs should collaborate in addressing all aspects of ADL functions, including sexuality. Additionally, COTAs should be aware of other team members' areas of expertise. Sexual dysfunction such as impotence, ejaculatory disturbances, anorgasmia (lack of orgasm), and pain during intercourse may be caused by side effects of medication. The physician and pharmacist must be notified about these concerns. Sexual dysfunction has a psychological component. Therefore the client should be referred for counseling with a social worker or psychologist who has expertise with elders who have disabilities and sexual dysfunction. In addition to the OT practitioner, some physical therapists and nurses may educate the client about sexual positioning. Speech therapists may assist elders who have communication difficulties (Lohman, Runyon, 1993).

ADDRESSING ELDER SEXUALITY IN A NURSING FACILITY

COTAs must be aware of laws and regulations for client rights in nursing facilities. Federal laws regulate privacy for institutionalized patients (Omnibus Budget Reconciliation Act, 1987; Laflin, 1990; Wallace, 1992) However, in spite of these regulations, elders living in nursing home facilities are sometimes interrupted or even reprimanded for engaging in some type of sexual activity (Mulligan, Modigh, 1991). Lyder (1991) found that nursing home staff members often violate clients' sexual rights by belittling an elders' attempts to flirt and look attractive and prohibiting elders from wearing sex-defining clothing. Other violations of sexual rights include not providing privacy during procedures and examinations.

In some institutional settings, envisioning elders being interested in sex is difficult. However, data suggests that institutionalized elders do in fact remain interested.

Mulligan and Palguta (1991) found that male elders in nursing home facilities displayed continued interest in sex and were sexually active if a partner was available.

Sexuality does not only include sexual intercourse. It also involves touching, hugging, and expressing the self as a sexual being (Lyder, 1991). COTAs participating in program planning can suggest dances and other social events that encourage romance and human touch. They can encourage elders through positive reinforcement to be well-dressed and well-groomed. In addition, COTAs should always be aware of respecting client privacy. Shutting a curtain between beds or going to another room for treatment with personal ADL functions helps preserve privacy rights (Figures 13-3 and 13-4).

Finally, education can help dispel myths and misconceptions about sexuality and elders (Lohman, Aitken, 1995). COTAs who have positive attitudes and are educated about sexuality and elders can help dispel the

ageist attitudes sometimes held by nursing home staff and family members.

EDUCATING AND COUNSELING THE ELDER CLIENT
The PLISSIT Model

Treatment models may help provide sexual education to elders. The permission, limited information, specific suggestions, and intensive therapy (PLISSIT) model developed by Annon (1974, 1976) is a useful format for presenting sexual education information (Box 13-2).

COTAs can employ the first, second, and third stages of this model during treatment. The elder must be assured of confidentiality throughout the educational process. In the first stage of the PLISSIT model, permission, the COTA applies therapeutic listening skills. The COTA's verbal and nonverbal body language must show comfort with the topic. COTAs can ask questions in a nonthreatening manner to encourage communication about sexual functioning during the ADL assessment (Goldstein, Runyon, 1993). In addition, the COTA can convey that sexuality is a normal part of every human's needs throughout a lifetime (Smedely, 1991). Sometimes, elders may cry because someone cares about this concern. Tears should not stop the discussion unless the elder indicates a desire to stop. Elders who are interested in discussing sexuality may have general questions about normal sexual changes with aging or common myths. The spouse or partner should be encouraged to join the discussion.

In the second stage of the model, the COTA can apply limited information by relating knowledge of sexuality gleaned from this chapter and other relevant sources. The COTA can provide specific suggestions in the third stage.

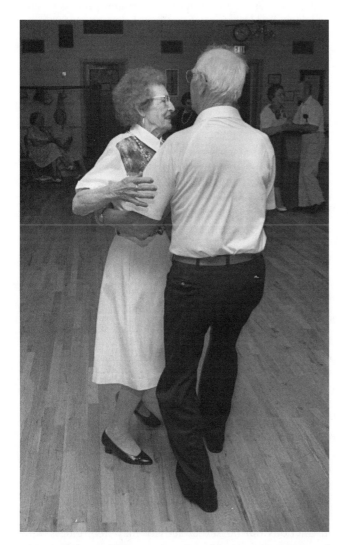

FIGURE 13-3 COTAs may suggest dances and other social events that encourage romance and affectionate touch.

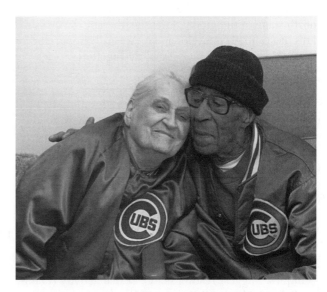

FIGURE 13-4 Sexuality involves touch, hugs, and other forms of expression.

BOX 13-2

The PLISSIT Model

P = Permission
This stage involves listening in a nonjudgmental, knowledgeable, and relaxed manner as the client discusses sexual concerns. General questions can be asked in an intake or screening evaluation (for example, "Do you have any concerns about the effects of your disease on sexual function?").

LI = Limited information
At this level the elder can be educated about normal physiological changes with aging, myths and stereotypes about the elder population, and sexuality and psychosocial factors that may inhibit or stress the elder.

SS = Specific suggestions
At this level, COTAs may make appropriate suggestions for improved sexual functioning. Elders may also need to be referred to specialists such as social workers, psychologists, and physical or occupational therapists.

IT = Intensive therapy
This level of counseling involves the expertise of a skilled social worker, psychologist, or psychiatrist.

Adapted from Lohman H, Runyon C: Counseling the geriatric client about sexual issues, *Sexuality Iss Counsel Ther* 1(5):1, 1995.

Many suggestions are discussed in this chapter to help elders who have disabling conditions and their partners maintain sexual function. The COTA should refer the elder who needs psychological support at any point of the education process to the appropriate counselor. The fourth stage of the model, intensive therapy, involves the skills of a trained counselor and is especially important for those elders experiencing sexual dysfunction.

The COTA's Role in Sexual Education

To provide elders with adequate sex education, COTAs must have a general knowledge about their medical conditions. Understanding the effects of a disease or disabling condition on sexual performance is necessary. COTAs must remember that the manifestations of a disease or condition differ with each person. The following are some general education suggestions:

1. Encourage elders to experiment with different sexual positions for comfort (Laflin, 1990).
2. Provide instruction on energy conservation techniques. Suggest resting before sexual activity (Hahn, 1989; Goldstein, Runyon, 1993).
3. Encourage elders with decreased energy to explore

other forms of sexual expression such as caressing, masturbation, and oral sex.
4. Reassure elders that once they are medically stable and their physician has approved resumption of sexual activity, further medical problems are unlikely (Hackett, Cassem, 1984; Burgener, Logan, 1989).
5. Talk with elders about any fears they may have about resuming sexual functioning (Goldstein, Runyon, 1993).

The specific sexual concerns of elders who have CVAs, heart disease; and arthritis are discussed in the following sections:

EFFECTS OF HEALTH CONDITIONS ON ELDER SEXUALITY

Cerebrovascular Accident

Cerebrovascular accident (CVA) is the diagnosis most frequently followed in occupational therapy (AOTA, 1990). COTAs assisting in the assessment process should address all ADL functions, including sexual function. COTAs should observe for motor abnormalities and other symptoms that can affect sexual function, including hemiplegia; perceptual, cognitive, and visual spatial disturbances; speech problems; emotional manifestations; and sensory deficits. For example, if elders are depressed, they may have no interest in sex. Anxiety may cause sexual performance problems such as male impotence and decreased female lubrication leading to painful intercourse. If elders have unilateral neglect, they may ignore one side of the body during sexual performance. Expressive aphasia may result in a difficulty stating sexual needs. Sensory deficits such as esthesia or hyperesthesia on the affected side may affect sexual pleasure (Zukas, Ross-Robinson, 1991). Motor disturbances such as muscle weakness or hypertonia can make sexual performance awkward (Zukas, Ross-Robinson, 1991). Chapter 24 provides a more in-depth discussion about CVA.

After identifying the symptoms that affect sexual performance, the OTR and the COTA should collaborate to develop specific treatment suggestions. For example, clients with hemiplegia are sometimes advised to lie on the affected side so that the unaffected arm is free to caress the partner (Burgener, Logan, 1989). Simple adaptations such as using pillows under the affected side, raising the headboard, and adding a bed trapeze can help with motor manifestations of the CVA (Zukas, Ross-Robinson, 1991). Touch and other forms of nonverbal communication are useful with elders who have expressive aphasia (Laflin, 1990). The partners of elders with visual field deficits should be encouraged to approach from the impaired side and use touch on both sides. Minimizing environmental distractions during sexual activity may help elders with cognitive deficits involving concentration (Neistadt, Freda, 1987).

Beyond the physical effects of a CVA, some elders may experience low self-esteem and depression. These symptoms can affect sexual desire and performance (Mooradian, 1991). Elders who are in some way dependent on a partner may feel ambivalent about resuming a sexual relationship because of role changes (Mooradian, 1991). In addition, elders may worry about sustaining another CVA (Burgener, Logan, 1989; Habot et al, 1989). Elders with these psychological manifestations may require counseling.

Heart Disease

Heart disease is one of the most common chronic ailments affecting the elder population (AARP, 1995). The possible sexual repercussions related to it should not be ignored. With physician approval, elders may resume a normal sex life after the acute phase of the condition has passed (Garner, Allen, 1988). According to Relf (1991), before receiving final approval from the physician, the elder will be assessed for "general health tolerance for physical activity before surgery; extent of myocardial damage; frequency and severity of angina, dyspnea, arrhythmias; wound healing; and operative factors."

The effect of a cardiac condition on sexual performance is usually more psychological than physical in nature (American Heart Association, 1990). The resumption of sexual activity after a heart attack is mistakenly believed to cause future cardiac incidents and even death (Garner, Allen, 1988; LoPiccolo, 1991; Relf, 1991). The elder needs to be assured that the physical demands of sexual activity are actually very mild (AHA, 1990). Some researchers have noted that intercourse is comparable to a brisk walk up two flights of steps (Hackett, Cassem, 1984; Relf, 1991). Relaxation is important because of the possible relationship between heart disease and stress (Garner, Allen, 1988). In addition, depression and anxiety are very common after a cardiac incident (Garner, Allen, 1988). COTAs can teach elders stress reduction techniques. Energy conservation techniques may also be helpful for those who are gradually building up their endurance.

Arthritis

Arthritis is another common chronic condition among elders. Elders with rheumatoid arthritis (RA), and those suffering from joint inflammation and pain may be particularly prone to sexual performance problems. A common treatment goal for people with RA is to maintain or increase functional abilities in all areas of life (Trombly, 1989), including sexual function. COTAs can make specific suggestions to help clients reduce joint pain and discomfort and preserve energy. Exercises to increase and maintain muscle strength affect the motor aspect of sexual performance. Elders should be encouraged to use a heating pad or tub bath before sexual activity to help decrease joint pain and inflammation. Elders and their partners may also experiment with various sexual positions that decrease joint pressure. Rest and energy conservation techniques may help make sexual performance less fatiguing (Goldstein, Runyon, 1993).

■ EXERCISE 13-4: ROLE PLAY

Addressing sexual concerns in treatment will become more comfortable for COTAs with practice. The purpose of this role-play exercise is to increase comfort levels when discussing sexual issues. It also serves as a review of chapter material. To begin the exercise, choose four people to be part of a radio talk-show panel made up of knowledgeable professionals who are experts on the sexuality of elders. Then choose people who will read the scenarios listed below. Members of the radio talk-show panel are allowed to consult notes and have a commercial break if they want to discuss a situation before responding.

Situations for Role Play: Radio Talk Show

- I am 78 years of age and have rheumatoid arthritis. Over the years, I have developed increasingly painful joints, particularly in my hips. I am presently a widow but will soon marry a wonderful man. I would like to enjoy my new sexual relationship. Do you have any suggestions?
- I am a 65-year-old man who recently had a heart attack 8 weeks ago. My doctor says that it is safe to begin sex again. Still, I have tremendous fears. Are these fears normal and what can I do about them?
- I am a nurse's aide who works in a nursing facility. I have recently noticed male and female patients taking an interest in each other. They are constantly holding hands and have been observed kissing. The other aides make fun of them and have told them to stop, but they continue openly expressing their affection. I feel that they have a right to express their romantic side. Who is right?
- I am an 82-year-old man. My wife and I continue to have a satisfying sexual relationship. However, I have noticed in recent years that my first erection is slower and it takes me even longer to achieve an erection the second time. I am afraid to ask my physician about this. Am I normal?
- I am a 64-year-old male who had a heart attack 2 years ago. I have suffered from impotence since getting out of the hospital. What should I do?
- I have a two-part question. I am 65 and have recently suffered a minor stroke. I am uncomfortable asking my physician about this. I have noticed over the years that sexual activity with my lover has become painful because of less vaginal lubrication. Is this normal, and is there anything I can do about it? Con-

cerning the stroke, my left side is impaired and weakened. Do you have any suggestions for sexual positioning?

▋CHAPTER REVIEW QUESTIONS

1 Discuss common myths related to elder sexuality.

2 Identify some of the normal age-related physiological changes for women and some simple treatment suggestions for them.

3 Identify some of the normal age-related physiological changes of men.

4 List the members of the treatment team and discuss ways the team can work together to address elders' sexual concerns.

5 Discuss the ways attitudes of health care workers in nursing home facilities affect elder sexuality.

6 Describe ways COTAs help facilitate elder sexual expression in a nursing home setting?

7 List and describe the parts of the PLISSIT model.

8 Describe ways COTAs may apply the PLISSIT model in treatment.

Answers to Exercise 13-3 1. T 2. T 3. F 4. T 5. T 6. F 7. T 8. F

REFERENCES

American Heart Association: *Sex and heart disease*, 1990, The Association.

American Association of Retired Persons: *A profile of older Americans*, Washington, DC, 1995, The Association.

American Occupational Therapy Association: *Member data survey*, Rockville, Md, 1990, The Association.

American Occupational Therapy Association: Uniform terminology for occupational therapy—third edition, *Am J Occup Ther* 48(11): 1047, 1994.

Annon JS: *The behavioral treatment of sexual problems: 1. In brief therapy*, Honolulu, 1974, Kapiolani Health Services (brochure).

Annon JS: *The behavioral treatment of sexual problems: brief therapy*, New York, 1976, Harper and Row.

Burgener S, Logan G: Sexuality concerns of the post-stroke patient, *Rehabil Nurs* 14(4):178, 1989.

Comfort A, Dial L: Sexuality and aging: an overview, *Clin Geriatr Med* 7(1):1, 1991.

Dorfman et al: Old, sad, alone: the myth of the aging homosexual, *J Gerontol Soc Work* 24(1/2):29, 1995.

Garner W, Allen H: Sexual rehabilitation and heart disease, *J Rehabil* 55:69, 1988.

Goodwin A, Scott L: Sexuality in second half of life. In Doress PB, Siegal DL, editors: *Ourselves growing older*, New York, 1987, Simon and Schuster.

Glass C, Dalton A: Sexuality in older adults: a continuing education concern, *J Cont Educ Nurs* 19:61, 1988.

Habot B et al: Sexual function among male hemiparetic post-CVA patients, *J Am Geriatr Soc* 37:1003, 1989.

Hackett TP, Cassem NH: Psychological aspects of rehabilitation after myocardial infarction and coronary artery bypass surgery. In Wenger NK, Hellerstein H, editors: *Rehabilitation of the coronary patient*, ed 2, New York, 1984, Simon and Schuster.

Hahn K: Sexuality and COPD, *Rehabil Nurs* 14(4):191, 1989.

Hammond D: Love, sex, and marriage in the later years. In Deichman ES, Kociechki R, editors: *Working with the elderly: an introduction*, Buffalo, NY, 1989, Prometheus Books.

Kaplan H: Sex, intimacy, and the aging process, *J Am Acad Psychoanal* 18:185, 1990.

Laflin M: Sexuality and the elderly. In Lewis C, editor: *Aging: the health-care challenge*, ed 2, Philadelphia, 1990, FA Davis.

Lohman H, Aitken M: Influence of education on knowledge and attitude toward older adult sexuality, *J Phys Occup Ther Geriatr* 13:51, 1995.

LoPiccolo J: Counseling and therapy for sexual problems in the elderly, *Clin Geriatr Med* 7:161, 1991.

Lohman H, Runyon C: An occupational therapy module to increase sensitivity about geriatric sexuality, *Phys Occup Ther Geriatr* 11(2): 57, 1993.

Lohman H, Runyon C: *Counseling the geriatric client about sexuality issues in counseling and therapy: lesson 5*, New York, 1995, Hatherleigh Company.

Lyder CH: Examining sexuality in long term care, *J Pract Nurs* 41(4):25, 1991.

Mulligan T, Palguta RF: Sexual interest, activity and satisfaction among male nursing home residents, *Arch Sexual Behav* 20(2):199, 1991.

Mulligan T, Modigh A: Sexuality in dependent living situations, *Clin Geriatr Med* 7(1):153, 1991.

Morrison-Beedy D, Robbins L: Sexual assessment and the aging female, *Nurse Pract* 14:36, 1989.

Mooradian AD: Geriatric sexuality and chronic diseases, *Clin Geriatr Med* 7(1):113, 1991.

Neistadt ME, Freda M: *Choices: a guide to sexual counseling with physically disabled adults*, Malabar, Fl, 1987, Robert E Krieger.

Omnibus Budget Reconciliation Act (OBRA): Health Care Financing Administration, Baltimore, Md, 1995.

Occupational Therapy Roles Task Force: Occupational therapy roles, *Am J Occup Ther* 47:1987, 1993.

Pfeiffer E, Verwoerdt A, Wang HS: Sexual behavior in aged men and women, *Arch Gen Psychiatry* 19:753, 1968.

Relf MV: Sexuality and the older bypass patient, *Geriatr Nurs* 12:294, 1991.

Smedely G: Addressing sexuality in the elderly, *Rehabil Nurs* 16:9, 1991.

Trombly CA: Arthritis. In Trombly CA, editor: *Occupational therapy for physical dysfunction*, ed 3, Baltimore, 1989, Williams & Wilkins.

Wallace M: Management of sexual relationships among elderly residents of long-term care facilities, *Geriatr Nurs* 13(6):308, 1992.

Zukas RR, Robinson-Ross L: Sexuality and the disabled woman, *Occup Ther Pract* 2:1, 1991.

Group Treatment With Elders

SUE BYERS-CONNON AND SHERRY HOFF

KEY TERMS

groups, facilitation, referral, therapeutic goals, psychosocial, closed groups, open groups, perceptual integration, cognitive function, therapeutic interaction, flexibility

CHAPTER OBJECTIVES

1. Discuss ways in which OT goals for elders can be addressed through groups.
2. Identify characteristics of elders for whom group participation is appropriate.
3. Describe group activities appropriate to meet the needs of elders in various settings.
4. Discuss methods of organizing internal and external environmental components, including staffing and safety.
5. Describe group facilitation skills used by COTAs.
6. Discuss components of group protocols.

Groups can be described in a variety of ways. Mosey (1970) provided a base: "A group is an aggregate of people who share a common purpose which can be attained only by group members interacting and working together." Group treatment has been a modality used by OT practitioners since the beginning of the profession. Meyer (1977) described hospitalized persons working at individual projects in a group setting. Anderson "first suggested that group projects should be designed with therapeutic goals for individual patients in mind" (Duncombe, Howe, 1995). Howe and Schwartzberg have "traced the historical development of occupational therapy groups since that time. They found that the following factors influenced the use of group treatment: (a) the enduring importance of occupation to health, (b) the ability to adapt group structures and goals

to the changing paradigms of treatment, (c) the importance of interpersonal relationships to wellness, and (d) the socioeconomic pressures that mold health care, such as the limited personnel or shrinking funds available to health care programs" (Duncombe, Howe, 1995).

Groups can be held anywhere. The most common sites for group treatment with elders are skilled nursing facilities, intermediate care facilities, adult day care programs, and assisted living facilities. This chapter demonstrates the use of groups in several settings where elders commonly gather. COTAs can apply the information in this chapter to use groups as a tool to meet individual goals for therapeutic programs. COTAs can also apply strategies for group planning, **facilitation,** and documentation.

BOX 14-1

Therapeutic Benefits of Groups

Power

The group is greater than the individual. By simple membership in the group, the participant gains strength.

Universality

As group members, participants realize they are not alone or totally unique. They are given the opportunity to acknowledge that they are "all in the same boat."

Sharing experiences

A group forum designed around member needs offers the opportunity for voluntary communication in a positive atmosphere. Members can easily learn about themselves and others.

Collective group identity

Attributes of each member blend together to form the group identity because members bring their positive and unique qualities to the group, making the group an aggregate. Members then reabsorb this positive sense of community membership.

Imparting information

Through verbal and nonverbal interaction, information is received and absorbed by members at their individual levels to meet their individual needs.

Instilling hope

Pessimistic and discouraged group members are encouraged as they observe improvement in others.

Unselfish concern for others

Through verbal and moral support exchanged between group members, participants can regain their sense of usefulness and importance.

Socialization and interpersonal learning

Through group interaction during nonthreatening tasks, members can practice offering positive rewards instead of negative judgment of others. Through role-modeling and practice, participants listen and respond to others in a manner that elicits the optimal response.

Expression of feelings

Group interaction allows members to openly express their thoughts and feelings.

Survivorship

Group membership helps participants feel satisfied that, despite all the pain and trauma they have endured in their lives, they are still alive and can be proud of themselves and their accomplishments.

Data from Burnside IM:*Working with the elderly: group process and techniques*, Monterey, Calif, 1984, Wadsworth.

MEETING INDIVIDUAL NEEDS WITHIN A GROUP SETTING

Many health care professionals have encouraged the use of groups for therapeutic activities. Irvin Yalom's work is the most prominent in group work and is often used as a basis for clinical application (Yalom, 1975). Burnside (1984), noted for her extensive work with elders, expanded Yalom's work on programs for elders. The principles identified by both Yalom and Burnside are helpful in providing motivation and justification for treating clients in groups (Box 14-1).

Referrals to Groups

Referral sources may include physicians, therapists, nursing staff, and others. Referral procedures for a specific group vary depending on the setting. A simple referral sheet can be used that includes the client's name, diagnosis, goals, and any other pertinent information such as safety issues (Table 14-1).

Groups can be planned and graded to accept elders with a wide range of physical and cognitive abilities. In many cases the more cognitively impaired participants require more staff assistance. If there is too wide a range in abilities, cognitively intact elders may either find a reason to leave the group or express displeasure with other participants. If the cognitively intact elders' confidence and attention cannot be regained by expanding their responsibilities, it may be more appropriate to excuse them from the group.

Setting Individual Goals Through the Group Process

Therapeutic goals of OT groups can be placed into three general categories: physical, cognitive, and **psychosocial.** Physical goals may be to increase mobility and range of motion and to improve strength and endurance. These goals may be met through group activities that require fine and gross motor movements. Cognitive goals such as improvement of memory and attention span, initiation of activity, orientation, and problem-solving can be addressed through reminiscence, games, and task groups. Appropriate social conduct, self-expression, and interpersonal skills are planned effects of the group interaction process. The added dimension of the social contact offered by groups cannot be duplicated in any other setting.

Even the simplest groups can provide positive individual therapeutic benefits for all members. With basic planning and appropriate facilitation, the leader orchestrates a setting and opportunities for interaction that are appropriate for all participants. For example, in a group of clients making wooden toys for underprivileged children, one elder could be working on increasing range of motion while sanding and reaching for heavy tools. Another elder could be working on increasing memory by

TABLE 14-1

Group Treatment Referral Form

			Cooking group	
Name	Diagnosis	Primary therapist	Safety precautions	Treatment considerations
R.W.	R CVA	Jan	Impulsive; Max A transfer; L neglect	Attend to L side. Use L hand for assistance.
G.H.	L CVA	Jan	Aphasic; flaccid R UE; no sensation	Follow 2-step directions. Maintain R arm in protected and functional position.
A.A.	Arthritis	Peter	Pain	Use joint protection techniques and adaptive equipment.
M.I.	R hip	Terri	Replacement posterior approach	Total hip precautions for posterior approach. Participate in meal preparation while maintaining full hip precautions.
H.L.	Diabetes R BK amp.	Sue	Decreased vision and sensation in fingers	Teach tactile discrimination and safety. Provide adaptations for decreased vision.

assembling a train engine. A third elder, whose goal is to learn to identify objects through touch to compensate for visual loss, may test whether the wood pieces are smooth enough to be safely handled by children. Yet another elder who is feeling hopeless may benefit from interaction and group process by sharing childhood experiences involving toys.

ORGANIZATION OF GROUPS WITH ELDERS
Open and Closed Groups

COTAs must make a distinction between **open groups** and **closed groups.** The setting generally dictates which type of group is used, and knowing the advantages of both types is helpful when planning activities.

Closed groups are most often found in adult day programs or long-term care facilities. The same members participate in each closed group session. Space is reserved for those who may occasionally miss a session. The advantage of closed groups is the progression of goals and growth of activities that can be planned. The internal development of personal attachments and friendships is an added benefit. An example of a closed group at a day program is one in which elders contribute to and publish a monthly newsletter. The group establishes the subject matter ahead of time and meets regularly to produce the monthly publication.

Open groups are common in almost every setting that includes work with elders. Open groups accept any appropriate elder who is available to attend. Each session changes in size and membership. These groups require reintroduction and discussion of purpose at each gathering. There is less opportunity to promote high interpersonal interaction. The ability to accommodate any available elders is an advantage of open groups.

Preparation for Groups

Group size is generally determined or limited by the number of COTAs and co-leaders available to help. A rule of thumb is one leader per four to five participants. Although one leader may be able to coordinate group tasks for more than four members, a group co-leader is necessary to handle unexpected demands such as lability or sudden illness. If a member creates a disturbance or departs from the group, the primary leader should continue with the group.

Space should be prepared before the group begins. The area should be well lighted and have wheelchair-accessible tables or space. All group members should have adequate space to move about. Elders with hearing impairments should be encouraged to sit closer to a leader so that information can be more easily heard or relayed. Another group member may also be relayed. (See Chapter 18 for detailed information on working with elders who have hearing impairments.)

All materials should be readily available. The leader should make adaptations before the session for elders who are unable to perform all parts of the task. Conversely, meeting the therapeutic goals of some higher-level participants may include using their help in preparing, planning, and setting up the group.

For a group whose goal is to prepare a fruit salad, a list of ingredients should be printed and enlarged or written on a wipe-off board. Ingredients should be gathered and prepared for assembly. For example, bananas are easy to peel but difficult to get started, so the leader may nick the ends of the bananas ahead of time. Appropriate equipment should be available, including nonslip placemats, cutting boards, melon ballers, and large-handled mixing spoons and knives. In anticipation of spills, COTAs should have a plastic tablecloth, washbasins, and plenty of towels available. In the case of any group activity involving food, COTAs should plan a hand-washing method for participants. For sanitary reasons, latex gloves may be used. As with any group, safety must always be considered. COTAs should also make sure that elders do not consume any contraindicated foods.

STAGES OF GROUP PROCESS

Group process is the organized interaction of a planned gathering of people for a set length of time. The five stages to organize group process, described by Ross and Burdick (1981), provide a solid basis for group organization.

1. Opening or introduction to the group. This stage can be lengthy because of the time required to assemble the members in the designated space. Small talk is exchanged, and members are introduced. In this stage the leader stays with the group. The co-leaders gather additional members, move chairs, and run last-minute errands. The leader determines when the group is sufficiently assembled and continues the opening in a more official manner, addressing the whole group. Opening phrases may include orientation statements such as, "Welcome to the News at Noon Group. This group meets every day just before lunch to discuss local, regional, national, and international news from the past 24 hours."

   The leader should introduce all members of the group. In open groups an effective method of gaining attention and providing visual focus on each individual is a balloon or ball toss. When the balloon comes to the members, they introduce themselves and tell a news item they would like to discuss. The balloon toss also provides a gentle warm-up and range-of-motion exercise.

2. Movement. This transitional phase can be graded to meet the needs of the group. Generally the movement should be purposeful and may have components of strengthening. Thus movement could be playing balloon volleyball or throwing weighted objects such as beanbags.

3. **Perceptual integration.** Perceptual activities include sensory stimulation and visual perceptual challenges. These activities are cleverly disguised as different games. Throwing or kicking balls at targets, such as a Hula-Hoop or wastebasket, can be fun and competitive. These skills can be generalized to daily living activities such as tossing laundry into a hamper.

4. **Cognitive function.** All therapy groups include the goal of organizing thought processes. Thus no group should lose the opportunity to challenge each member cognitively. Again, this is easily blended with goals from the movement and perceptual integration stages. All forms of games, crafts, discussion, reading, and writing require cognitive attention.

5. Closing. Closing provides a summary or wrap-up. It can be as simple as thanking the participants for coming or as complex as a verbal summary that includes a plan for the next group. Closing may also involve an activity. As this stage evolves, group members may finally become aware that they are participating in a process. An example of closing a group after a balloon toss could be to ask each member to choose a color of balloon that represents a positive attribute of another member. As with any stage, closing is an important time for the leader to make observations. Group members will likely be alert and relaxed. They will feel comfortable with each other and their accomplishments. This is when the leader can set up **therapeutic interactions** between members. If additional time is beneficial to particular members, the leader can stay with them, allowing the co-leaders to help the other group members leave.

COTAS AS GROUP FACILITATORS WITH ELDERS

COTAs must observe, listen to, and make eye contact with each group member. Members feel included and important when they receive individualized attention, even if it is brief. COTAs can observe for distractions, decreased interaction, and nonverbal signs of decline in participation such as droopy eyes. A gentle touch or question can redirect participants to the group.

Flexibility is the key to successful group management. Although an agenda may be planned well ahead of time, any number of events can force changes in the plan. For example, one member may make a suggestion for an activity the leader had not anticipated. Astute COTAs may recognize this as a more valuable activity and welcome the idea. The planned activity can be diverted or modified accordingly, with a better outcome for the group. For example, COTAs may have planned a task group to assemble a puzzle when a group member comments that he has received an absentee voter ballot that is due soon. He requests the group discuss the voter pamphlet for clarification of the issues. A current events discussion may be desirable with this group, and the puzzle could easily wait for another day. COTAs should quickly assess the group's goals and determine whether all members would benefit from the change in task if members are agreeable.

If switching from a task group to a discussion group such as in the above example does not seem appropriate, a good response may be to validate the needs of the requesting member. Those issues can be addressed in a later discussion group or during a one-to-one interaction. The successful group leader keeps in mind that all group processes and activities are for the benefit of the participants. Group leaders are motivators and should remain open and flexible without a personal agenda (Stoedefalke, 1985).

The COTA must understand the interaction of the group leader and the co-leader. For the benefit of individual group members, the designated leader directs the group agenda. The co-leader is available to assist as needed. The co-leader may assist in adding and removing supplies, helping participants with difficult tasks, or taking a group member to and from the restroom. When group leaders are aware of each other's leadership strengths and styles, leading groups becomes smooth, effortless, and fun. Co-leaders are often helpful in large groups. Unfortunately, sometimes a co-leader is not available, and COTAs must be prepared to adapt the task, modify the goals, exclude some members, or refuse to lead a group that may present an unsafe situation.

Recruiting Group Participants

Cooperation for OT groups begins during the evaluation process. At that time the OT practitioner should explain the ways that each group can help elders meet personal goals. The practitioner should also inform group members and facility staff of the group schedule ahead of time to avoid conflicting appointments. Group notices and schedules can be posted on bulletin boards and in newsletters. Large letters and good color contrast help attract attention to the sign and allow elders with vision impairment to read it.

Verbal reminders can provide an opportunity for additional social interaction between leaders and members. A delicate balance exists between encouraging elders to participate and honoring their rights to refuse. Good clinical reasoning is necessary to determine why an elder refuses to participate. Is the elder depressed or afraid of failure? Has the elder been offended by the leader or other members? Is the task meaningless to the elder? Does the elder prefer solitary activities? Is the elder ill? COTAs should not make assumptions regarding the refusal and should confirm their conclusions with the elder.

Often a positive approach is the most successful way to encourage group participation. For example, a statement of fact such as "The activity group starts in an hour," may be met with more positive reception than a closed-ended question, such as, "Would you like to come to group?" In addition, emphasizing the elder's particular contribution to the group may be helpful, such as, "We are looking forward to your artistic touch on our collage," or, "We need a strong arm to churn the butter." Participants should always be treated with integrity and as individuals. Even the most cognitively disabled person can detect infantilizing treatment.

TYPES OF GROUPS

Groups may be focused on tasks or discussion. In task groups, also known as *activity groups*, participants create or prepare something. Discussion groups, also known as *verbal groups*, emphasize cognitive activity. Current events or reminiscence groups are examples of this type of group. Both types of groups should be designed to meet participants' therapeutic goals (Box 14-2).

BOX 14-2

Ideas for Groups

Sports
  Olympics
  Wheelchair olympics
  Balloon volleyball
  Stretching
Woodcrafting
  Toys
  Picture frames
  Transfer boards
Pets
Music
  Piano or guitar sing-alongs
  Rhythm band
  Name that tune
Sensory
  Fragrances
Circus
Celebration/holidays
  Masks
  Pumpkin carving
  Labor Day (jobs)
  Weddings
Food
  Apples: pie, sauce, carved, dried figures
  Taffy
  Pizza
Gardening
  Flowers, herbs
  Digging in the dirt
Puzzles
Stamping
  Rubber stamp, potato stamp
Tea parties (or espresso)
Community skills
Relaxation
Discussion
  Current events
  Politics
  Reminiscence
  Life review
  What's this old thing? (antique store item)
  Occupations

Task Groups

Task groups vary in complexity according to participants and settings. Ideas for tasks include meal preparation, gardening, sewing, and other crafts. Group projects such as preparing butter, ice cream, jelly, bread, and soup are highly successful with elders, who remember participating in these activities when they were younger. The demand for sequencing of these familiar tasks increases the level of arousal and attention, thus improving cognition. In addition, participants may take on more of a leadership role when they are familiar with the task.

Task groups, which include fabricating gifts for others, can help meet psychosocial goals. Cookie making and gardening can yield meaningful gifts and allow participants to give of themselves.

Discussion Groups

Discussion groups need less equipment and advance preparation time than activity groups. They also require a different style of leadership. Discussion groups work best if kept small to allow participants to hear each other and to decrease the sense of vulnerability that might inhibit sharing. Verbal groups can be easily dominated by one person, so COTAs have to gently redirect questions to those participants who are reluctant to speak. Some groups begin with a general discussion of a current news item and progress to a comparison with past or similar news items. Newspapers often carry summaries of news from 25 or 50 years ago. Another option is to begin with a selected topic such as an upcoming holiday or sporting or political event. The group can even watch and discuss a clip from an old movie.

COTAs must remain patient and allow participants time to think of answers and respond (Hesse, 1983). If elders do not have sufficient time to respond, they may no longer attempt to participate, thereby losing the benefit of the interaction. The group leaders are responsible for knowing each group member's name and engaging each member at an appropriate level (Figures 14-1 and 14-2).

Group Protocols

According to Early (1993), the four main purposes of group protocols are as follows: "To communicate with other staff who may refer elders to the group; identify elders who might benefit from the group; clarify goals, methods, and the COTA's role as leader; and measure achievement of individual goals which may or may not be realized by the end of the group." These protocols can be as simple or complex as needed to meet the demands of the members, setting, and group leaders. Group protocols should include the title of the group, source, description rationale, group goals, selection criteria, group structure, environment, equipment, leader's role, session formation, variations, and expected outcome (Box 14-3).

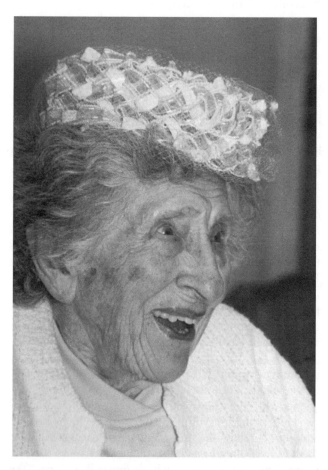

FIGURE 14-2. Participation in group tasks has the potential to arouse an elder's attention. This elder, who is participating in a Hat Group, enjoys seeing herself in a hat similar to one she wore as a younger woman. (Courtesy Yvonne Laulainen.)

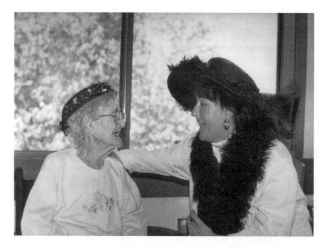

FIGURE 14-1. The COTA (right) must participate in the group task (in this case, a Hat Group), along with members. (Courtesy Yvonne Laulainen.)

BOX 14-3

Group Protocol Example

Title of group
Hat group

Source
Sherry Hoff

Description rationale
By selecting and donning vintage hats, group participants receive physical, cognitive, social, and emotional stimulus. The selection of a hat involves concentration and decision-making skills. Placing the hat on the head and adjusting it to the right angle requires upper extremity function, especially shoulder flexion. Discussion of the chosen hats and others the participants might have worn in the past evokes memory and reminiscence. Participants can be encouraged to attend to their appearance by looking at themselves in the mirror, adjusting the hat, and fixing their hair. Strange hats prompt laughter if worn by persons such as the group leader, and all hats promote social interaction.

Group goals
1. Group members will use functional upper extremity motor tasks to retrieve hats from a table and place them on their heads.
2. Group members will make cognitive choices in their selection of appropriate hats, including color, size, and shape.
3. Group members will demonstrate environmental spatial relationships as they place the hats on their heads and then adjust the angle.
4. Group members will use long-term memory to recall hats worn by themselves and others.
5. Group members will address their own self-expression by visualizing themselves in the mirror wearing the hats and commenting on their feelings.
6. Group members will interact socially through nonverbal communication, acknowledging others in their hats.
7. Group members will exercise appropriate social conduct while waiting their turns to try on hats.

Selection criteria
This activity can be used with elders in all settings with a large or small group. Group members who are able to speak or use their upper extremities can feel and look at the hats on their heads.

Group structure
Size: Five group members for every COTA or co-leader.
Length of session: 50 to 60 minutes or as tolerated.
Duration: Single session repeatable with seasonal changes.

Environment
Well-lighted room with space for participants and wheelchair mobility. Hats are placed on tables for easy viewing or hidden and brought out one at a time.

Equipment
Twice as many assorted hats as male and female participants. Several mirrors, the larger the better.

Leader's role
The leader (who is wearing a hat) is in the group space when the first elder arrives. The leader engages all participants with one another as they are brought in by other staff. Interaction may be in the form of conversation or balloon or ball toss. When all participants arrive, or when the leader decides the time is right, the leader opens the session by welcoming the participants, and explaining the course of events. The leader facilitates the co-leaders in helping participants try on various hats and examine themselves in the mirror. The leader promotes conversation by prompting talk about individual hats and similar hats the elders may have worn.

Session format
Co-leaders bring the participants into the area where the group is to take place. They are seated in a circle or around tables. The session continues as described above. The co-leaders help elders place hats on their heads and view themselves in the mirror. The co-leader facilitates conversation among the group members. Co-leaders are available to meet unexpected needs of the group participants. Food may be offered, such as punch and cookies, if appropriate.

Co-leaders assist the elders from the group space. Active conversation among co-leader, leader, and participant can continue after the session is over.

Variations
The hat group can also be in an Easter Parade format and works well with large groups. The leader introduces elders individually and describes the hats being worn, like in a fashion show. The leader may choose to describe the hat by comparing it with a hat worn in a famous movie (for example, *Casablanca*, *The African Queen*, *and Mary Poppins*). Applause is encouraged at each presentation.

Expected outcome
Elders will be able to respond to hats of other eras of their lives. They will be able to use their normal body movements to pick up the hats and place them on their heads. They will adjust the hats using mirrors. Elders will communicate their thoughts about the hats and interact with one another.

SUMMARY

The use of groups as a modality for treating elders is not only in keeping with the basic philosophy of the profession but offers the opportunity to address a wide range of treatment goals. COTAs as leaders and guides can demonstrate creativity and flexibility in helping participants meet their individual goals in a setting of empowerment and community.

■ CHAPTER REVIEW QUESTIONS

Della, a 78-year-old widow, has been depressed and withdrawn. She is brought to an adult day center three times a week by her daughter, who wants her mother to be around other elders of her age. Before Della's retirement, she worked as a cook at a grade school for 30 years.

1 Using Yalom's principles, identify two therapeutic factors that would provide justification for Della's participation in a cooking group.
2 How could Della benefit from a closed group?
3 One of the COTA's roles as group facilitator is to motivate clients. How would you motivate Della to participate if she seemed hesitant?
4 Della has been attending the cooking group on a regular basis. She indicates interest in attending a discussion group that focuses on life review. A participant who regularly attends this group is a recent widow who cries frequently and has been disruptive in the past. How would you encourage Della to support that other participant?

5 Identify four activities that would be appropriate for a closed group and explain your choices.
6 Identify four activities that would be appropriate for an open group and explain your choices.
7 Why is it important for COTAs and co-leaders to communicate effectively?
8 Explain how a written group protocol can benefit COTAs and other staff members.

REFERENCES

Burnside IM: *Working with the elderly: group process and techniques,* Monterey, Calif, 1984, Wadsworth.

American Occupational Therapy Association: Occupational therapy roles, *Am J Occup Ther* 47:1087, 1993.

Duncombe LW, Howe M: Group treatment: Goals, tasks, and economic implications, *Am J Occup Ther* 49(3): 199, 1995.

Early MB: *Mental health concepts and techniques for the occupational therapy assistant,* New York, 1993, Raven Press.

Hesse KH: Motivating the geriatric patient for rehabilitation, *J Am Geriatr Soc* 31(10): 586, 1983.

Meyer A: The philosophy of occupational therapy, *Am J Occup Ther* 31: 639, 1977.

Mosey AC: *Three frames of reference for mental health,* Thorofare, NJ, 1970, SLACK.

Ross M, Burdick D: *Sensory integration,* Thorofare, NJ, 1981, SLACK.

Stoedefalke KG: Motivating and sustaining the older adult in an exercise program, *Top Geriatr Rehabil* 1(1): 78, 1985.

Yalom ID: *The theory and practice of group psychotherapy,* ed 2, New York, 1975, Basic Books.

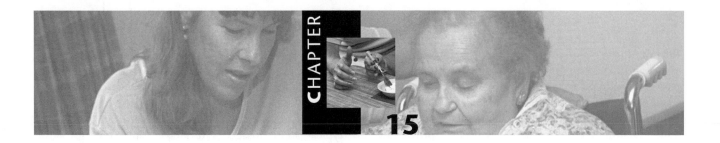

CHAPTER 15

Use of Medications by Elders

BARBARA **F**LYNN AND **B**RENDA **M**. **C**OPPARD

KEY TERMS

self-medication, over the counter (OTC), PRN, polypharmacy, delirium, adverse drug
reactions (ADRs), drug interactions, pill box, medication diary

CHAPTER OBJECTIVES

1. Define polypharmacy and identify recommended interventions to diminish drug-related problems of polypharmacy in elders.
2. Identify factors that predispose elders to adverse drug events and discuss strategies to detect medication problems.
3. Identify classes of medications commonly associated with adverse drug reactions in elders.
4. Identify common symptoms of adverse drug reactions in elders.
5. Identify and describe skills needed for safe self-medication.
6. Explain the ways that adaptive devices help compensate for skills needed for safe self-medication.
7. Describe elder and caregiver education needs regarding self-medication.

Holly, a COTA working in a long-term care facility, asked the facility's consulting pharmacist to review one of the client's medications. The client, Miss Albert, had been falling frequently and seemed tired and confused. Holly wondered if any of Miss Albert's medications might be causing problems.

The pharmacist reviewed Miss Albert's chart and found that the medications were contributing to her falls and changes in mental status. Holly was wise to be concerned about Miss Albert's medications, especially because one of her falls resulted in a hip fracture. Elders tend to be very sensitive to drug effects. If Miss Albert's medications had not been adjusted, her progress in OT may have been hindered.

COTAs often work with elders on a daily basis in a variety of treatment settings. Because COTAs spend a considerable amount of time with the elder population, they are a valuable asset in addressing medication routines. COTAs also may convey vital information regarding medications and side effects to the health care team. Common medications and medication-related problems encountered by elders are discussed in this chapter. Skills for **self-medication** and intervention programs for elders and caregivers are also discussed. More specific medication information is available from textbooks such as *Physician's Desk Reference* and *Physician's GenRx*.

Elders have many chronic and debilitating illnesses. Therefore they use many medications to manage these conditions. It is estimated that elders consume more than 40% of all **over-the-counter (OTC)** medications (Lucas, Noyes, Stratton, 1995). Elders living in long-term care facilities tend to take more medications than those residing in the community. For example, elder women residing in the community have been estimated to use five routinely administered and three as needed (prn) medications daily (Lucas, Noyes, Stratton, 1995). Elders in long-term care facilities may take seven to eight routinely administered medications and several prn medications (Avorn, Gurwitz, 1995).

MEDICATIONS COMMONLY PRESCRIBED FOR ELDERS

COTAs should always check the medication sections of elders' medical records to determine which medications are being used. This information helps COTAs be aware of possible side effects and drug interactions that might be observed in clinical treatment. COTAs should contact the elders' physicians and pharmacies with any medication-related concerns or questions. (Common drug-related abbreviations and definitions are listed in Table 15-1.)

Medications commonly prescribed for elders include those used to manage chronic diseases such as high blood pressure, diabetes, arthritis, and depression. Cardiovascular drugs (digoxin, diuretics, high blood pressure medications, medications for chest pain, and blood thinners), hypoglycemic agents (insulin and oral agents), gastrointestinal agents (antacids, laxatives, and antiulcer medications), and analgesics and antiinflammatory agents are commonly prescribed (Hussar, 1991). Antianxiety and antipsychotic medications are frequently used to manage behavioral disturbances such as psychosis, anxiety, and dementia caused by Alzheimer's and other diseases. Psychosis is thought to affect up to 38% of elders who live in long-term care facilities. In addition, 20% to 50% of these elders are estimated to receive an antipsychotic medication (Frederickson, Boult, 1995).

TABLE **15-1**

Common Drug-Related Terminology	
Abbreviation	**Definition**
po	By mouth
qd	Once daily
bid	Twice daily
tid	Three times daily
qid	Four times daily
prn	As needed
IM	Intramuscular (injection into the muscle)
IV	Intravenous (injection into the vein)

Inappropriate Medication Use

One of the most frequently overlooked aspects of drug therapy is periodic reevaluation. Often medications intended for short-term therapy are not discontinued. With elders, drug dosages may be excessive. Some elders benefit from starting with one third to one half of the typical adult dosage. The adage "start low, go slow" certainly applies to initiating medications with elders.

Elders *must* know the medical reason for every medication they are receiving. Surprisingly, this basic information frequently is not conveyed to elders, their families, or other members of the health care team. Some medications are prescribed for multiple diagnoses. Diuretics, for example, have multiple indications for use. Is the individual receiving a diuretic for high blood pressure or to manage congestive heart failure? The medical reason for use of the drug is vital information to all persons involved in the elder's care.

Polypharmacy

Polypharmacy is the term for the use of many medications by one person. It not only increases the cost of drug therapy dramatically but also increases the incidence of adverse side effects. Polypharmacy may occur when several physicians are caring for one person and communication between them is limited. Confused elders may not be able to give accurate medication-related information. Polypharmacy may also result when elders misunderstand directions about the use of medications. For example, when a currently prescribed medication is ineffective and a new drug is initiated, elders may not understand that they are to stop taking the initial medication.

Adverse Drug Reactions

Given the complexity of drug regimens, it is not surprising that elders are prone to **adverse drug reactions** (ADRs) and **drug interactions.** Lucas, Noyes, and Stratton (1995) estimated that 39% of persons hospitalized for ADRs and 51% of deaths caused by ADRs occurred in elders older than 60 years of age. (Medications and common side effects are listed in Table 15-2.)

Many factors are involved in the increased incidence of drug toxicity in elders. With aging, kidney and liver functions decline. Many medications are excreted by the kidney and metabolized, or degraded, by the liver. Therefore changes in organ function may frequently lead to increased drug accumulation in the body. This accumulation leads to ADRs, which in elders are commonly manifested by constipation, incontinence, confusion, memory loss, restlessness, falls, and depression. Movement disturbances, which are called *extrapyramidal syndromes,* may also occur in elders receiving antipsychotic medications.

Elders are more sensitive to the effects of certain medications such as narcotic analgesics, blood thinners, and heart medications. Any medication that has central nervous system side effects may become problematic because of this increased sensitivity in elders.

Many medications prescribed for elders may impair functional capabilities. Drug-induced **delirium,** for example, is characterized by an acute and reversible confusion state (DeMaagd, 1995). Because of the prevalence of this side effect, OT practitioners must be familiar with drugs that may cause delirium in elders. COTAs should discuss any mental changes they witness with the other members of the health care team. Medications reported to cause delirium include antihistamines, antipsychotics, antianxiety agents, antidepressants, and seizure medications. High blood pressure medications, analgesics, antibiotics, cardiac drugs, drugs used to treat or prevent ulcers, and drugs used in managing Parkinson's disease may also induce drug delirium. Delirium usually resolves with discontinuation of the involved medication.

The risk for falls is greatly increased because of medications commonly prescribed to elders. Many of these medications cause dizziness, mental confusion, sedation, and changes in blood pressure, thereby predisposing elders to falls. The clinical consequences of falls can be very serious. (Refer to Chapter 16 for further discussion of the consequences of falls.)

Drug-Drug Interactions

Drug interactions may also affect functional status. Although common in elders, not all interactions are clinically significant. Drug interactions occur for several reasons. Interactions are more commonly based on the number of prescriptions and over-the-counter medica-

TABLE 15-2

Disease States, Medications, and Common Side Effects

Disease state	Medication	Common side effect

Hypertension	Diuretics
	    Bumex, Lasix
	Antihypertensives
	    Cardizem, Levatol, Lopressor, Procardia
		Dizziness, low blood pressure, fall risk, changes in electrolyte levels

Arthritis	Nonsteroidal antiinflammatory drugs (NSAIDs) Advil, Ascriptin, Feldene, Motrin, Naprosyn, Orudis	Stomach upset, ulcers, mental confusion, fluid retention
	Narcotic analgesics Darvocet, Darvon, Demerol, Empirin with codeine, morphine, Percocet, Tylenol with codeine, Tylox	Mental confusion, constipation, stomach upset
Depression	Antidepressants Anafranil, Asendin, Desyrel, Elavil, Norpramin, Pamelor, Prozac, Sinequan, Tofranil, Wellbutrin, Zoloft	Dizziness, low blood pressure with posture changes, mental confusion
Congestive heart failure	Digoxin, Bumex, Lasix, Aldactone, Dyazide, Maxzide	Mental confusion, weakness, slow heart rate, arrhythmias
Diabetes	Insulin Oral hypoglycemics Diabeta, Diabinese, Glucotrol, Humulin, Micronase, Orinase	Low blood sugar, dizziness

Anxiety/insomnia/
    psychosis/behavioral
    disturbances
	Antianxiety drugs
	    Atarax, Ativan, Buspar, Serax, Tranxene, Valium, Vistaril, Xanax
	Sedatives
	    Dalmane, Halcion, Restoril
	Antipsychotics
	    Clozaril, Compazine, Haldol, Loxitane, Mellaril, Navane, Prolixin, Risperdal, Stelazine, Thorazine
		Falls, sedation, unsteady gait, confusion, blood pressure changes

```
┌─────────────────────────────────────────────────────────────────┐
│  Resident: _____  Room #: _____  │
│  Consult requested by: _____  Date: _____  │
│  Therapeutic problem: _____ │
│  Consult completed by: _____  Date: _____  │
│  Could problem be drug related?  No _____                       │
│                                                                   │
│                                  Yes _____  (See recommendations)│
│  Recommendations:                                                 │
│  Drug therapy interventions (dosage reduction, drug discontinuation, switch to │
│  different drug, or other): _____ │
│                                                                   │
│  _____ │
│  Laboratory monitoring: _____ │
│                                                                   │
│  _____ │
│  Nursing monitoring: _____ │
│                                                                   │
│  _____ │
│  Other recommendations: _____ │
│                                                                   │
│  _____ │
│                                                                   │
│  Should you have any further questions, please contact the pharmacist completing │
│  this evaluation. Thank you.                                      │
└─────────────────────────────────────────────────────────────────┘
```

FIGURE 15-1. Interdisciplinary drug therapy consult form.

tions taken by elders. Age-related changes that predispose elders to adverse outcomes from drug interactions may also play a role.

Drug interactions occur by many different mechanisms. Some interactions involve cumulative effects when medications with similar side effects are used simultaneously. For example, antianxiety agents and narcotic analgesics both possess sedative properties, which may lead to excessive sedation if used together. Another drug interaction results when medications with opposing actions are used together. For example, use of an antiinflammatory medication such as Advil may cause fluid retention, thereby counteracting the diuretic effect of Lasix. Drug interactions may also result from declining organ capabilities in elders. Decreased liver and kidney function have already been mentioned. Other drug interactions involve depletion or accumulation of electrolytes such as potassium.

Detection of Medication Problems in Elders

Mental confusion is probably the most common medication side effect in elders. Other common side effects include dizziness, weakness, stomach upset, constipation, and difficulty with urination. Many disease states also may present with these symptoms. Clinical differentiation between disease and medication-related problems can be challenging. For example, mental confusion caused by medications can be misdiagnosed as Alzheimer's disease.

Detailed questioning about an elder's compliance with the drug regimen is critical. This questioning can be part of the OTR and COTA team's evaluation of activities of daily living (ADL) functions (American Occupational Therapy Association (AOTA), 1994). Many elders may customize their drug regimens without consulting a health care professional because of cost concerns or drug side effects. Elders should be questioned about the exact manner in which the medication is taken because many do not follow the directions printed on labels.

COTAs should consult other health care professionals about medication-related concerns. Optimal care involves a multidisciplinary approach. Such consultation may be initiated verbally or by written consultation when a pharmacist is not available (Figure 15-1).

SKILLS REQUIRED FOR INDEPENDENT SELF-MEDICATION

Even though medication routine is a performance area listed in "Uniform Terminology for Occupational Therapy" (AOTA, 1994) a person's ability to self-medicate is rarely addressed (Potts, 1994). This is evident in the lack of literature on self-medication programs and OT interventions with medication routines. Instruction in proper use of medication should be dealt with as part of ADL routines (Lewis, 1989). The performance area of medication routine includes "obtaining medication, opening and closing containers, following prescribed schedules, taking correct quantities, reporting problems and adverse effects, and administering correct quantities by using prescribed methods" (AOTA, 1994).

Various skills and abilities are needed for elders to medicate themselves safely and efficiently. In addition to a normal swallow (if needed), these skills may include manual dexterity, vision, hearing, memory, problem solving, motivation, ambulation/transportation, and communication.

Manual Dexterity

Usually a great deal of fine motor coordination, finger dexterity, and some degree of strength are needed to open and close medication containers. Fine grasp patterns are required when picking up pills or tablets. Therefore elders with conditions such as rheumatoid arthritis may have difficulty opening childproof containers.

Vision and Visual Perception

Visual perception skills may be required by elders who take multiple medications. Visual perception skills include color discrimination, depth perception, and figure-ground perception. Visual acuity and perception are required to distinguish between different containers of medication and to read instruction labels. If needed, glasses should be worn when elders self-medicate. Adaptations may be used to assist elders who have visual impairments (Figure 15-2). Magnifying lenses and large type or contrasting print may be helpful. For severe visual impairments, different size, different shape, or multicolor containers can be used for medication storage. Instructions for administration can be tape recorded to relay information that cannot be read. Depth perception skills are needed to obtain pills in a multipartition container. Figure-ground perception is also needed to see white pills in a white **pill box.**

Hearing

Approximately 31% of elders older than 65 years of age have hearing impairment (American Association of Retired Persons, 1994). COTAs should remember this when educating elders, family members, and caregivers. The ability to hear is important for elders to understand medication dosages and changes. COTAs should give both verbal and written instructions when educating elders. For example, Kathy, a COTA, meets with Vladimir, who has difficulty hearing, to review his discharge program. She first checks to make sure Vladimir is wearing his hearing aid and reviews the information in his client education packet. Kathy speaks slowly and clearly. She also frequently asks Vladimir whether he has any questions.

Memory

Both long- and short-term memory are required for independent self-medication. Elders need long-term

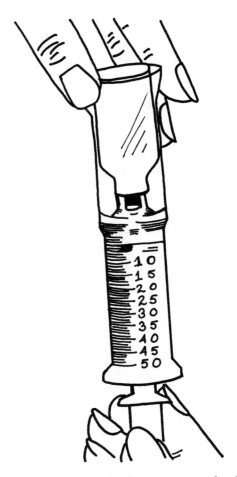

FIGURE 15-2. This magnifier device consists of a plastic cylinder in which the medication and syringe fit at each end and permit elders with visual impairments to view amounts easily.

memory to understand which condition is being treated. Understanding and remembering the nature of the regimen is also required for self-medication. Elders also need long-term memory to remember where the medication is stored. Short-term memory is needed to avoid under medication or overmedication. This frequently occurs when elders do not remember whether they took a medication. Various devices such as alarms and pill storage boxes can aid self-medication.

Problem Solving

A great deal of problem solving is needed to properly self-medicate. Elders must decide whether to contact the physician when changes in a condition occur. For example, Ken goes to his physician because he wonders whether his frequent headaches indicate that his blood pressure medication is not working or whether he needs a new prescription for his glasses. Problem-solving is also needed to determine when refills need to be obtained and how to safely store medication.

Motivation

Elders must be motivated to comply with their medication regimen. Depression, uncertainty, misunderstanding, financial worries, lack of confidence, side effects, and social or cultural taboos are all factors that may contribute to a lack of motivation. For example, Hazel, a 74-year-old woman with a history of angina and high blood pressure, sometimes takes her Procardia tablets only once a day instead of three times a day as prescribed. Hazel does this when she feels "better" to save money.

Ambulation and Transportation

Elders taking medications need to have a way of getting prescriptions filled on a regular basis. Elders who do not drive or are wheelchair-bound may seek community resources to obtain rides to medical appointments and the pharmacy. Some pharmacies will deliver medications for a fee. In addition, some communities have volunteer programs to provide this service at no cost. For example, Antonio is unable to drive because of his poor vision, but he is able to renew prescriptions by using a free transportation service provided by his church.

Communication

Elders must be able to communicate about their medication regimen with health care providers and caregivers. Health care providers must reciprocate communication in an effective manner. Demonstration, verbal, and written formats can be used for communication. Elders may find it helpful to keep names, phone numbers, and addresses of health care providers and agencies in a regular place so they are available for emergencies. For example, Greta has been deaf since birth but is able to communicate by using a notebook that contains information regarding her past and present medical condition. She stores this notebook in a drawer in the night stand by her bed. She has also notified family members where the notebook is located in case of an emergency.

ASSISTIVE AIDS FOR SELF-MEDICATION

Many commercial or homemade aids can assist individuals with self-medication (Meyer, 1993). Each aid has advantages and disadvantages.

Commercial Aids

Calendars. Calendars are helpful for tracking medication schedules. A pocket calendar or a calendar hung near the place where medication is taken can be used to mark each time medication is taken. At the end of the day, marks are counted to make sure the medication schedule was followed. The advantages of using a calendar are that the medications are stored in their original containers and remain properly labeled. Calendars are also inexpensive.

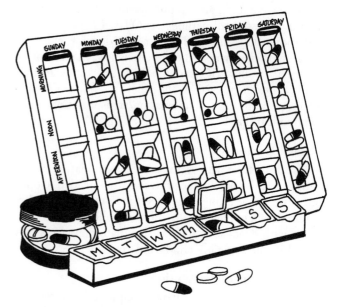

FIGURE 15-3. Various pill boxes are available with compartments for single or multiple daily and weekly doses.

The disadvantage of using a calendar is that it requires some basic reading, comprehension, and memory skills to mark the calendar each time medication is taken (Meyer, 1993).

Pill storage boxes. Storage boxes are containers with compartments in which to put medications (Figure 15-3). Storage pill boxes are available to organize medications for one day, one week, or one month. Pill boxes require manual dexterity skills to open and close and manipulate pills. Visual discrimination is also required to identify desired pills. Pill boxes usually do not provide tight storage for medications that require tight containers. In addition, the pills are no longer in labeled, childproof containers.

There are advantages and disadvantages for using daily and seven-day pill boxes (Meyer, 1993). An advantage of a daily pill box is a better chance of taking all daily doses. Any errors made in setting up this pill box would be experienced for only one day. A disadvantage of a daily pill box is that each compartment could contain several unlabeled pills. The elder would have to identify the medication by physical appearance. This is a serious safety concern if pills are similar in size or shape, especially if the elder has impaired vision or is easily confused.

Weekly pill boxes store medication for seven days. The design of some pill boxes allows separation of multiple daily doses. These boxes often consist of four rows and seven columns. The four rows are marked with times of the day (morning, noon, evening, bedtime), and the seven columns are marked with the day of the week. The advantage of using a seven-day pill box is that setup is required only once a week. The disadvantage is that setup

TABLE 15-3

	Contents of a Medication Diary
Section	**Information**
Section 1: Demographics	Name
	Date
	Address
	Phone number
	Date of birth
	Medication allergies: date of occurrence and type of reaction
	Vaccinations (year, date)
	Flu shots (year, date)
Section 2: Health care providers	List names and phone numbers of all health care providers (tape their business cards here).
Section 3: Past medications	List all medical conditions that required treatment with medication over the years.
	List all medical conditions that currently require treatment with medication.
Section 4: Special equipment	List all adaptive or special equipment required (such as a nebulizer, ostomy products, incontinence products). Include the brand, size, and model and the supplier's name and phone number.
Section 5: Recent medications	Enter the name of new medications used, the date, the reason the medication is being used, the strength of the medication, and how often the medication is taken each day.
	Keep track of any dosage changes, discontinuation, date, and the reason for the change or discontinuation.
Section 6: Over-the-counter medications	List any OTC medications used for the eye, ears, skin, and other organs and tissues.
	Enter how often it is used.
Section 7: Questions for health care providers	List any questions to ask the doctor or pharmacist.

requires more accuracy (Meyer, 1993). If there is a mistake, it may occur seven times.

A pill boxes with an alarm is an option for elders who must take their medication on time. The advantage of this type of pill box is that it alerts elders of the medication schedule. A disadvantage is that elders must be able to read, understand, and follow in-depth instructions. These devices often need to be programmed and may require very fine manipulation to set the clock or the alarm. If the device breaks, repairs may be difficult and expensive. Another disadvantage is the risk of not hearing the alarm when it sounds.

Homemade Aids

Medication diary. A **medication diary** is another aid for tracking medication use (Table 15-3). COTAs may assist elders in making a diary, which can be kept in a notebook.

Storage cups. Storage cups can be made at home by using small plastic or paper cups that are stacked and ordered according to the number of times the medication must be taken throughout the day. The cups should be marked in relation to when medications are taken (for example, morning, noon, dinner, and bedtime) (Figure

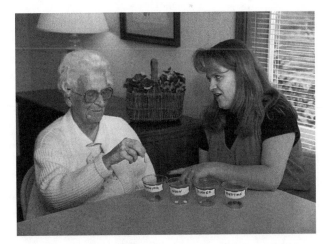

FIGURE 15-4. Storage pill cups can be made at home by simply using small plastic or paper cups.

15-4). After the morning medication is taken, the "morning" cup is moved to the bottom of the stack. This allows the next medication dose to be on the top. A similar system can be made using egg cartons. For liquid or powder medications, a system can be set up using small,

BOX 15-1

Guidelines for Caregivers Who Administer Medications

Elders most at risk to experience problems with medications are:

- Seeing many physicians
- Taking many medications
- Using many pharmacies

Keep track of the following information on the elder(s) you are caring for:

- *All* the prescription drugs the elder is taking
- *All* the nonprescription (OTC) drugs the elder is taking
- *All* other medicinal items the elder uses from a health food store or supermarket
- When and how much medicine to give
- What results to expect from the medicine
- Any physical or mental change in the elder (report to physician)
- What to do if a dose is missed

Prescriptions

The need for the medications should be reevaluated at least every 3 to 6 months. Do not save unused medication for future use without the physician's approval. Flush unused medication down the toilet. Do not share medications with anyone.

Do *Not* be satisfied with directions such as:

- Take as directed
- Take before meals
- Take as needed
- Take 4 times a day

Ask the pharmacist to put the specific directions on the label and to tell you exactly how to follow them

- What does 4 times a day really mean?
- Does it mean every 6 hours? Does it mean with meals and at bedtime?
- Can this medicine be taken with other medications?

To reduce the risk of aspiration and swallowing problems, *Never* give tablets or capsules while the elder is lying down. *Always* give medications with plenty of fluids to reduce stomach upset unless directed otherwise.

Medication storage

Store medications properly. If you count or measure medications, keep them in a cool, dry place, away from the sunlight and away from children. Keep the label on the medication container until all medicine is used or destroyed. If traveling, take the original medicine container with you in case of an emergency.

Take precautions with the following:

- Chewable tablets: Elders often do not like chewable tablets because they can interfere with dentures.

One option is to have the elder suck on the tablet to dissolve it. Chewable tablets should not be swallowed whole.

- Crushing tablets or opening capsules: Many pills should not be crushed because they are designed to be long-acting. Other pills should not be crushed because the contents may cause stomach upset.

Always check with the pharmacist. Occasionally a liquid substitute is available.

- Liquid medications: Because liquid medications are difficult to measure accurately, ask the pharmacist for a measuring device to ensure the correct dose.
- Applying ointments: Because medications applied to the elder's skin will have an effect on your skin, wash hands after each application. Use gauze or gloves to apply.
- Applying patches: Always remove old patches. Know how often and where to apply the patch on the body. Notify the pharmacist if the skin becomes irritated or the patch does not stick.
- Giving injections: Practice administration techniques with a nurse or pharmacist. Always draw up the dose in advance.
- Tube feedings: Tube feedings with medication require special instructions. Contact the pharmacist to know exactly how to give the medication.

Discharge plans from the hospital or nursing home

This can be a very confusing time! Medications often change while the elder is in the hospital. Everyone must know which medications to take and which *not* to take.

- Know about any generic drugs. Tablets or capsules may look different and have a different name, but the medications contain the same ingredient in the same amount. Know exactly what each generic medication is. Keep an accurate list or bring all the medications when visiting every doctor. Shop at one pharmacy to avoid medication duplication. If moving to another area, ask the pharmacist to forward your prescription records to your new pharmacist.
- Monitor the elder's nutrition, diet, and fluids. Pay attention to the elder's appetite and notify the physician if there are any concerns such as, weight gain or loss. Know whether the elder requires a special diet, including foods/liquids to avoid and to encourage. Administer medication by offering plenty of liquids, unless otherwise instructed.

Data from Simon GI, Silverman HM: *The pill book*, New York, 1986, Bantam Books; Parke-Davis Center for the Elderly, Elder Health Program, University of Maryland School of Pharmacy: *The caregiver's medication guidelines*, Morris Plains, NJ, 1995, Parke-Davis Elder Care Program.

labeled, air-tight containers. Using a homemade system is simple and inexpensive. However, using a homemade system may cause medication to be exposed to improper storage conditions (Meyer, 1993). Also, pills in open view may tempt small children who live in or visit the home. This risk can be reduced by storing the medication out of view.

SELF-MEDICATION PROGRAM

A formal self-medication program may help prevent problems with polypharmacy (Potts, 1994). The program is designed to (1) use an interdisciplinary team approach, (2) educate elders about their medications, (3) develop elders' motor skills for proper administration, (4) offer practice opportunities to elders, (5) assess elders for any adaptive devices that may be useful, and (6) evaluate elders' skills in medication administration before discharge.

The elder's treatment plan should include interventions to maximize independence with self-medication. Depending on elders' limitations and deficits, COTAs should engage them in simulated medication tasks. An example of such a task is using small colored candy pieces to practice color discrimination and fine prehensile patterns. Reading and comprehending general labels can aid in reading medication labels. Opening and closing medication containers should be practiced. In addition, elders should master any adaptive aids before being discharged from OT.

Relatives, friends, and home care personnel who assist in the delivery of medications have often not been included in discussions of medications (Wieder, Wolf-Klein, 1994). Family and caregivers should be able to name the elder's medications, describe the purpose of each medication, and describe any precautions associated with each medication (Box 15-1).

CASE STUDY

Polly Smith is an 83-year-old woman living at home with her 85-year-old husband. Polly is currently under the care of two physicians: her primary medical physician and a psychiatrist. A few weeks ago Polly fell and fractured her hip. Her mental status fluctuates. Her husband is in charge of administering medications. Her problems and medications are listed as follows in the table below:

Disease state	Medication
High blood pressure	Lasix (diuretic, or water pill)
Insomnia and anxiety	Ativan (antianxiety)
Rheumatoid arthritis	Aspirin (pain reliever)
Depression	Prozac (antidepressant)
Insomnia	Benadryl (nonprescription sleep aid)

CHAPTER REVIEW QUESTIONS

1 Which medication-related problems might be of concern to COTAs?
2 Could any of Polly's current medical problems be caused by her medications? If so, which medications cause which side effects?
3 What other factors may place Polly at risk for polypharmacy and medication-related problems?
4 The COTA is concerned about the frequency of Polly's falls and the risk of another hip fracture but is unsure whether any medications are contributing. What is a reasonable course of action to address this plausible medication-related concern?
5 What skills for safe self-medication are affected in Polly's case?
6 What assistive devices may help with her medication routine and why?
7 Who should be involved in a self-medication program to help Polly with her medications?
8 Considering the information in this chapter, explain why the COTA is an important player in the health care team to address medication issues with elders.
9 What are some reasons for polypharmacy among elders?
10 What is one side effect of each of the following: diuretics, NSAIDs, narcotic analgesics, antidepressants, digoxin, insulin, antipsychotics?
11 What is a common symptom of elders having adverse medication reactions?
12 What resources and personnel are available to address COTAs' concerns or questions about medications?
13 Explain eight skills needed for safe self-medication.
14 What aids are available to elders with poor vision, memory, or hearing, or lack of transportation?
15 What should be included in a medication diary?
16 What are some essential components to a self-medication program?
17 What information should COTAs provide to educate caregivers?

REFERENCES

American Association of Retired Persons: *A profile of older Americans,* Washington, DC, 1994, The Association.
American Occupational Therapy Association: Uniform terminology for occupational therapy—third edition, *Am J Occup Ther* 48:1047, 1994.
Avorn J, Gurwitz JH: Drug use in the nursing home, *Ann Intern Med* 123:195, 1995.
DeMaagd GA: Review of the pharmacologic causes of delirium in the elderly, *Cons Pharm* 10:461, 1995.
Frederickson TW, Boult C: Federal regulation and the use of antipsychotic medications in nursing homes, *Nurs Home Med* 3:41, 1995.

Hussar DA: *Drug interactions in the elderly*, East Hanover, NJ, 1991, Sandoz Pharmaceutical Corp.

Lewis SC: *Elder care in occupational therapy*, Thorofare, NJ, 1989, Slack.

Lucas DS, Noyes MA, Stratton MA: Principles of geriatric pharmacotherapy, *Clin Cons* 14, 1995.

Messner RL, Gardner SS: Drug interactions we all overlook: start with the medicine cabinet, *RN* 56(1):50, 1993.

Meyer ME: *Coping with medications*, San Diego, Calif, 1993, Singular Publishing Group.

Parke-Davis Center for the Elderly, Elder Health Program, University of Maryland School of Pharmacy: *The caregiver's medication-guidelines*, Morris Plains, NJ, 1995, Parke-Davis Elder Care Program.

Potts JM: Developing a patient self-medication program for the rehabilitation setting, *Rehabil Nurs* 19:344, 1994.

Simon GI, Silverman HM: *The pill book*, ed 3, New York, 1986, Bantam Books.

Wieder AJ, Wolf-Klein GP: When medications change, tell the caregiver, too, *Geriat* 49:48, 1994.

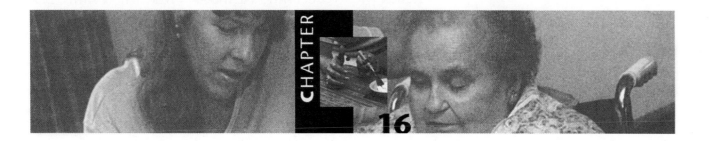

Considerations of Mobility

PART 1 **Restraint Reduction** KAI GALYEN
PART 2 **Fall Prevention** SANDRA HATTORI OKADA
PART 3 **Community Mobility** PENNI JEAN LAVOOT

KEY TERMS

restraints, restraint reduction, environmental adaptations, psychosocial approaches,
activity alternatives, fall prevention, aging in place, environmental hazards, mobility,
transit, driving, pedestrian, paratransit

CHAPTER OBJECTIVES

1. Discuss Omnibus Budget Reconciliation Act (OBRA) regulations pertaining to the use of physical restraints.
2. Describe steps in the establishment of a restraint reduction program.
3. Describe the role of the COTA in restraint reduction.
4. Identify three reasons that elder adults are at a higher risk for falls than the general population.
5. Identify environmental, biological, psychosocial, and functional causes of falls.
6. Describe the process of obtaining a fall history using the acronym "SLIPPED" to collect information.
7. Describe recommended interventions to prevent falls.
8. Discuss ways elders may gain access to public transportation.
9. Describe ways elders may become safer pedestrians.
10. Describe a driving evaluation, and identify criteria for this assessment.
11. Describe visual and physical changes in elders that may affect their ability to drive.

KAI GALYEN

PART 1   Restraint Reduction

HISTORY

Physical **restraints** have been used in this country since the 1700s to manage psychotic behavior. More recently, restraint use has been associated with cognitive impairment (Atkins, 1996). Until the late 1980s, use of restraints was almost universal in nursing homes (Eigsti, Vrooman, 1992). This practice was based on institutional tradition rather than on demonstrated benefit (Donius, Rader, 1994).

The literature indicates that restraints are essentially ineffective in eliminating serious injury secondary to falls and that they cause agitation, behavioral difficulties, and a myriad of problems associated with immobility (Rader, 1995; Stolley, 1995) (Box 16-1). Concern among health care professionals, consumers, and advocates for elders about these detrimental effects and the right of elders to self-determination, mobility, and dignity led to a movement for **restraint reduction** that contributed to the historical Nursing Home Reform Act, part of the Omnibus Budget Reconciliation Act (OBRA) of 1987 (Sullivan-Marx, 1995).

OBRA Regulations

OBRA was drafted to protect elders from abuse and promote choice and dignity. The ultimate goal is that each person reach his or her highest practical level of well-being. A reduction in the use of restraints is only a small part of this intent. OBRA requires caregivers to develop an individualized plan of care that supports each elder in the least restrictive environment possible (Health Care Financing Administration [HCFA], 1995). COTAs should become familiar with OBRA guidelines regarding restraints.

Two types of restraints are used: chemical and physical. Chemical restraints are drugs prescribed to control mood, mental status, and behavior for purposes of discipline or convenience rather than management of a medical condition. Physical restraints are any method, device, material, or equipment that is difficult to self-remove and restricts freedom of movement or normal access to one's

Acknowledgement: I wish to acknowledge Joanne Rader, RN, MN, FAAN, my mentor of "compassionate care," for her major contribution to the knowledge of individualized care. Gratitude to Joanne, Rod Galyen, RN, MN, and Maggie Donius, RN, MN, for their insightful perspectives and support. Also, a big thank-you to all my cohorts in OT, as well as to the administration of the Benedictine Nursing Center who made it possible for me to participate in this project.

body. Restraints are permitted only when they enable greater functional independence, restrict the elder from interfering with the provision of life-saving treatment, or are necessary because less restrictive devices have failed. A documented medical need and physician's order for restraints must exist. Clients must be released at least every 2 hours, and the restraints can be used only as a temporary intervention (HCFA, 1995).

In spite of these guidelines, improper use of restraints continues in the United States. COTAs have an ethical and legal obligation to report elder abuse, which includes using restraints as punishment for patients or as

BOX 16-1

Negative Effects of Restraints	
Psychosocial	**Physical**
Depression	Hazards of immobility
Lethargy	Incontinence
Withdrawal	Constipation
Anxiety	Disturbed sleep pattern
Distress	Loss of balance
Fear	Falls
Panic	Pressure ulcers
Anger	Bone demineralization
Agitation	Loss of muscle tone
Increased aggression	and mass
Reduced opportunity	Respiratory difficulties
for social contact	Pneumonia
Threat to identity	Infection
Embarrassment	Thrombophlebitis
Humiliation	Dehydration
Demoralization	Impaired circulation
Decreased feelings	Respiratory problems
of dignity	Orthostatic hypo-
Decreased sense of	tension
self-esteem	Decreased appetite
Decreased autonomy	Decreased ability to
Helplessness	care for self
Dependence	Abrasions
Regression	Cuts
Increased confusion	Bruises
Increased disorientation	Decreased functional status
Increased disorganized	Loss of freedom
behavior	Death caused by suffoca-
Broken human spirit	tion or strangulation

a convenience to staff. COTAs should also participate in educating others about restraints and may wish to initiate a restraint reduction program in their own facility.

ESTABLISHING A RESTRAINT REDUCTION PROGRAM

The move toward eliminating the use of restraints must be done in a gradual, planned, systematic way. Factors to consider include gaining administrative support, training staff, and developing strategies to assure that restraints become an unacceptable option in the facility.

Philosophy

A fundamental philosophical concept in the care of elders is the empowerment of both elders and staff. This empowerment is expressed in collaborative solutions to problems. The ability to contribute to solutions allows elders dignity and adds meaning and quality to their lives (Kari, Michels, 1991). Making choices, including the choice to take a risk, is an essential part of life and contributes to maintaining self-respect. Caregivers must recognize that decisions concerning risk must include input from even cognitively impaired elders (Rader, 1995). Caregivers have been indoctrinated with the concept that safety automatically includes the use of restraints (Mason, O'Connor, Kemble, 1995). After years of viewing restraints only as safety devices, caregivers find it difficult to accept that these measures are often unsafe. Caregivers may also have trouble accepting that freedom and choice precede safety in importance. We need to become elder centered rather than system or task centered (Kapp, 1991).

Policy

Administrative stability, involvement, and demonstration of support by the clear articulation of policy are essential to the success of any restraint elimination program (Mahoney, 1995). Research indicates that reducing restraints is cost effective, especially because of decreased medical complications from immobility and fewer serious falls (Bradley, Siddique, Dufton, 1995). Studies also indicate that reduction of restraints is usually accomplished with no additional staff (Bloom, Braun, 1991). Because restraints have been shown to be potentially harmful, litigation is more likely to occur from applying restraints than from withholding them. In addition, Medicare and Medicaid sanctions (such as decertification and even delicensure of the facility) are more likely to result from imposing restraints than from removing them (Kapp, 1991).

Education

Practitioners must teach these new concepts not only because they have been mandated by federal regulation but because, as Brungardt (1994) indicates, elders' func-

tion cannot improve "if they are tied down or drugged up." We should recognize that even those of us without dementia would not react positively to being restrained, even for our own good (Rader, 1995). Sullivan-Marx (1995) has likened the symptoms resulting from the trauma of restraint to post-traumatic stress disorder, learned helplessness, or battered-woman syndrome. Including the teaching of such concepts in a restraint reduction training program creates disequilibrium, which is necessary to change belief systems. Another teaching strategy is to provide practical and applicable information (Strumpf et al, 1992). Including an experiential component, such as applying a variety of restraints to participants, also adds to the effectiveness of the training. Few individuals can imagine choosing restraints as an appropriate intervention for themselves. Feeling the helplessness and degradation of being restrained sensitizes staff to the use of restraints on elders. Education should use and affirm participants' life experiences. Including board members, volunteers, and all facility employees (kitchen workers, bookkeepers, administration, chaplains, maintenance workers), in this educational program has been identified as a factor leading to decreased reliance on restraints (Janelli, Kanski, Neary, 1994). Kapp (1991) recommends mandatory training sessions provided on a continuing basis and introduction to this subject in orientation material.

Steps for Success

All members of the team, including families, staff from each shift, consultants, contract personnel, ombudsmen, state surveyors, physicians, and elders themselves, should be included in all stages of the program. Dialogue between these participants from the beginning makes the transition to restraint-free care much smoother. All team members play an important role. Family members can, for example, describe the elder's previous routines and preferences. Kari and Michels (1991) assert that Certified Nursing Assistants (CNAs) have essential knowledge of elders and that their usual lack of influence in decision making negatively affects the quality of care. CNAs may be the team members who first notice behavioral changes and the need for removal of restraints in elders (Janelli, Kanski, Neary, 1994). Strumpf et al (1992) indicate that respect for the dignity of their work is vital for any significant reduction in the use of restraints. An interdisciplinary team assessment of the need for restraint is helpful in reducing reliance on restraints (Mion, Mercurio, 1992).

A procedure outlining steps for implementing use of any restraint in a variety of situations should be developed. A committee should be formed to review existing and new requests for restraints (Atkins, 1996). In addition, restraints should be removed from the unit so that they are unavailable without consultation (Rader, 1995).

Most successful restraint-free programs have adopted

permanent staffing (Rader, 1996). This model assigns daily a "primary" CNA (and RN, housekeeper, therapist, etc.) to each elder. When these staff members are not working, they should have regular replacements. Permanence in staffing fosters relationships between elders, families, and staff that contribute to feelings of safety and connectedness and are particularly important to elders with cognitive impairment.

Interventions to eliminate restraint use should be individualized to produce a safer and more comfortable environment for elders. Individualized interventions are paramount to the quality and success of restraint elimination programs (Burgener, Shiver, Murrell, 1993). Mion and Mercurio (1992) suggest starting with an elder who has been identified as a good candidate for removal of restraints. Success will help staff members feel confident about continuing restraint reduction. Finally, each individualized intervention should be reassessed on a regular basis (Janelli, Kanski, Neary, 1994).

Rader (1995) has found that the biggest obstacles to eliminating restraints are our fears, biases, and unwillingness to change. She proposes that caregivers, clients, advocates, and regulators work together to create new interventions based on the elder's perspectives and wishes. Reducing restraints should be only the beginning of providing safe care in a dignified and less restrictive environment that promotes the elder's abilities (Werner et al, 1994).

ROLE OF THE COTA

In collaboration with an OTR, COTAs may assess the need for restraints, consult with staff about alternatives to restraint, and provide intervention to eliminate restraint use. Before restraints are used, supportive documentation is required regardless of the reason for restraint or the person who identified the need.

Assessment

Once need for intervention is documented and an occupational therapy order has been received, the OTR/COTA team performs an evaluation. Specific assessments of posture, alignment, balance, strength, and visual acuity are necessary. Assessments of head control, trunk stability, upper extremity support, and ability to self-propel are added to evaluate seating needs (Ericson, 1991). Perceptual and cognitive assessments should be included only as appropriate. Practitioners should not embarrass or agitate cognitively impaired elders by assessing areas already documented as deficient. However, before elders with multiple sclerosis can receive electric wheelchairs, they must demonstrate cognitive and perceptual skill adequate to operate the chair safely.

Consultation

The assessment often reveals minimal intervention needs, perhaps only consultation. Patterson, Strumpf, and Evans (1995) include the roles of advocate, observer, teacher, information specialist, team problem-solver, and identifier of resources and alternatives in their definition of *consultant*. They also report that the combination of consultation with formal restraint reduction training significantly reduces the use of restraints. COTAs are uniquely qualified to function as consultants in developing alternatives to restraints, especially if they are familiar with restraint reduction principles, OBRA regulations, and the basic principles of positioning. For example, an elbow air splint may be all that is necessary for an elder who continually scratches at sutures on a healing incision. Although an air splint certainly is restrictive, it allows more movement than wrist restraints, thereby meeting the criterion for "least restrictive environment." Because wound healing is temporary, the air-splint is a temporary measure. A protocol for use of the air splint should be provided. The care plan should document the reason that the splint is being used, the way it will be used, and the way it will be reassessed by nursing staff.

COTAs may recommend other environmental, psychosocial, and activity-related alternatives (Box 16-2). The alternatives outlined are not a complete list. Options are limitless, depending on the COTA's creativity. Each measure considered should provide as much free choice and control as possible for elders. Eigsti and Vrooman (1992) claim that the basic ingredient in reducing restraint use is teaching staff to understand and believe that alternatives exist.

Environmental Adaptations

Environmental adaptations are an important source of restraint alternatives. For example, many different styles of chairs are found in nursing homes. The one selected must be comfortable both physically and emotionally for the elder. However, replacing a belt or vest restraint with a reclined chair from which the elder is unable to rise is not an acceptable alternative. An inexpensive and less restrictive alternative for the confused elder who rises unsafely from a chair might be a personal alarm. Several such alarms are on the market. They do not prevent the elder from rising, but they do alert staff. An elder's attempt to rise usually occurs for a reason and warrants attention from the caregiver.

A wrap-around walker with a seat is an alternative device that allows independent ambulation for some elders who would otherwise require assistance (Kerr, 1994) (Figure 16-1). It can provide a means for safe and comfortable ambulation, allowing an elder who previously sat alone all day the opportunity to engage in social interaction and exercise. With supporting documentation, this walker should be interpreted as a beneficial orthotic device. If it makes the elder feel confined or agitated, however, it is considered a restraint.

Many facilities have discovered that nursery intercoms are an inexpensive and effective way to monitor safe

BOX **16-2**

Alternatives to Restraints

Environmental adaptations

Chairs
Deep seats
Tilted
Recliners
Rockers
Gliders
Bean bag
Adirondack type
Customized

Monitoring systems
TV monitoring
Enclosed courtyards
Alarms
  Exit alarms
  Door buzzers
  Nursery intercom
  Personal alarms
    Pressure sensitive pads
    Positional alarms
    Limb bracelet alarms

Signs
Directional
Stop or Keep Out
Identifying (elder's name)

Safety adaptations
Nonskid surfaces
Low bed
Mattress or sleep mat on floor
¾ to ½ length bed rails (instead of full length)
Lowered or no bed rail
Accessible call lights
Safe furniture arrangement
Accessible light switches
Safe walking routes
Encouraged use of handrail
Bedside commode or urinal
Items within reach
Shoes or non-skid socks worn in bed

Personalized room
Familiar furniture
Familiar objects to hold
Meaningful pictures and photographs

Other adaptations
Bean bags (different sizes)
Pillows
Foam
Nonslip mats
Firm wheelchair seats
Air-splints
"Wrap-around" walkers with seats

Psychosocial approaches

Behavioral strategies
Remotivation
Reality orientation (if helpful)
Frequent reminders
Active listening
Responding to agenda behavior

Decrease or increase
Interactions
Visiting
Sensory stimulation (especially noise such as that from
  overhead paging, TV, radio, etc.)
Identification of antecedent to the unwanted behavior and
  appropriate measures to address

Activities

Structured daily routines
Self-care
Permit or encourage wandering and pacing
Exercise
  Bowling
  Nature walks
  Wheelchair aerobics, dances, ballgames.
Ambulation Programs
Toileting every two hours
Night-time activities

Volunteer and family assistance
Buddy system
Activity kits
Diversional opportunities
Relaxation techniques
Massage
  Therapeutic touch
  Warm bath
  Music specific to elder

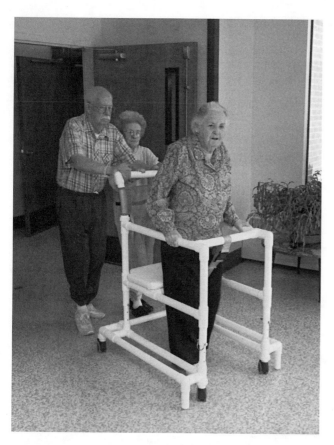

FIGURE 16-1 A wrap-around walker allows independent ambulation for this elder who would otherwise need assistance.

behavior provides a sense of identity and promotes feelings of belonging, safety, and connectedness, diminishing the elder's need to seek those feelings elsewhere. Further incidences of wandering are subsequently decreased or eliminated. Brungardt (1994) adds that this method works well if the elder's welfare is considered before the needs or routines of the facility.

Activity Alternatives

Providing meaningful **activity alternatives** can decrease behavior such as restlessness that has traditionally led to the use of restraints. An activity kit, perhaps in the form of a sewing basket, briefcase, fanny pack, or tackle box, may be helpful. The kit may be assembled by family members who are familiar with the elder's interests. (Rader, 1995). The idea is to provide something familiar, comfortable, and safe that engages the elder's attention.

Treatment

Although not all referrals require intervention beyond consultation, the assessment may identify a need for ongoing treatment. Examples of treatment to eliminate the need for restraint include development of self-care techniques, upper body positioning, and seating adaptations.

Because restraint use is associated with the inability to perform self-care, elders and their caregivers should be taught strategies for accomplishing this goal. Determining the routines the elder followed in the past to maintain a sense of continuity and predictability is particularly important. Because part of the objective is to reduce anxiety and agitation, self-care must be done according to the elder's agenda and routine rather than those of the COTA or facility.

Elders with hemiplegia are often provided with lapboards to assist with upper body positioning. Because these elders need the best support possible for their upper extremities, this is one of the few cases in which it may be advantageous to begin with the most restrictive device, a full lapboard, and adapt if necessary. If a full lapboard causes agitation or seems too restrictive (perhaps the elder is unable to use a urinal independently), a swing-away half laptray may be used. Another solution is a foam wedge or cylindrical bean bag, which can extend the width of the armrest for safe positioning without a lapboard. As with any restrictive device, however, less-than-perfect positioning may be necessary to accommodate the elder's choice.

Another specific occupational therapy intervention aimed at reducing the need for restraints is a positioning assessment for elders who are wheelchair bound. Ill-fitting wheelchairs contribute to restraint use, either of which can lead to abnormal sitting posture and eventual loss of function (Greenburg, 1996). For example, wheelchairs usually found in nursing homes were not designed for independent mobility or long-term sitting. Necessary

ambulators who wander. Directional signs may help these elders locate their rooms and deter them from entering someone else's room. Families should be encouraged to help elders decorate their rooms with familiar objects, pictures, and even furniture, which help elders feel more connected to their surroundings and reduce the likelihood of wandering.

Psychosocial Approaches

Psychosocial approaches to reduce restraint use are very important. Rader, Doan, and Schwab (1985) define *agenda behavior* as the plans and actions of cognitively impaired elders that result from an effort to fulfill physical, emotional, or social needs. The authors indicate that such behavior often follows feelings of loneliness or separation. Wandering or attempts to get up from a chair may be part of an elder's agenda behavior and lead to agitation if the elder is restrained. Rader (1987) indicates that the keys to responding successfully to agenda behavior are to allow elders to act on their plans, identify a point at which they may accept a suggestion or guidance, and allow them to keep their dignity throughout an incident. The important difference in the result of this approach compared with others is that allowing the elder to play out the adaptations for comfort and function include dropping the seat so that elders can reach the floor with their feet, replacing the sling seat with a firm seat and cushion, and replacing the sling back with a firm back. A narrower chair may help elders propel themselves more comfortably (Jones, 1995). Knowledge of the principles of positioning is essential. (Basic alignment principles applicable to any elder are outlined in Chapter 21.) Once adaptations have been designed and implemented, the elder's verbal, behavioral, and postural response must be observed. The system should be reassessed and adapted as necessary until the positioning goals have been met. Documentation should accompany every step of this process, especially if the elder declines the intervention. With very difficult cases, consultation with a seating expert may be helpful. However, even the nonexpert can make many "low-tech" foam supports.

Relatively inexpensive foam is available in large sizes at the local building or craft store and can easily be cut and shaped with an electric knife. This type of foam works well for the addition of width to an armrest, fabrication of forearm wedges to elevate edematous upper extremities, or provision of lightweight lateral trunk support. Egg crate foam is another inexpensive material suitable for limited purposes. Neither of these low-density foams are adequate to support entire body weight while sitting or during episodes of spasticity. For long-term positioning, manufactured cushions of mixed density foam, gel, or air

cushions are more durable and are recommended for both comfort and maintained skin integrity. The therapeutic role of orthotic devices in achieving proper body position, balance, and alignment and improving overall functional capacity without the potential negative effects of restraint use is recognized by HCFA (1995). This recognition does not provide license to use wedges, reclining chairs, or seat belts as restraints, even for cognitively intact elders. However, it does allow the legitimate use of positioning devices to increase function, given a demonstrated necessity. Any adaptation should maintain the dignity of elders and augment their quality of life.

CONCLUSION

COTAs have a responsibility to clearly state their professional opinion and recommendations. Clients must choose whether to act on that advice. True restraint reduction requires an examination of our attitudes about the rights of elders, especially those with cognitive impairment, to make choices and take risks. We must be willing to become advocates for elders. An understanding of OBRA regulations and positioning principles and the ability to be flexible and creative within a team framework permit COTAs to contribute effectively to restraint elimination programs. If we have honestly attempted to increase function and honor the dignity of the elders we serve, we will have followed not only the letter of the law but the intent and spirit as well.

SANDRA HATTORI OKADA

PART 2 **Fall Prevention**

COTAs must be aware of the high risk of falls among the elderly and the importance of **fall prevention**. Falls can be a major cause of immobility, premature nursing home placement, and even death. Some risk factors include a history of falls, neurological illness, multiple medications, poor eyesight, deconditioning, and age-related changes such as decreased protective responses. More importantly, delicate balance exists between biological and psychosocial factors and common environmental hazards. Therefore even a small disruption in this dynamic system can lead to a devastating fall.

Elders over the age of 75 suffer falls more frequently than any group except infants and toddlers. However, elders face a significantly greater risk of sustaining a severe or fatal injury. Accidents are the sixth leading cause of death for those over the age of 65, and falls are the leading type of accidents in the home (Hettinger, 1996).

Once a fall occurs, one elder out of 40 will be hospitalized (Campbell et al, 1981). Of those elders hospitalized after a fall, only about half will be alive 1 year later (Gryfe, Amies, Ashley, 1977; Rubenstein, Robbins, 1989).

Many falls may not be reported because of memory impairments and a lack of witnesses. Elders may fear being judged incompetent and sent to a nursing home. In addition, some elders may not consider stumbling and sliding off furniture actual falls or may think that falls are simply part of normal aging.

CAUSES OF FALLS
Environmental Causes

Accidents related to the environment are the primary cause of falls among elders (Tideiksaar, 1987; Rubenstein, Robbins, 1989). Approximately one third of falls occur in the home (Hettinger, 1996). About 30% of older adults

Knowing the location of the next step and judging its depth can become a big challenge. It is not surprising that 85% of all deaths resulting from stair accidents involve elders. The fact that 75% of all stair accidents occur while descending the stairs, most in the second half of the flight, is also noteworthy (Brummel-Smith, 1990). New bifocals or trifocals may require adjustment time, and looking down stairs requires constant head and eye adjustments.

Medical conditions affecting vision include macular degeneration, cataracts, diabetic retinopathy, glaucoma, and stroke. These conditions may manifest as scotomas (blind spots), which impair safety in mobility. Objects on the floor, such as pencils and telephone cords, may not be apparent. Elders with visual impairments may also run into furniture.

A disorder involving spatial organization or figure ground may cause an elder to perceive a change in rug color or flooring as a stair, and glare on the linoleum as spilled liquid. A dark stairway may be perceived as a ramp. Misinterpreting this information may cause a misjudged step and a fall. (Chapter 17 provides more detailed information on age-related changes in vision and recommended adaptations.)

Neurological/Musculoskeletal. Conditions that affect posture and body alignment cause changes in center of gravity, gait, stride, strength, and joint stability, all of which increase the risk for falls. Age-related changes in postural control include decreased proprioception, slower righting reflexes, decreased muscle tone, and increased postural sway. Changes in gait include decreased height of stepping. Men tend to have a more flexed posture and wide-based, short-stepped gait, whereas women tend to have a more narrow-based, waddling gait (Kane, Luslander, Abrass, 1994). Medical conditions that affect instability include degenerative joint disease, deconditioning, malnutrition, dehydration, and neurological disorders such as neuropathy, stroke, Parkinson's disease, and dementia (Brummel-Smith, 1990; Kane, Luslander, Abrass, 1994). Elder women are more susceptible to brittle bones, with a higher incidence of osteoporosis after menopause. In the case of brittle bones, it may be a fractured bone that causes the fall rather than vice versa.

To compensate for changes in gait and decreased balance, elders may "furniture glide" by holding on to furniture for support while they walk (Figure 16-3). They may also drag a foot or lose their balance toward their weaker side (stroke), have a shuffling gait (Alzheimer's disease), or fall forward (Parkinson's disease) during ADL training. Older adults may hold onto faucets to get into the tub or shower or lean against the shower wall for stability while bathing.

Cardiovascular. Age-related changes include orthostatic hypotension, which affects approximately 30% of the elder population (Brummel-Smith, 1990). Other medical conditions that cause blood pressure changes

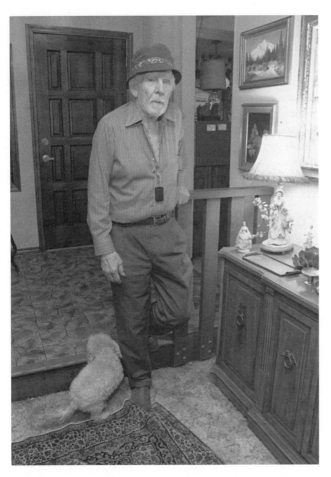

FIGURE **16-2** Common potential hazards that may cause falls include rugs and pets underfoot.

are **aging in place** (growing old at home), a 32% increase from 13 years ago (AARP, 1995). A poorly kept home or yard may be an environmental sign of age-related changes. As people age, they may lose the endurance, strength, and cognitive ability to structure tasks and deal with their environment. Common **environmental hazards** in the home include poor lighting or glare, uneven stairs, lack of handrails by stairs, and uneven or unsafe surfaces (frayed rug edges, slippery floors in the shower and tub, cracks in cement, high doorsteps, etc.). Other hazards may involve old, unstable, or low furniture (chairs, beds, or toilets), pets, young children, clutter or electric cords in walkways, inaccessible items, and limited space for ADL functions (Figure 16-2). New, used, or improperly installed equipment and unfamiliar environments may also be hazardous.

Biological Causes

Sensory. Age-related changes that may influence falls include decreases in depth perception, peripheral vision, color discrimination, acuity, accommodation, and hearing. Stairs may become more difficult to maneuver.

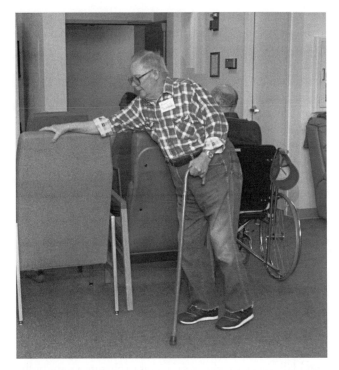

FIGURE **16-3** Elders often "furniture glide" by holding on to furniture to compensate for changes in gait and decreased balance.

include hypertension, neuropathy, and diabetes. In addition, these changes can occur as side effects of certain medications. Arrhythmias may cause up to 50% of syncopal episodes in elders (Brummel-Smith, 1990). Elders may experience a higher incidence of dizziness or light headedness, with lower cardiac output, autonomic dysfunction, impaired venous return, and prolonged bed rest. Together with extrinsic, or environmental, factors, these biological, or intrinsic, factors are the primary causes of falls among elders (Tideiksaar, 1987; Rubenstein, Robbins, 1989).

Psychosocial Causes

Psychosocial risk factors that may influence falls include poor judgment, insight, and problem-solving skills; confusion; and inattention resulting from fatigue, depression, and dementia. Other factors may include reactions to psychotropic medications, fear of falling, unfamiliarity with a new environment or caregiver, and a strong drive for independence. Elders and their families may not comply with recommended safety modifications because of cultural or personal preferences, aesthetic values, and limited financial or social resources. Consequently, both the caregiver and the client are at higher risk of suffering a fall.

Functional Causes

Performing ADL functions becomes increasingly challenging for elders. In 1986, 23% of the elder population

Work-up for Falls
S   Safety judgment
L   Length of time at residence
I   Important activities to continue doing
P   Performance; how the activity was done
P   Personal assistance, time left alone
E   Environmental hazards
D   Devices used or not used

living in the community had difficulties with one or more ADL functions and 28% had difficulty with one or more instrumental activities of daily living (IADL) functions (AARP, 1995). Functional mobility problems that may lead to falls include difficulty with performing transfers (to or from lounge chair, bed, toilet, tub or shower, wheelchair, and car), dressing and bathing (especially the lower body), reaching, and sitting, standing, and walking unsupported. Other factors may include the lack of assistive aids for ambulation or an inability to use them. Elders with dementia may forget where they left a cane or walk carrying their walker rather than using it for support. Old, lost, borrowed, or smudged glasses may impair vision. Poorly fitting shoes, loose pants with dragging hems, and flimsy sandals with nylons can affect balance. Falls most commonly occur in places where elders perform most self-care activities: by the bed and in the bathroom (Tideiksaar, 1987).

FALL PREVENTION

The interdisciplinary team must obtain an accurate history of falls to prevent their future occurrence. Team members, including the COTA, can help identify the frequency and location of the falls, the medical history and symptoms, medications taken and their side effects, and gait analysis (Tideiksaar, 1989). The acronym *SLIPPED* can be used to collect information (Box 16-3).

When asking about functional status, COTAs should not only ask whether the elder is able to perform ADL functions but also observe the way these are done. For example, when the COTA asked Mr. Owen if he could get off the toilet by himself, he responded that he was independent with toileting. When the COTA asked him to demonstrate this transfer, Mr. Owen hooked his cane on a towel rack to pull himself off the toilet. The COTA was able to determine a high risk for falling only because the transfer was observed. If the COTA had simply accepted Mr. Owen's report of independence, she would not have been able to recommend a raised toilet seat and toilet rails or replacement of the towel racks with sturdy grab bars.

COTAs should encourage elders to wear sturdy,

comfortable, rubber-sole footwear (for example, tennis shoes) to help obtain a more secure footing. When dressing, elders should pull pant legs above their ankles before standing. Pants should be pulled down *after* transferring from the wheelchair to the toilet to avoid tripping.

Fogel (1992) observed that elders with a reach of less than 6 to 7 inches were also limited in their mobility skills and were the most restricted in ADL activities. Older adults who have difficulty reaching and carrying objects may require reachers, extended handles on bath brushes or shoe horns, carts, walker trays or bags, and sock aids. COTAs can also help problem solve: for example, they can determine the best way to attach the reacher to the walker or rearrange items around the living space so they are within reach. Higher electrical outlets could also be recommended to limit the need to reach and bend.

Difficulty with transfers and **mobility** during ADL functions may require safety training with the cane, walker, or wheelchair. This is particularly important because many falls occur in **transit** during transfers. Elders with nocturia, a normal age change involving increased frequency of urination at night, have a particular need for night lights and a clear passage to the toilet. Before rearranging furniture to provide wider walkways, COTAs must first make sure elders do not need the furniture for stability when ambulating. A consultation with a physical therapist may help clarify the most appropriate and safe assistive device for ambulation.

Bathroom modifications may include a tub or shower bench with arm rests and back, a hand-held shower hose, grab bars, and a raised toilet seat. Throw rugs should be removed, or nonskid backing should be applied under them. Nonskid stripping or rubber mats can be placed on tub or shower floors. Sliding glass doors should be removed to allow for wider access into the tub. Heat-sensitive safety valves can also be installed to prevent scalding. If the elder uses a wheelchair and the door to the bathroom is too narrow, a rolling shower bench or commode chair with wheels may help. Placing a commode chair by the bed may eliminate unsafe night transfers to the bathroom toilet. A three-in-one commode chair is an inexpensive solution. This type of commode is light and can be used at bedside, over the toilet, or in the tub or shower. Caregivers should remember, however, that emptying the commode bucket and lifting and relocating the commode can be difficult for elders. They should be discouraged from using soap dispensers, towel racks, and toilet-paper holders for support. Hygiene items should be placed within reach. Mirrors may be tilted or lowered for better viewing during ADL functions. Doors under the sink should be removed to give the elder more leg room while sitting in front of the sink.

Similar precautions should be taken in the kitchen. Step stools should be avoided, and frequently used utensils and dishes should be rearranged so they are within safe reach. Use of energy conservation techniques during meal preparation may decrease the risk of falling because of fatigue or orthostatic hypotension. General strengthening programs incorporated in the elder's daily routine can help decrease deconditioning, especially that caused by a sedentary lifestyle.

The height of seats (beds, sofas, chairs) can be increased with firm cushions. Worn mattresses or cushions should be rotated. Chairs with arm rests are recommended to facilitate rising from the chair. Chairs with wheels should be avoided, and the brakes of wheelchairs and commodes must be secured before transfers are attempted. Elders should lean forward in the wheelchair only when both feet are flat on the floor (not on the footrests).

Caregivers must ensure that stairs are well lit, with no glare, and equipped with railings running along the entire length of the stairwell on both sides. Stripping of various colors can be used at the edge of each step to distinguish them from each other. Light switches should be within reach at both the top and bottom of the stairway. COTAs should discuss with elders safe ways to change a light bulb. User-friendly, touch-sensitive, and motion-sensor light switches are also available.

Interventions to compensate for visual loss include increased lighting with limited glare, improved contrast for steps and furniture, decreased clutter in walkways, and well maintained flooring. COTAs should anticipate elders' performance at different times of the day, with varied natural lighting and indoor lighting. Referrals to vision specialists may be appropriate to make sure elders are wearing the appropriate eyewear.

Elders who complain of dizziness with a change in position may be experiencing a drop in blood pressure that could result in a fall with or without syncope. Blood pressure should be monitored, and elders should be allowed to make slow transitions from supine to sitting or sitting to standing positions. A few minutes may be necessary to allow the blood pressure to accommodate to the change in head position. By teaching elders different techniques for dressing and bathing and instructing them in the use of long handle devices, COTAs can help elders limit and modify their bending. The rest of the health care team should be informed of complaints of dizziness and unstable changes in blood pressure.

Gradual increases in activity are recommended for people with conditions that affect endurance (such as cardiac conditions and deconditioning). Strategically located sturdy chairs may be useful for elders who require rest periods when going from one room to another. Sitting while bathing and avoiding long hot baths are also recommended. A commode chair by the bed may save energy. Activities that involve straining and holding one's breath (such as during toileting, strenuous transfers, or exercise) can cause light-headedness and should be monitored.

COTAs, elders, family members, and caregivers should work together to identify activities important to elders that can be modified to prevent falls. Family members should be included because elders may depend on them to help with preparation and assistance. Elders may prefer to perform toileting activities independently but not mind assistance with feeding. COTAs should identify personal and shared spaces in the elder's living environment. If family members do not want to modify the only bathroom in the home with a raised toilet seat and grab bars, a commode chair by the elder's bed may be appropriate. COTAs should help elders and their family members address safety concerns and practice giving assistance in a safe environment.

COTAs should make sure that strategies exist for emergency situations. Typical questions include the following. If a curtain is not drawn, will the neighbor know that this may be an indication of trouble? If an elder falls, will he or she know the proper way to get up from the floor if no injuries are apparent? Is a telephone within reach? Are emergency phone numbers listed by the phone? If the elder is at home alone, are there emergency alert systems available to signal for help? Is a telephone reassurance program available in which a volunteer calls daily? Is it safer to soil clothes than risk an unassisted transfer to the toilet? All these questions should be addressed to assure the elder's safety before discharge from occupational therapy.

PENNI JEAN LAVOOT

PART 3 Community Mobility

Most elders prefer the freedom of traveling by automobile (Figure 16-4). Driving is an important factor in their independence and mental health (Malfetti, Winter, 1986). By the year 2000, one out of every three drivers in the United States will be 55 years of age or older. A total of 15.7 million elders were licensed drivers in 1994, an increase of 45% from 1984. Elder drivers make up approximately 9% of all licensed drivers and 13% of all traffic fatalities (U.S. Department of Transportation, 1994). Elders may experience age-related changes that can negatively affect their ability to drive, including decreased visual acuity, color discrimination, and peripheral vision and increased sensitivity to glare (Okada, 1990). Other factors that may influence driving and mobility include unrecognized disease processes, deconditioning, psychosocial issues, medications, dementia, and environmental issues such as small print on signs.

Age-related changes affect the mobility of elders, whether they are pedestrians, drivers, or users of public transportation. For example, pedestrians may have difficulty stepping up or down from curbs or crossing streets within the time allotted by crossing signals (Figure 16-5). Drivers may have difficulties merging, yielding the right of way, negotiating intersections, backing up, handling quick maneuvers, reading traffic signs, and making left turns (Okada, 1990). Physical barriers may make public transportation inaccessible. All these challenges may rob elders of the freedom and independence they may have enjoyed throughout their lives.

A common goal of occupational therapy is to assist elders in being as independent as possible in their homes and communities. As with most adults, elders regularly go to the doctor's office, grocery store, and pharmacy. These places may be around the corner or many miles from the elder's home. The COTA's role in helping identify realistic goals and treatment plans for elders often includes increasing their ability to move in the community. To do this effectively, COTAs must explore as many

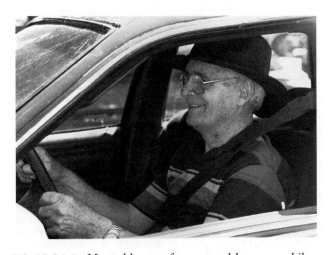

FIGURE 16-4 Most elders prefer to travel by automobile.

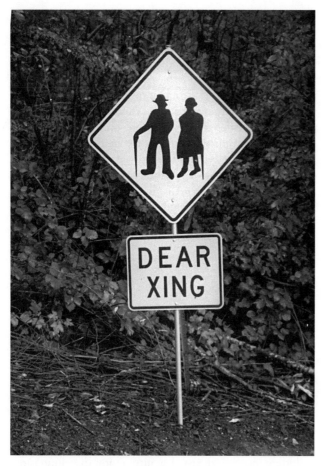

FIGURE 16-5   Elder pedestrians may need more time to cross streets than other people.

options for community mobility as possible (Box 16-4). Community transportation options vary greatly among rural areas and cities.

PEDESTRIAN SAFETY

Walking safely is an important factor in community mobility. Elders account for 18% of all **pedestrian** fatalities (U.S. Department of Transportation, 1994). COTAs should evaluate the ability of elders to walk outdoors. Box 16-5 lists precautions for safe walking.

Elders who use wheelchairs, walkers, and scooters usually have more difficulty and require more time conquering crosswalks, curbs, and uneven sidewalks. These elders need training to negotiate cut-out curbs because electric scooters or wheelchairs may overturn when descending. Electric scooters with three wheels tend to tip more often than those with four wheels. A mobility expert should conduct an evaluation to determine the type of equipment needed. This evaluation should take into consideration the elder's cognition, physical impairments, home environment, and seating and positioning needs and the progression of disease. Whenever possible, COTAs should provide safety train-

ing with the exact type of mobility equipment that elders will be using in the community. COTAs can also help elders advocate for curb cuts or longer crossing times at various intersections to ensure independence and safety in the community. To this end, the city's Traffic Commission or the Architectural and Transportation Compliance Board can be of assistance.

Elders who fatigue easily or are unable to walk long distances may consider using an electric scooter or wheelchair (Figure 16-6). Golf carts can be especially helpful for elders who live in a planned retirement

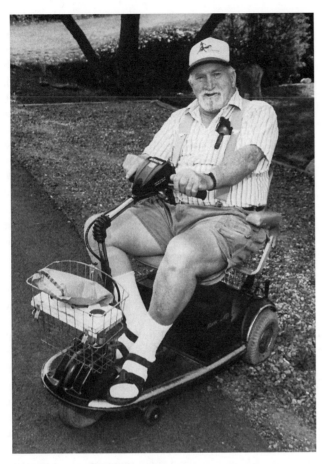

FIGURE 16-6 Elders may use electric scooters to move around freely in the community.

community and stay within the closed community area. An obstacle course can be set up to determine the elder's ability to maneuver before this expensive device is purchased. An evaluation by a specialist in wheelchair and scooter prescriptions is also recommended before purchase.

If elders need to transport a wheelchair or scooter in their personal vehicle, community mobility becomes much more complicated. Electric wheelchairs should only be transported in a van fitted with an electric lift of the appropriate size and weight. A driver rehabilitation professional should evaluate each case before a van or lift is purchased to prevent expensive mistakes such as incompatible equipment. A driver rehabilitation professional takes into account many factors, including the type of wheelchair or scooter that must be transported, whether the person needing this equipment will be a driver or passenger, and the length of time this equipment will be needed. The diagnosis of the elder is also important. An elder with a progressive illness has different needs than an elder who does not have a progressive illness. A driver rehabilitation professional can be found by contacting ADED or using the AAA

Mobility Guide (AAA, 1995). Refer to the appendix for these and other resources.

The driver rehabilitation professional can also provide resources for vendors who install adaptive equipment for vehicles in a particular geographical area. Before an electric lift or scooter carrier is purchased, the prospective user should demonstrate an ability to perform the entire loading process using the recommended equipment. COTAs can assist elders by providing information on driver rehabilitation specialists in the area.

In contrast to electric wheelchairs, electric scooters can be transported in a variety of ways. They can be stored in the trunk of some cars or on the back of the vehicle. The elder and caregivers must practice *every* step of this process before the equipment is purchased. The mobility device and personal vehicle must be compatible for safety reasons. Checking with the manufacturer of the vehicle to see whether it can handle the extra weight of a scooter carrier is necessary.

COTAs can assist the elder driver in applying for a disabled parking placard, usually issued by the Department of Motor Vehicles (DMV) of each state. This entitles the driver of the car to park close to buildings and may also include assistance at the gas station. Some elder drivers do not apply for this placard because they do not understand the application procedure. Other elders may not apply because of a perceived social stigma.

ALTERNATIVE TRANSPORTATION

When planning occupational therapy intervention, COTAs must take into consideration the individual's lifestyle and needs. This is especially true for elders who have never driven, are now unable to drive because of impairments, voluntarily decided not to drive, or want the option of using community transportation in addition to their personal vehicle. Elders who relied on others for transportation may need to learn to drive, especially if those people are no longer available. COTAs should investigate community transportation resources available where the elder currently resides or is planning to live. Information on alternative transportation can be obtained by calling city hall, a local senior citizens' center, the local DMV, local transportation agencies, the area's Office on Aging, and the local American Association of Retired Persons offices. Independent living centers in the community may also be good sources of information. When calling these agencies, COTAs must obtain information about application procedures, cost, distance traveled, eligibility requirements, and the type of additional equipment available on the vehicles.

Title II of the Americans with Disabilities Act (ADA) addresses many needs of elders with disabilities. This act states that no qualified individual with a disability shall, by reason of that disability, be excluded from participating in or be denied the benefits of the services, programs, or activities of a public entity. According to the ADA, a *qualified individual* is defined as a person with a disability who meets the essential eligibility requirements for receiving services or participating in programs or activities provided by a public entity. The individual may meet these qualifications with or without reasonable modifications to rules, policies, or practices. They may also qualify with or without the removal of architectural barriers or the provision of auxiliary aids and services. *Public entity* refers to any state or local government or instrumentality of a state or local government. The **paratransit** and other special transportation services provided by public entities are designed to be usable by individuals with disabilities, be they physical or mental, who need the assistance of another individual to board, ride, or disembark from any vehicle on the system. Individuals for whom no fixed and accessible route transit (usually public bus) is available are also eligible for paratransit and special transportation services. However, fixed, accessible route transit should be used if available (West, 1991) (Figure 16-7).

Elders who have impairments that prevent them from traveling to or from a boarding location for fixed transportation may also be eligible for special services. Under the law, any individual accompanying the person with the disability may be eligible for paratransit services provided that space is available and other people with disabilities are not displaced (West, 1991) (Figure 16-8). This means that if elders with a disability cannot use the available bus system, another transportation system that can pick them up directly from their home must be provided. COTAs working with elders who have a disability must know the ADA as it relates to transportation and accessibility. COTAs should also become knowledgeable about the paratransit services in the local community.

As good as paratransit services may be, they almost never help elders in leaving their homes. Regardless of whether elders are using a bus, paratransit service, or personal vehicle, their ability to exit their homes safely is of critical importance and must be evaluated to determine whether available services should be used. The elder may be unable to climb stairs or even unlock or lock the door. COTAs should consider these factors and include them when training in the use of transportation services.

Some elders find the process of applying for special transportation services overly complicated and confusing. COTAs should have applications available and know the eligibility requirements for these services. If possible, COTAs should schedule an outing with elders to use particular services and help them resolve any difficulties that arise. Elders may need encouragement to be assertive when they require assistance. If the outing is successful,

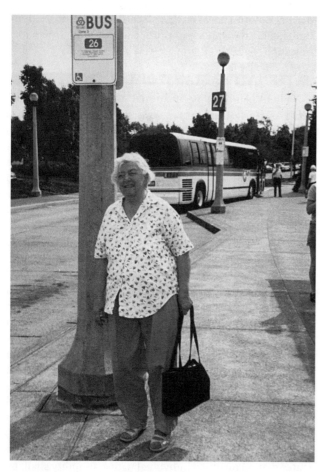

FIGURE 16-7 Elders may need to learn to use community transportation in addition to their personal vehicle.

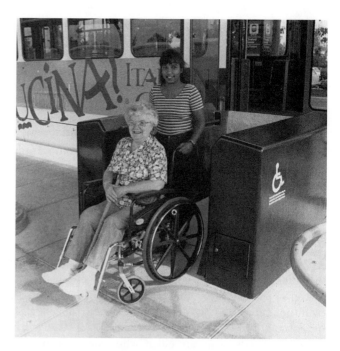

FIGURE 16-8 Public transportation may be a viable option for elders who may no longer be able to drive.

elders are more likely to use the service independently or with a friend or family member.

SAFE DRIVING

Aging is a highly complex process that varies tremendously among individuals. Chronological age alone is not a good predictor of driving performance. The physical effects of aging in combination with a disability make driving safety an important issue. Although driving may seem simple because so many people do it, it is an extremely complex occupation that requires constant attention and concentration (Malfetti, Winter, 1991). Driving involves a number of abilities. The abilities of sensing, deciding, and acting are critical in operating a vehicle. Drivers must perform a series of coordinated activities with their hands and feet while using input from their eyes and ears. Drivers must make many decisions based on what they see and hear in relation to other vehicles on the road, other drivers, traffic signs, signals, and road conditions. These decisions result in the actions of braking, steering, and accelerating or a combination of all three to maintain or adjust the position of the vehicle in traffic. Because fluctuations in traffic occur quickly, the coordination between decisions and actions must be smooth. Drivers make about 20 decisions for each mile traveled, demonstrating that the occupation of driving is complex and fast paced (Malfetti, Winter, 1991). Age- or disability-related decreases in sensorimotor skills may compromise driving safety by reducing the speed with which an elder can sense, decide, and act in traffic.

The sense dimension of driving includes visual acuity, visual accommodation, field of vision, dark adaptation, color vision, visual searching, and hearing. Glare and illumination, as well as certain diseases of the eye, may also affect the way the driver senses environmental changes. Integrity of muscles and joints and reaction time are also intimately related to driving. Elders may not perceive, interpret, and react to sensory stimulation as acutely or quickly as younger people do.

Vision is usually defined as visual acuity or the ability to see fine details. Static acuity (such as looking at an eye chart) is tested in driver licensing examinations. Dynamic acuity (subject or target moving) is more closely related to traffic accidents but seldom tested. Up to ages 40 or 50, little change in visual acuity occurs, but after so, visual acuity declines markedly (Malfetti, Winter, 1991). By age 70, most elders have poor acuity without correction. The implications of this decline for driving are that drivers find distinguishing between objects increasingly difficult and need to be closer to objects to clearly perceive them. To compensate for this, elders may drive slowly to distinguish hazards on the road in time to avoid them. Some diseases of the eye, such as macular degeneration, can be improved with devices such as bioptic lenses. However, in some states driving with these lenses is illegal.

Accommodation is defined as the ability to focus the eyes on nearby objects. With aging, changes in the lenses of the eyes and in the muscles that adjust them decrease their capacity for accommodation. For this reason, many elders need bifocal or trifocal eyewear, which affects driving because more time is required to change focus from near to distant objects, such as when looking from the instrument panel to the road and vice versa. A younger person can change focus in about 2 seconds, whereas adults over age 40 take 3 seconds or more. This delay is potentially hazardous.

The retina of the normal eye receives about one half as much light at age 50 as at age 20, and about one third as much at age 60 as at age 20 (Malfetti, Wintter, 1991). This change is primarily due to a decrease in the size of the pupil. Elders who complain of night blindness have good reason not to drive at night, because less light is available. Choosing well-lighted highways and instrument panels and keeping headlights, windows, and eyeglasses clean are helpful measures.

Field of vision decreases with age and can contribute to the possibility of collisions. For example, people who can see only directly ahead confront a greater risk of accidents at intersections because they cannot see vehicles approaching from the sides. Compensations for a decreased field of vision can include the use of special panoramic mirrors and the habit of turning the head more often to check for traffic. Many elders may also not be aware of their blind spot on the side of the vehicle. Reminders to look over the shoulder before all lane changes may be necessary.

Glare occurs when too much light or light from the wrong direction or source is present. If excessive light shines on a highway sign, the elder may not see it. Quick recovery from oncoming headlights is necessary for safe driving. In the elder driver, eye recovery is slower and sensitivity to glare increases.

Dark adaptation is the process whereby eyes adjust for better vision in low light. Elders not only see less clearly in darkness but also require more time to accommodate to it. This can be a particular problem when driving in and out of tunnels. Many elders decide on their own not to drive at night for this reason.

Elders may not identify the color of traffic signs or signals as well as younger people, especially when the light is dim or glare is present. This can be a problem because elders require additional time to read road signs, which diverts their attention from the road and traffic (Malfetti, Winter, 1991). According to the AARP (1992), elders may be able to compensate for some visual limitations. They should have their vision checked at least yearly and avoid eyeglass frames that obstruct peripheral vision. Learning the general meaning of traffic signs by their shapes and colors and avoiding driving at night whenever possible are useful precautions.

Approximately 30% of people over the age of 65 experience some hearing loss (Brenton, 1986). This loss can cause problems during driving because horns, sirens, and train whistles may be difficult to hear. It may also prevent elders from realizing that the turn signal indicator is on when no turns are being made. Elders should have their hearing tested by a qualified professional. When adjusting to any hearing assistive devices, elders should keep the volume of the car radio as low as possible, leave the air conditioning or heating units on the lowest possible setting, and visually check turn signals. (Resources for drivers with hearing difficulties are listed in the appendix.)

The aging process also affects muscles and joints in ways that may affect driving. Elders may experience back pain, making it difficult to sit for long periods. Special cushions may be helpful. Arthritis may cause stiffness in the neck, which makes turning to check for traffic painful. Fatigue and discomfort are also problems that may distract elders and lessen their awareness of traffic conditions. Power steering and power brakes can help tremendously. A wide variety of mirrors are available to compensate for stiffness in the neck. Using tilt steering and arm rests may also help.

Reaction time is extremely important in safe driving. Reaction time is the time required by the eyes to see and the brain to process, decide what to do, and transmit the information to the proper body parts. For example, after seeing that the traffic ahead has stopped, a driver extends the right leg and pushes on the brake pedal. The ability to respond quickly may decrease with age, but specific safety measures can be used to compensate for the loss. One strategy is to maintain a safe distance from the car ahead. When stopping, the driver should be able to see the tires of the car in front. Other strategies are to avoid rush-hour traffic and to take someone else along, especially when traveling to a new destination. If elders are upset or ill, they will probably have a slower reaction time. Education on compensatory techniques can help the elders to change unsafe habits. The AARP and the AAA offer various programs and courses for elder drivers (Figure 16-9). However, these classes do not include behind-the-wheel testing. COTAs should discuss concern about the elder's ability to drive safely with the supervising OTR and physician whenever possible.

A behind-the-wheel evaluation is the best method for determining driver safety. A driving evaluation program that specializes in working with persons with disabilities can determine safety and equipment needs. The Handicapped Driver's Mobility Guide (AAA, 1995) and the Association of Driver Educators for the Disabled can assist COTAs in locating driver evaluation programs. These programs can also instruct COTAs in the proper procedures for reporting unsafe or questionable drivers to

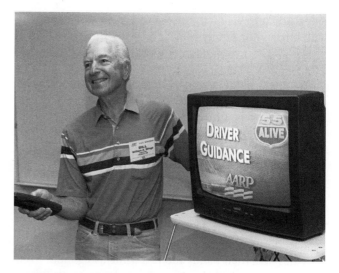

FIGURE **16-9**   There are various programs and courses in the community to assist elder drivers.

the DMV of each state. COTAs should clearly document all recommendations to elders. For example, if the COTA recommends that an elder's driving ability be evaluated after a stroke, this recommendation must be clearly stated in the medical chart. To demonstrate thorough care, COTAs are advised to document the names of at least three resources given to the client.

A wide variety of equipment is available to help elders continue driving. This equipment is available from a variety of sources, including equipment catalogs, vendors, and automobile manufacturers (Table 16-1). Refer to the appendix for addresses of organizations to contact for additional resources.

CASE STUDY

Mr. Thomas is 62-years-old. He had a right cerebrovascular accident (CVA) 1 year before requesting a driving evaluation and has a nonfunctional left upper extremity. For long distances, he uses a manual wheelchair, which he pushes with his right lower extremity. For short distances; he is able to slowly ambulate using a quad cane. Other medical conditions include a seizure disorder controlled by medication and a left hip joint replacement that causes pain and discomfort with prolonged sitting. A former physical education teacher, Mr. Thomas enjoys working with students at the high school level and is anxious to return to work in some capacity. His wife works full time, but he receives occasional assistance in transportation from friends. He believes he is ready to drive, but his wife is very concerned for his safety.

Mr. Thomas received a driving evaluation, whereupon he exhibited difficulties such as weaving out of the lane and forgetting to turn off his turn signal. After driving for 20 minutes, he drifted across two lanes and lost concentration. The driving instructor had to take over the steering wheel to pull the car over to the side of the road. Mr. Thomas stated that his "leg hurt."

After the evaluation the deficits observed during driving

TABLE 16-1

Adaptive Equipment Ideas		
Difficulty	**Effect on driving**	**Resources to assist elder drivers**
Decreased neck ROM or pain when turning head	Limited scope of view of traffic around car	Install panoramic mirrors (Brookstone) or convex mirrors (can be installed by vendors), refer to driving program for evaluation; instruct client in use of head support
Decreased shoulder ROM or pain in shoulders	Difficulty steering, reaching for seat belt, and adjusting rear-view mirror	Use arm supports already in vehicle; automobile upholsterer can build up existing arm supports to support elbows, which usually decreases client shoulder pain; client may need effort of steering reduced, which can be determined by driving evaluation (driving program can refer to appropriate vendor for this modification); instruct elder in use of stick to adjust rear view mirror and tilt steering wheel
Decreased ROM or pain fingers and hands	Difficulty turning key, opening door, adjusting radio, air conditioning, etc; possible difficulty holding onto steering wheel safely	A wide variety of key holders and door openers are available from medical supply catalogs; knob extensions can be made by car vendors; refer client for driving evaluation to determine need for steering device or built-up steering wheel
Back pain	Decreased concentration caused by pain; difficulty turning to check traffic	A wide variety of cushions and lumbar supports are available from medical supply companies and vendors; these should be tried before purchase; driving programs can also evaluate and provide resources
Impairment or loss of both lower extremities	Inability to operate gas and brake pedals	Refer to driving program for evaluation of ability to use hand controls
Impairment or loss of right lower extremity	Difficulty using gas and brake pedals	Refer to driving program for evaluation of ability to use left foot accelerator
Impairment or loss of left upper extremity	Difficulty using turn signal and turning	Refer to driving program for evaluation of ability to use right cross-over directional and spinner knob
Impairment or loss of right upper extremity	Difficulty steering, shifting gears in automatic or manual cars	Refer to driving program for evaluation of ability to use spinner knob
Hearing impairment	Inability to hear emergency sirens; failure to turn off turn signal	Elder drivers can purchase equipment to amplify sound of blinker; hearing aids can help clients hear sirens better.
Cognitive impairment	Decreased judgment and decision making; slow reaction time; unsafe driving	Refer to driving program for detailed evaluation; discuss concerns with OTR; document recommendations clearly
Visual impairment	Compromised ability to read signs; overly slow driving; generally unsafe driving skills	Refer to optometrist for vision check-up; if elder has low vision, refer to opthalmologist who specializes in low vision.

(ROM; Range of motion.)
Adapted from Lillie S: Evaluation for driving. In Yoshikawa TT et al, editors: *Ambulatory geriatric care*, St. Louis, 1993, Mosby.

were discussed. Mr. Thomas demonstrated insight into his difficulties and expressed the desire to begin training to improve his driving skills. Equipment needs included a spinner knob to allow him to steer with one hand and a right cross-over directional device that enabled him to use his right hand for directional use. Training strategies included asking Mr. Thomas to tell the driving instructor when he was starting to have pain in his leg and pull over when it was safe. He was reminded to turn off his directional signal after use and to look ahead while driving. After three

training sessions, Mr. Thomas was able to demonstrate safe driving skills. He received a driving test from the DMV and passed. He is now able to return to part time work and independent living.

CHAPTER REVIEW QUESTIONS

1 Explain the reason that OBRA regulations involving use of restraints were drafted and discuss related requirements for health providers.

2 Explain the steps to be taken in establishing a restraint reduction program.

3 Explain the role of the COTA in consultations regarding use of restraints.

4 Describe at least three environmental adaptations that may help reduce the use of restraints.

5 Identify psychosocial approaches to reducing the use of restraints with an elder who wanders.

6 Explain the ways activity aids in the reduction of restraints.

7 Identify three reasons that many falls go unreported.

8 Explain the reason that some elders and their family members are reluctant to change the environment when personal safety and prevention of falls are a concern.

9 Explain the need for assessment of an elder's nighttime toileting skills.

10 Describe ways the home can be modified to prevent falls if elders have vision impairments and poor standing balance.

11 Identify three emergency strategies for an elder who lives alone and has a history of falls.

12 List the issues that must be considered when recommending community transportation.

13 Describe strategies to alleviate the elder's fear of using transportation.

14 Describe the actions of the COTA when the client's ability to be a safe driver is in question.

15 Considering the case of Mr. Thomas, identify some relevant recommendations for driving if he had experienced a spinal cord injury rather than a CVA.

16 Identify alternatives for transportation appropriate for Mr. Thomas if he had failed the driving evaluation.

REFERENCES

American Association of Retired Persons: *A profile of older Americans*, Washington, DC, 1995, The Association.

American Association of Retired Persons: Older driver skill assessment and resource guide, Pub No. 4994, Washington, DC, 1992, The Association.

American Automobile Association, Traffic Safety and Engineering Department: *The disabled drivers mobility guide*, Heathrow, Fla, 1995, The Association (brochure).

American Automobile Association, Traffic Safety and Engineering Department: *Walking through the years*, Heathrow, Fla, 1993, The Association (brochure).

Atkins C: Teamwork is the real key to reduced use of restraints, *Adv Occup Therapists* 12(1):5, 1996.

Bloom C, Braun J: Restraints in the 90's: success with wanderers; *Geriatr Nurs* 12(1):20, 1991.

Bradley L, Dufton B: Breaking free, *Canadian Nurse* 91(1):36, 1995.

Bradley L, Siddique CM, Dufton B: Reducing the use of physical restraints in long-term care facilities, *J Gerontol Nurs* 21(9):21, 1995.

Brenton M: The older person's guide to safe driving, Public Affairs Pamphlet No. 641, Falls Church, Va, 1986, AAA Foundation for Traffic Safety.

Brummel-Smith K: Falls and instability in the older person. In B Kemp, K Brummel-Smith, and JW Ramsdell, editors: *Geriatric rehabilitation*, Boston, 1990, College Hill Press.

Brungardt G: Patient restraints: new guidelines for a less restrictive approach, *Geriatrics*, 49(6):43, 1994.

Burgener SC, Shiver R, Murrell L: Expressions of individuality in cognitively impaired elders, *J Gerontol Nurs* 19(14):13, 1993.

Campbell AJ et al: Falls in old age: a study of frequency and other related factors, *Age Ageing*, 10:264, 1981.

Donius M, Rader J: Use of siderails: rethinking a standard of practice, *J Gerontol Nurs* 20(11):23, 1994.

Eigste DG, Vrooman N: Releasing restraints in the nursing home: it can be done, *J Gerontol Nurs* 18(1):21, 1992.

Ericson LL: Restraints in the nursing home environment, *Occup Ther Forum* 6(4):1, 1991.

Fogel BS: Simple balance measure proven effective (measure frailty), *Brown Univ Long Term Care Quality Letter*, 1992.

Greenberg D: Geriatric seating and positioning: definitely a therapy task, *Gerontol Special Interest Section Newsletter* 19(3):1, 1996.

Gryfe CI, Amies A, Ashley MJ: A longitudinal study of falls in an elderly population: incidence and morbidity, *Age Ageing* 6:201, 1977.

Health Care Financing Administration Interpretive Guidelines Rev. 250: *Part II Guidance to Surveyors for Long-Term Care Facilities*, Tag #s f221–241, pp 44–53, April 1995.

Hettinger J: Encouraging activity in older adults. *OT Week* 15, Feb 8, 1996.

Janelli LM, Kanski GW, Neary MA: Physical restraints: has OBRA made a difference? *J Gerontolog Nurs* 20(6):17, 1994.

Jones DA: Seating problems in long-term care. In EM Tornquist, editor: *Individualized dementia care: creative compassionate approaches*, New York, NY, 1995, Springer.

Kane RL, Luslander JG, Abrass IB: Instability and falls. In JD Jeffers, M Navrozov, editors: *Essentials of clinical geriatrics*, New York, NY, 1994, McGraw-Hill.

Kapp MB: Reduce legal risks through restraint reduction plan, *Provider* 17(8):48, 1991.

Kari N, Michels P: The Lazarus project: the politics of empowerment, *Am J Occup Ther* 45(8):719, 1991.

Kerr T: Making 'merry walkers' of once-restrained residents, *Adv Occup Ther* 10(6):42, 1994.

Lillie S: Evaluation for driving. In Yoshikawa TT et al, editors: *Ambulatory geriatric care*, St. Louis, 1993, Mosby.

Mahoney DF: Analysis of restraint-free nursing homes, *Image: J Nurs Schol* 27(2):155, 1995.

Malfetti J, Winter DJ: *Drivers 55 plus: Test your own performance: A self rating form of questions, factors and suggestions for safe driving*, Falls Church, Va, 1986, American Automobile Association Foundation for Traffic Safety (brochure).

Malfetti J, Winter DJ: *Concerned about an older driver? A guide for families and friends*, Washington, DC, 1991, Safety Research and Education Project and AAA Foundation for Traffic Safety (brochure).

Mason R, O'Connor M, Kemble S: Untying the elderly: response to quality of life issues, *Geriatr Nurs* 16(2):68, 1995.

Mion LC, Mercurio A: Methods to reduce restraints: process, outcomes, and future directions, *J Gerontol Nurs* 18(11):5, 1992.

Okada S: Should Miss Daisy drive? *Geriatr Rehabil Prev* 2(3):1, 1990.

Patterson JE, Strumpf NE, Evans LK: Nursing consultation to reduce restraints in a nursing home, *Clin Nurse Specialist* 9(4):231, 1995.

Rader J: A comprehensive staff approach to problem wandering, *Gerontologist* 27(6): 756, 1987.

Rader J: In Tornquist Em, editor: *Individualized dementia care: creative, compassionate approaches*, New York, NY, 1995, Springer Publishing.

Rader J: Personal communication, 1996.

Rader J, Doan J, Schwab Sr. M: How to decrease wandering, a form of agenda behavior, *Geriatr Nurs* 6(4):196, 1985.

Rubenstein LZ: NSC home safety check list. In US National Safety Council in cooperation with the American Association of Retired Persons: *Falling - the unexpected trip: a safety program for older adults, leader's guide*, Washington, DC, 1982, USCPSC.

Rubenstein LZ, Robbins AS: Falling syndromes in elderly persons, *Comp Ther* 15:6, 1989.

Stolley JM: Freeing your patients from restraints, *Am J Nurs* 12(3): 27, 1995.

Strumpf NE et al: Reducing physical restraint: developing an educational program, *J Psychol Nurs* 33(6):20, 1992.

Sullivan-Marx EM: Psychological responses to physical restraint use in older adults, *J Psycholog Nurs* 33(6):20, 1995.

Tideiksaar R: Fall prevention in the home, *Top Geriatr Rehabil* 3:1, 1987.

Tideiksaar R: Geriatric falls: assessing the cause, preventing recurrence, *Geriatrics* 44(7):57, 1989.

U.S. Department of Transportation (1994).

Werner P. et al: Individualized care alternatives used in the process of removing restraints in the nursing home, *J Am Geriatr Soc* 42(3):321, 1994.

West J: *The Americans with Disabilities Act*, New York, NY, 1991, Milbank Memorial Fund.

Working With Elders Who Have Vision Impairments

REBECCA PLAS BOTHWELL

KEY TERMS

cataracts, glaucoma, retina, lens, macular degeneration, diabetic retinopathy, visual acuity, contrast sensitivity, visual cognition, visual memory, pattern recognition, scanning, visual attention, oculomotor control, visual fields, eccentric viewing

CHAPTER OBJECTIVES

1. Describe the typical physiological changes affecting vision that occur with aging.
2. Name and describe the major ocular diseases affecting vision in elders.
3. Describe the common vision deficits resulting from neurological insult in elders.
4. Identify general principles to enhance vision and increase independence in elders with low vision.
5. Identify general principles in the treatment of vision dysfunction after brain insult.

The aging process causes many changes in visual function that increase the likelihood of elders developing some type of vision impairment. In addition to these normal changes, many specific ocular diseases can affect an elder's vision. An estimated 3 million elders have low vision, which is vision that cannot be fully corrected with surgery or conventional optical aids (Castor, Carter, 1995). Vision loss is ranked third, below arthritis and heart disease, as one of the most common chronic conditions requiring assistance in activities of daily living (ADL) in elders (LaPlante, 1988). In addition, elders are also at risk for cerebrovascular accidents (CVAs), which often result in vision impairment.

PSYCHOLOGICAL IMPLICATIONS OF VISION LOSS

Most people think of vision loss as total blindness; however, most individuals with low vision are not totally blind. In the United States, only 80,000 of the 14 million individuals with low vision are totally blind (Seligmann, 1990), while the rest have some degree of residual vision. These individuals with partial vision disabilities also find it difficult to complete daily living tasks and must adjust to learning new work methods or finding other interests they can pursue. People with partial sight do not have fewer adjustment problems than those who are totally blind (Mehr, Mehr, Ault, 1970). Research shows that people with partial vision disabilities have more adaptation problems, because individuals with normal vision are unsure of the capabilities of persons with low vision. Persons with normal vision often do not want to cause embarrassment by giving unrequested assistance, but they also are often uncomfortable watching a vision-impaired individual struggle with a particular task. This discomfort produces anxiety, which may lead to avoidance of anxiety-producing situations. For this reason, individuals with low vision often have a reduced self-image and may eventually become isolated when friends and family members disengage.

EFFECTS OF THE NORMAL AGING PROCESS ON VISION

An elder's ability to perform daily living tasks independently is significantly affected by changes in vision. This is partly explained by the fact that some specific ocular conditions such as **cataracts** and **glaucoma** occur more frequently in elders, but the aging process itself brings about significant visual changes (National Institute on Aging, 1988).

The **retina** is a multilayered lining of neural tissue on the innermost part of the eye (Figure 17-1). It contains cells that respond to visual stimuli by a photochemical reaction. The central area of the retina, or macula, has a concentration of cone cells that enable color vision and fine-detail discrimination. Rod cells that are extremely light sensitive are scattered throughout the periphery and are responsible for light and dark adaptation (Bennett, 1992). As the retina ages, it gradually loses neurons. Central or peripheral vision may be affected, depending on which retinal neurons die. The rate of retinal deterioration and the resultant visual field loss varies among individuals, but generally, elders experience a shrinkage of the peripheral field, experience difficulty

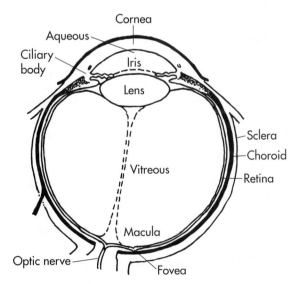

FIGURE 17-1 Anatomy of the eye.

with light and dark adaptation, and require an increased time to recover from glare (Bennett, 1992). Because the pupils also decrease in size with age, elders require more illumination for fine-detail tasks. For example, a 30-year-old individual typically requires a 100-watt lamp for good visibility on near-vision tasks, whereas a 70-year-old person will likely require a 300-watt lamp for the same tasks (Cristarella, 1977).

Changes may also occur in the **lens** of the eye with age (see Figure 17-1). The lens is responsible for properly focusing the image on the retina. It does this by changing shape according to the distance of the object being viewed. As the lens ages, it loses some of its elasticity, making shape change or accommodation more difficult. This condition, called *presbyopia*, affects focal ability at near distances, making it difficult to read print or perform close-vision tasks (National Institute on Aging, 1988). The greatest change occurs between the ages of 45 and 55 years. Reading glasses or bifocals are often prescribed at this time.

In addition to this loss of elasticity, the lens also becomes more yellow. This deeper yellow affects the ability to differentiate between colors. After age 30, the deep yellow of the aging lens restricts violet, blue, black, and green colors from entering the eye, thereby contributing to difficulty differentiating between them (Cristarella, 1977) (Table 17-1).

SPECIFIC OCULAR PATHOLOGIES

In addition to the natural aging process, several specific pathological conditions have a more profound effect on functional abilities. Four major conditions that affect an elder's vision are **macular degeneration,** cataracts, glaucoma, and **diabetic retinopathy.** These conditions often occur in isolation, but they commonly co-exist in elders, creating greater challenges for elders to remain independent (see Table 17-1).

Macular Degeneration

Macular degeneration is the most common cause of vision loss in elders (Fletcher, 1991). The macula is the central portion of the retina where the clearest vision is found. Because of decreased circulation, the macula may degenerate, resulting in a loss of the central field of vision (Bennett, 1992). This loss rarely extends into the periphery, so total blindness resulting from macular degeneration is unlikely.

However, because the vision affected by macular degeneration is in the most sensitive area of the retina, this disease can have a significant effect on performance of ADL functions. Macular vision is used for reading, recognizing acquaintances, doing needlework, matching clothing colors, and writing. Any activity that requires fine-detail discrimination and color perception may become impossible for persons with macular degeneration.

TABLE 17-1

Functional Outcomes of Ocular Conditions		
Condition	**Cause**	**Functional outcome**
Cataract	A protein degeneration in the lens results in opacification	Hazy, blurred vision Increased sensitivity to glare Difficulty with night driving Difficulty finding appropriate lighting
Glaucoma	An increase in pressure inside the eye results in damage to the tissues, especially the optic nerve	Decreased peripheral vision Difficulty adjusting to changes in lighting Shadowlike halos around lights Increased sensitivity to glare
Diabetic retinopathy	Hemorrhaging of blood vessels and/or formation of microaneurysms results in damage to the retina	Fluctuating, blurred vision Change in focal ability Loss in visual field, peripheral or central
Macular degeneration	The central portion of the retina undergoes a deterioration, in some cases brought on by hemorrhaging blood vessels	Central field loss Decreased acuity

Macular degeneration typically involves the bleeding of small blood vessels in the retina, leaving scar tissue on the surface. These areas result in small scotomas, or blind spots, in the central visual field.

Treatment of macular degeneration in some individuals may involve photocoagulation. In this procedure, a laser seals retinal hemorrhages to prevent further bleeding (Bennett, 1992). Photocoagulation is not always an option, however, because bleeding may be too profuse. Laser treatments also often leave small scarred areas on the retina, which can result in blind spots. Therefore treatment of macular degeneration usually involves simply slowing the progression of the disease if possible. Complete correction of the condition is not yet an option.

Cataracts

With aging, the lens may undergo a protein degeneration resulting in opacification, or clouding, which is known as a *cataract*. Cataracts prevent an adequate amount of light from reaching the retina. Individuals with cataracts have hazy or blurred vision, increased sensitivity to glare, difficulty with night driving, and difficulty finding the correct type and distance of lighting necessary for close work such as reading and sewing (Bennett, 1991).

Cataracts can usually be treated successfully by surgically removing the entire lens. As a substitute, individuals may wear eyeglasses with a thick convex lens or wear a contact lens. However, the most common procedure is to replace the opacified lens with an intraocular lens implant. This plastic lens functions much like the individual's

natural lens, thereby eliminating adjustment to wearing thick-lens eyeglasses or inserting a contact lens (Bennett, 1991).

Glaucoma

Glaucoma is a disease in which the pressure inside the eyeball is so great that it damages the tissues of the eye, resulting in some loss of vision. The most common form of the disease, called *open-angle glaucoma*, progresses slowly. Typically, a change in the fluid flux in the eye occurs, which produces a buildup of aqueous humor, the gel-like substance in the anterior chamber of the eye. This buildup causes an increase in the pressure inside the eyeball, which may eventually damage structures of the eye, especially the optic nerve. The first indication of the disease is usually a loss of peripheral vision, which is often not noticed or ignored. If left undetected and untreated, this loss can lead to total blindness. Elders should be encouraged to have routine ophthalmologic visits so glaucoma may be diagnosed at an early stage. When the diagnosis is early, individuals respond well to medication and, if necessary, surgery (Whitmore, 1986).

Closed- or narrow-angle glaucoma is less common. This type of glaucoma progresses rapidly and symptoms are immediately apparent. Nausea, headaches, severe redness of the eye, and pain may be symptoms of an acute attack of narrow-angle glaucoma (Jose, 1985). Emergency surgery is often required to reduce the intraocular pressure. Unfortunately, because central vision is the last to be affected, individuals are often unaware of their reduced vision and often ignore the symptoms.

The functional implications of glaucoma vary greatly depending on the severity of the disease, which is usually related to its time of diagnosis. When diagnosis is early, glaucoma can be treated and many people may have little need to adjust their lifestyles. If the disease is allowed to progress, individuals may notice decreased peripheral vision, difficulty adjusting to changing light, fluctuating and blurred vision, shadowlike halos around lights, and an increased sensitivity to glare (Bennett, 1991, 1992). Individuals with undiagnosed glaucoma may lose all of their vision beginning with their peripheral field and eventually extending into their central vision.

Diabetic Retinopathy

Diabetic retinopathy, one of the complications of diabetes mellitus, is another leading cause of visual impairment in elders. Diabetic retinopathy is also the leading cause of blindness in all age groups in the United States (Jose, 1985). Of all individuals with diabetes mellitus, 90% will experience some degree of change in their vision as a result of diabetic retinopathy (Faye, 1984).

Diabetic retinopathy occurs in two stages: background and proliferative diabetic retinopathy. In background retinopathy, microaneurysms form but are reabsorbed by the retina. **Visual acuity,** which is sharpness or clarity of vision, may fluctuate in this stage but usually remains better than 20/200. However, with proliferative retinopathy, visual acuity is less than 20/200 and may eventually result in either light perception only (LPO) vision or no light perception vision (NPO), or total blindness. The term *proliferative* is used to indicate the new blood vessels that grow throughout the retina during this stage of retinopathy. These vessels easily rupture and produce bleeding into the eye, often resulting in scotomas, or blind spots in the central visual field. When scar tissue forms near the retina, retinal detachments may also occur (Bennett, 1991, 1992).

The functional implications of diabetic retinopathy, like glaucoma, vary depending on early diagnosis and severity of the disease. Some individuals may have a mild degree of retinopathy and may not need to make any adaptations in their lifestyles. Others, however, may need to make major life changes as their disease continues to progress. They may eventually need to learn the techniques of blind people for all ADL functions. Symptoms may include fluctuating and blurred vision, a change in focal ability, and eventually losses in visual field (Bennett, 1992).

Diabetic retinopathy may be treated either by photocoagulation or a procedure known as *vitrectomy*. Photocoagulation with a laser to treat diabetic retinopathy is similar to the procedure used to treat macular degeneration. A vitrectomy may be performed to remove blood and scar tissue from the vitreous if photocoagulation does

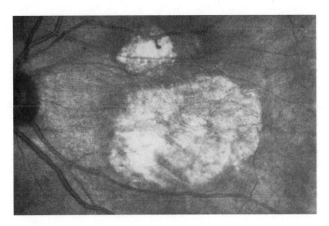

FIGURE 17-2 This photograph, which was taken with a scanning laser opthalmoscope, shows the deterioration of a retina (white areas) in an elder client who has macular degeneration. Blood vessels extend from the optic disk (dark circle).

not stop the bleeding or when it is not an option (Bennett, 1992).

PRINCIPLES OF TREATMENT

An evaluation by an ophthalmologist or optometrist who is a low vision specialist is helpful in guiding treatment of elders with low vision. Information can be gathered on several vision functions, and recommendations can be made accordingly.

Knowledge of an elder's visual acuity, or sharpness of vision, is helpful in determining the size of letters necessary to read printed signs and materials. Many low-vision specialists give both a far and a near acuity score. Far acuity scores are usually given in Snellen equivalents such as 20/200. This score, for example, means that an individual has to be at 20 feet to see the same size letter that someone with no visual impairment can see at 200 feet. Near acuity scores may be given in "M" units. An elder client with low vision may be able to read only letters at a near distance that are 3M units in height. Newspaper print is 1 M, so this elder would need print three times that size.

Low-vision specialists may also provide valuable information about an elder's visual field status. Individuals with macular degeneration who have a central field loss would likely have difficulty reading standard print, because the central blind spot would obscure their view (Figure 17-2). Individuals with glaucoma who have a peripheral field loss would likely not have any difficulty reading print because their central field is intact, but they might have difficulty ambulating safely as a result of the restricted peripheral field (Figure 17-3).

Some low-vision specialists also test **contrast sensitivity.** This is the ability to differentiate between very subtle shades of the same color. Although acuity charts are

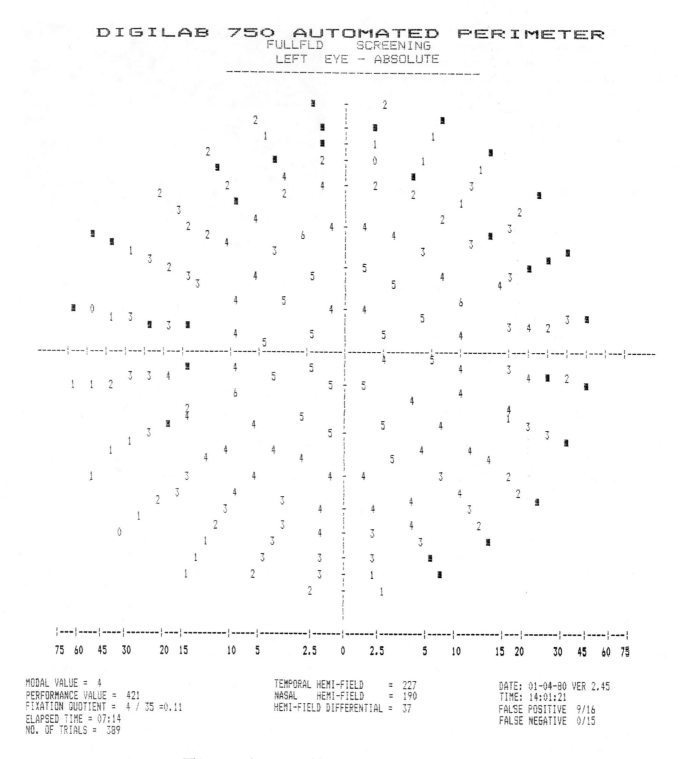

FIGURE **17-3**   This map indicates visual loss in points marked with black squares. Note the peripheral distribution.

helpful, they are only an indication of an individual's visual capability when presented with black and white objects. In daily life, good contrast sensitivity is needed to see a gray car against a concrete building under cloudy sky conditions. Contrast sensitivity also allows discrimination

of the subtle contours on people's faces, thereby facilitating recognition. This function is often affected in elders with low vision.

Many low-vision specialists make recommendations for special optical devices if an elder's acuity is impaired

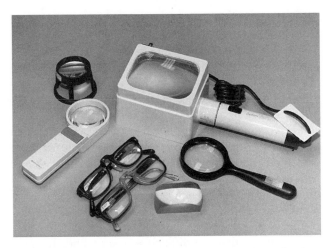

FIGURE **17-4**   Some common optic aids used by individuals with low vision.

and the elder cannot read standard print or view distant signs. A wide variety of assistive devices is available. By using these devices, many individuals with low vision can pursue daily activities that were once difficult, such as reading, sewing, and viewing distant objects and events. However, these devices are often very foreign to elders, and without proper training, prove to be too cumbersome and difficult. COTAs may find it beneficial to familiarize themselves with the most commonly used devices (Figure 17-4).

When working with elders with low vision, COTAs can make specific adaptations according to the individual's level of ability, lifestyle, and interests. However, some general principles should be considered when helping elders with low vision to maximize their independence.

Proper lighting is usually critical for optimal performance. Most elders with low vision require increased illumination. However, some individuals may also be photophobic, or light sensitive, a condition that presents a challenge in finding appropriate lighting. Halogen lighting is often used with elders with low vision because it provides more illumination than regular incandescent bulbs, but tends to be more tolerable for individuals who are sensitive to glare. Good room lighting is necessary for ease and safety in ambulating. A directional, focal type of light source, such as a gooseneck lamp, is recommended for fine-detail tasks such as reading and sewing. Proper positioning of the lamp must be considered to avoid glare. Directing the light from behind the elder's shoulder so the glare source is not in the eyes and from a position opposite the dominant hand to avoid shadows when writing usually works best (Figures 17-5 and 17-6).

Another technique to adapt the environment for elders with low vision is to enhance contrast wherever possible. For persons with low contrast sensitivity, the world often loses its definition, and objects seem to blend together.

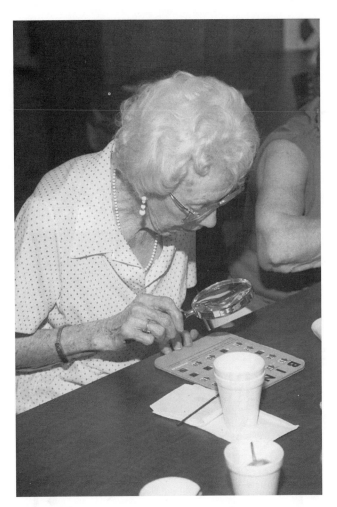

FIGURE **17-5**   This elder is able to pursue a hobby by using a low-tech device.

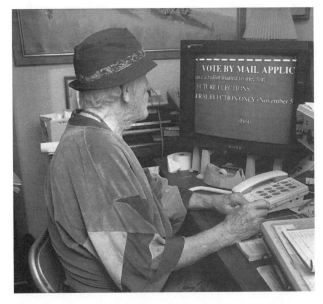

FIGURE **17-6**   This elder would be able to function in his environment more effectively if the clutter was removed.

BOX 17-1

Examples of Modifications Using Contrast in the Environment

- Use a black felt tip marker for writing.
- Add strips of contrasting tape (usually orange or yellow is best) to the edge of steps.
- Use a white coffee cup so the level of coffee can be seen against the white background when pouring.
- Use a black and white reversible cutting board and slice light-colored items, such as onions, on the black side and vice versa.
- Mark light switches with contrasting fluorescent tape to increase visibility.

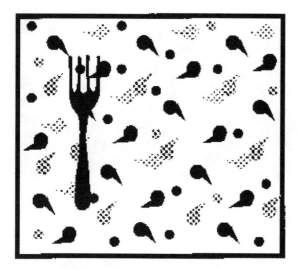

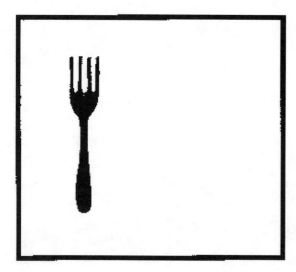

FIGURE 17-7 A patterned background can make it difficult to locate objects.

Many items used in daily activities can be changed to add more contrast and definition (Box 17-1).

Another factor that may interfere with an elder's visual function is clutter. When there is a lot of design or pattern in the background, the elder with low vision may have difficulty identifying needed objects. A patterned background can "draw objects in" even with good color contrast (Figure 17-7). In daily life, finding a pill dropped on a "busy" floral tablecloth might be difficult for those with good vision, but would be nearly impossible for those with low vision. Simple, solid colors should be used throughout the home, and care should be taken to avoid unnecessary clutter.

Elders should use an organization system to help identify items that are difficult to see or find. Keeping things in their assigned places becomes critical for elders with low vision. Their ability to search the environment effectively is often compromised by reduced acuity, contrast sensitivity, and visual field loss. Organizing canned goods in a specific manner can aid the elder in identifying them. Keeping reading glasses or special devices in the same place when not in use eliminates the need to search.

All the above principles are guidelines to maximize elders' visual functions and thus their abilities to function in daily life. However, many individuals have such low vision that these methods are ineffective. COTAs should also learn basic vision substitution techniques for ADL functions to teach those elders who have no functional vision. The next section lists some professionals who may be able to provide some training in these techniques or who may be able to direct OT practitioners to appropriate training seminars and literature.

RESOURCES

Low-vision rehabilitation is becoming a specialty area in the field of occupational therapy. Those who work in this area receive specialized training in addition to their basic OT skills. Fortunately, there are already many professionals working in low-vision rehabilitation who can serve as a resource or who can supplement the OT program. These professionals include low-vision specialists (ophthalmologists or optometrists), rehabilitation teachers, vision teachers, and orientation and mobility specialists. It would be beneficial to become familiar with local low-vision clinics or state rehabilitation programs and the services they offer so an exchange of information can occur that would benefit elders being treated.

There are many assistive devices for individuals with low vision such as talking clocks; large-print playing cards and bingo cards; insulin-drawing devices with raised numbers for diabetics; large-print or raised-letter measuring spoons, cups, and oven dials; and closed circuit televisions to enlarge print. (Catalogs and other resources can be obtained from organizations listed in the Appendix.)

VISUAL DYSFUNCTION AFTER NEUROLOGICAL INSULT

The discussion of visual impairments in elders thus far has focused on impairments as a result of ocular conditions. However, the visual system is not composed of the eyeballs alone. To perceive visual information, the data must travel through a complex nervous system and be processed by appropriate cerebral centers. In addition, effective control of eye movements depends on proper impulses from the brain. Thus successful adaptation to the environment through the visual sense requires the proper functioning of both ocular and neurological components.

Causes of brain insult include trauma, cancer, and multiple sclerosis; however, elders are particularly at risk for cerebrovascular accidents (CVAs), or strokes. The vision system is vulnerable to strokes or other types of brain insult (Warren, 1993).

Homonymous hemianopsia, or loss of visual field in the corresponding right or left half of each eye, is a frequent result of strokes (Leigh, Zee, 1983). The presence of a visual field loss has been directly associated with a decline in functional daily activities, including dressing, driving, reading, and returning to work (Warren, 1981; Gianutsos et al, 1983; Hier, Mondlock, Caplan, 1983; Johnson, Keltner, 1983; Grosswasser, Cohen, Blankstein, 1990).

Oculomotor dysfunction, or an impairment in eye movement control, may occur through either a disruption of cranial nerve function or a disruption of central neural control. Injury to cranial nerves results in paralysis or paresis of extraocular muscles. When this occurs, the two eyes are unable to work together, resulting in diplopia, or double vision. Other types of oculomotor dysfunction occur when damage is not to the cranial nerves, but to other complex cortical and subcortical structures. Damage to the cerebellum may affect the direction, extent, force, and timing of eye movements. Parietal lobe injuries may result in difficulty initiating saccades (shifts in gaze from one target to the next). Injury in the frontal eye field region may cause unorganized or incomplete scan patterns (Warren, 1993). These structures do not comprise the complete list of the cortical components involved in the visual system, but this system is clearly complex.

FRAMEWORK FOR ADDRESSING VISUAL DYSFUNCTION

Because of the complexity of the visual system, a framework for evaluation and treatment of visual impairments, whether ocular or neurological in nature, may be helpful. Warren (1993) suggests a developmental model that conceptualizes vision abilities in a hierarchy (Figure 17-8). The abilities at the bottom of the figure form the foundation for each successive level. Higher-level abilities depend on the complete integration of lower-level abilities for their development.

The highest vision ability in this model is **visual cognition.** Visual cognition is the ability to mentally

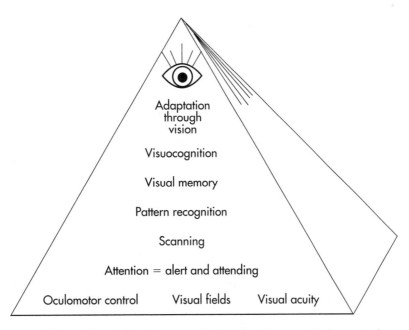

FIGURE 17-8 Hierarchy of visual perceptual skills development in the central nervous system. (Adapted from Warren ML: A hierarchical model for evaluation and treatment of visual perceptual dysfunction in adult acquired brain injury, part 1, *Am J Occup Ther* 47:42, 1993.)

manipulate visual information and integrate it with other sensory information to solve problems, formulate plans, and make decisions. This ability is required for reading, writing, and solving mathematical problems.

Visual memory is the ability directly after visual cognition. Visual cognition depends on visual memory because mental manipulation of a visual stimulus requires the ability to retain a mental picture (Ratcliff, 1987).

To store a visual image, individuals must be able to recognize a pattern. **Pattern recognition,** the next ability level, involves identification of the salient features of an object (Jules, 1981, 1985). An individual must not only be able to identify the holistic aspects of an object such as its shape and contour but also specific features of an object such as its color detail, shading, and texture.

The ability to scan the environment is necessary for effective pattern recognition. **Scanning,** therefore, is a foundation ability for pattern recognition. The eye must record all the details of a scene systematically and follow an organized scan path.

The ability directly below scanning is **visual attention.** Engagement of visual attention is necessary for proper scanning to occur. If individuals are not attending to visual stimuli in a specific space, they will not initiate scanning into that area. A classic example is of the elder with a CVA with left hemineglect who requires constant cueing to scan to the left to avoid colliding with objects.

Visual attention and all the higher-level abilities depend on three primary visual abilities that form the foundation for all vision functions: **oculomotor control, visual fields,** and visual acuity. Oculomotor control enables efficient and conjugate eye movements, which ensure completion of accurate scan paths and "teaming" of the eyes for binocular vision. The visual fields register the scene and ensure that the central nervous system has a complete picture.

Evaluation and Treatment of Visual Dysfunction

Evaluation and treatment of visual dysfunction should begin with a thorough examination of the foundation abilities followed by an assessment of the next higher-level abilities, visual attention and scanning. The majority of deficits occur in these areas (Warren, 1993). When deficits are observed, the treatment focus can be directed at correcting or compensating for these deficient abilities. Elders who have a visual field loss may be taught to compensate for this loss in daily activities. The first step, however, is to increase the elder's awareness of the visual field loss. Having accurate information on the extent and location of field loss is critical for teaching elders proper methods of compensation. Elders who have central field loss, such as that seen with macular degeneration, must learn to compensate by directing their gaze to the side of the target rather than directly at the target. This technique, called **eccentric viewing,** enables the indi-

vidual to place the target outside of the blind spot so it can be seen. This requires a conscious effort on the elder's part to override the natural tendency to direct the fovea, the most central area of the retina, to the target. An elder with a homonymous hemianopsia occurring after CVAs may also be taught to compensate for this loss of half the visual field by systematically training them to turn the head and scan into the impaired field.

Compensating for reduced visual acuity can also be accomplished through special optical devices as mentioned previously in the discussion of ocular impairments. Proper training in the use of these devices is crucial because elders are not usually used to working with "gadgets" and may be intimidated by these occasionally-awkward devices. Large-print materials and writing larger by using a felt tip pen are also helpful techniques to compensate for reduced acuity.

Treatment for oculomotor dysfunction may involve more of a remediation approach. After careful analysis to determine which ocular muscles are affected, therapy may be directed at strengthening specific muscles and improving oculomotor control so that single binocular vision is once again possible.

Initial treatment of deficits in visual attention and scanning often involves increasing the elder's awareness of the deficit followed up with appropriate compensation and/or remediation techniques. Research has shown that individuals with left visual neglect may be trained to reorganize their scanning strategies by beginning the scan path in the impaired space (Weinberg et al, 1979). This is accomplished through activities that require and encourage a systematic left-to-right scan pattern with an anchor placed to the left as a cue if necessary.

SUMMARY

Visual impairments in elders may result from either ocular or neurological pathology. Normal physiological changes that may occur with aging include a shrinkage of the peripheral field, increased time required to recover from glare, difficulty with light and dark adaptation, increased need for illumination, loss of elasticity in the lens, and yellowing of the lens. The most common ocular diseases that may occur in elders are macular degeneration, cataracts, glaucoma, and diabetic retinopathy. Elders are also at risk for CVAs, which may disrupt any of several neurological components necessary for effective visual functioning.

COTAs can play vital roles in helping elders with low vision learn to function as independently as possible. By providing education about a particular vision loss, COTAs may be able to provide the first sense of security these individuals have had since being diagnosed as visually impaired. COTAs may also provide instruction in the techniques for compensating for vision loss in daily activities. Finally, COTAs may make assistive adaptations to the elder's environment, which may enable the elder to function more independently.

The loss of vision in elders is a common occurrence, whether it results from the natural aging process, ocular disease, or disruption of neurological components. Vision loss itself has significant functional implications and can complicate the elder's rehabilitation process with other physical impairments. This emphasizes the need for COTAs to familiarize themselves with the causes and types of vision loss as well as effective treatment techniques, whether they are working in low-vision clinics, general rehabilitation centers, or acute care hospitals.

CASE STUDY

E.M., a 78-year-old widow, is admitted to the rehabilitation unit of an acute care hospital after surgery involving a right total hip replacement. The surgery was necessary after she fell and broke her hip. The COTA finds that E.M. has difficulty reading the hospital handout on the precautions necessary after hip replacement. E.M. wears glasses with bi-focals but states that she has had difficulty reading for the past couple months. This bothers her because she had been an avid reader. When the COTA asks E.M. to sign her name on a loan policy for assistive equipment, E.M. starts to sign on the line, but her name drifts down below it. During her usual daily living activities, E.M. pulls out a pair of socks from her drawer, but one is navy and the other is black. When asked about how she fell, E.M. states that she was going to cross a street and accidentally stepped off the curb. She states she could not see the subtle changes in color between the curb and the street because it was an unmarked curb. When asked if she has seen an eye doctor recently, E.M. re-plies that she saw one last year, who told her that he noticed the beginning of "some kind of disease" in the back of her eye, but she could not remember its name. The eye doc-tor asked her to return in a year for a follow-up or sooner if she noticed any significant changes in her vision. She had been meaning to set up that appointment, but had not got-ten around to doing it yet. E.M.'s daughter appears to be supportive and is anxious to learn anything she can that will help her mother. She inquires whether her mother's vision problem could have anything to do with the fact that she seems to lose things all the time even though she has an amazingly good memory.

▮ CHAPTER REVIEW QUESTIONS

1 Referring to the Case Study, what ocular disease does E.M. likely have?
2 State some effective principles to incorporate into E.M.'s treatment.
3 E.M. will be discharged relatively soon. What rec-ommendations could the COTA make for further services or assistance?
4 Why is it of particular importance that this client learn low-vision compensatory techniques?
5 Referring to the total chapter, what are the func-tional implications of macular degeneration on daily activities of elders?

6 What are the primary vision abilities that form the foundation for all other vision abilities?
7 What are typical symptoms of narrow-angle glaucoma?
8 What is the difference between background and proliferative diabetic retinopathy?
9 What changes may the lens undergo during the natural aging process?
10 What other vision changes may occur with the natural aging process?
11 What are some possible vision problems following a CVA?
12 Of the four ocular diseases discussed, which has the most successful outcome from medical or surgical management?

REFERENCES

Bennett, SH: Visual changes associated with aging: influence on practice, *Occup Ther Prac* 3(1):12, 1991.

Bennett, SH: Low vision: clinical aspects and interventions. In Rothman J, Levine R, editors: *Prevention practice strategies for physical therapy and occupational therapy*, New York, 1992, WB Saunders.

Castor TD, Carter TL: Low vision: physician screening helps to im-prove patient function, *Geriatrics* 50(2):51, 1995.

Cristarella MC: Visual functions of the elderly, *Am J Occup Ther* 31: 432, 1977.

Faye EE: *Clinical low vision*, Boston, 1984, Little, Brown.

Fletcher D et al: Low vision rehabilitation: Finding capable people behind damaged eyeballs, *West J Med* 154:554, 1991.

Gianutsos R et al: Visual imperception in brain injured adults: multifaceted measures, *Arch Phys Med Rehabil* 64:456, 1983.

Grosswasser Z, Cohen M, Blankstein E: Polytrauma associated with traumatic brain injury: incidence, nature, and impact on rehabili-tation outcome, *Brain Injury* 4:161, 1990.

Hier DB, Mondlock J, Caplan LR: Behavioral abnormalities after right hemisphere stroke, *Neurol* 33:334, 1983.

Johnson CA, Keltner JL: Incidence of visual field loss in 20,000 eyes and its relationship to driving performance, *Arch Ophthalmol* 101: 371, 1983.

Jose RT: The eye and functional vision. In Jose RT, editor: *Under-standing low vision*, New York, 1985, American Foundation for the Blind.

Jules B: Texton, the elements of texture perception and their interac-tions, *Nature* 290(12):91, 1981.

Jules B: Preconscious and conscious processing in vision. In Chagas C, Gattass R, editors: Pattern recognition mechanisms, *Exper Brain Res* 11(suppl 11): 333, 1985.

LaPlante MP: Prevalence of conditions causing need for assistance in activities of daily living. In *Data on disability From the National Health Interview Survey, 1983–1985-Info Use Report*, Washington, DC, 1988, US National Institute on Disability and Rehabilitation Research.

Leigh RJ, Zee DS: *Neurology of eye movements*, Philadelphia, 1983, FA Davis.

Mehr HM, Mehr EB, Ault C: Psychological aspects of low vision re-habilitation, *Am J Optom* 47:605, 1970.

National Institute on Aging: *Aging and your eyes*, US Department of Health and Human Services Pub No 88-195, Washington DC, 1988, US Government Printing Office.

Ratcliff G: Perception and complex visual processes. In Meier MJ, Benton AL, Diller L, editors: *Neuropsychological rehabilitation*, New York, 1987, Guilford.

Seligmann J: Making the most of sight: a brighter future for the millions of Americans with "low" vision, *Newsweek* April 6, 92, 1992.

Warren ML: Relationship of constructional apraxia and body scheme disorders to dressing performance in adult CVA, *Am J Occup Ther* 35:431, 1981.

Warren ML: A hierarchical model for evaluation and treatment of visual perceptual dysfunction in adult acquired brain injury, part 1, *Am J Occup Ther* 47:42, 1993.

Weinberg, J et al: Visual scanning training effect on reading-related tasks in acquired right brain damage, *Arch Phys Med Rehabil* 60: 479, 1979.

Whitmore LA: *Living with and understanding glaucoma: a reference guide for patients and their families*, San Francisco, 1986, Foundation for Glaucoma Research.

CHAPTER 18

Working With Elders Who Have Hearing Impairments

SHARON STOFFEL

KEY TERMS

sensorineural hearing loss, presbycusis (sensory, neural, mechanical), conductive hearing loss, cochlear implants, tinnitus, hearing aid, assistive listening device (ALD), audiologist

CHAPTER OBJECTIVES

1. Describe sensorineural and conductive hearing losses.
2. Describe ways that presbycusis interferes with functional communication.
3. List environmental modifications that reduce background noise in homes and institutions.
4. Describe possible safety recommendations for home and institutional environments where hearing-impaired elders reside.
5. Describe the effect of age-related hearing losses on socialization and its possible contribution to feelings of isolation for hearing-impaired elders.
6. List suggestions for improving communication with a hearing-impaired elder.
7. Describe possible behaviors that may indicate hearing impairment.

The voice of a loved one, the chimes of a grandfather clock, a violin concerto—these are sounds many people not only enjoy, but take for granted. For elders who have hearing impairments, these sounds may be either misinterpreted or missed altogether. Hearing impairments may also be associated with ambulation difficulties, balance problems, and increased incidence of falls (Kinderknecht, Garner, 1993; Tobias et al, 1990). Hearing impairments can contribute to social isolation. Safety related to hearing impairments may become a concern when elders are unable to hear alarms and other warning signals.

Hearing loss is more prevalent than any other chronic condition (DiDomenico, Ziegler, 1994; Luey, 1994; Rieske, Hostege, 1996). By the year 2050, 26 million people are expected to have a hearing impairment (Kinderknecht, Garner, 1993; Riekse, Hostege, 1996). Although persons of all ages experience hearing impairments, elders are primarily affected (Hooper, 1994). Elders between the ages of 65 and 74 years experience an estimated 25% hearing loss. This percentage increases to 40% for those over 75 years of age, and some studies indicate that 85% to 90% of nursing home residents have hearing impairments that limit function (Hooper, 1994).

Even though hearing impairments are more prevalent than vision losses, they are often more difficult to distinguish. Levels of "normal" hearing for elders have never been clearly defined (Hooper, 1994; Kinderknecht, Garner, 1993). Because changes in hearing are often subtle and occur gradually, elders, family members, and health care personnel may not recognize hearing losses. Some may accept the loss as an inevitable and unalterable aspect of aging.

Because elders seldom seek assistance or plan interventions to enhance their hearing, COTAs must be able to distinguish the various types of hearing impairments. In addition, COTAs should be aware of interventions, services, devices, and activities that can enhance functional performance for elders who are hearing impaired. This chapter provides an overview of the most common types of hearing losses that affect elders. The possible psychosocial effects that a hearing impairment may have on elders, their families, and their friends are also addressed. Rehabilitation considerations are discussed, including communicating with an elder who has a hearing impairment, methods for modifying home and institutional environments, and recommendations for assisting elders in the use of hearing aids and assisted listening devices.

HEARING CONDITIONS ASSOCIATED WITH AGING

An elder who has a hearing loss should see a physician to determine cause and rule out or treat other underlying pathologic processes (Kinderknecht, Garner, 1993). Generally, hearing losses are divided into the three following areas: sensorineural, conductive, and mixed. These conditions may affect one or both ears.

The most common type of hearing loss in elders is the result of sensorineural damage to the hearing organ itself or to the peripheral or central nervous system (or both). Although elders rarely have just one type of **sensorineural loss,** the most common type of loss is caused by hair cell damage or loss of the sensory hair cells of the cochlea. As individuals age, these hair cells are slowly lost, and the ability to hear high-frequency sounds is diminished. In elders, this type of high-frequency hearing loss is referred to as **presbycusis,** which means "old hearing" (Perlmutter, Hall, 1992).

Elders living in areas with low noise levels may experience less high-frequency hearing loss than those living in noisy, industrial areas. Some high-frequency loss eventually affects elders regardless of environmental conditions. However, continued exposure at any age to loud noises for long periods, such as listening to head phones at high volumes, may cause permanent damage, resulting in premature presbycusis (Perlmutter, Hall, 1992).

Distinguishing age-related presbycusis from other types of hearing impairments can be complicated by the presence of other symptoms, a reduction in certain auditory nerve cells, and damage to the middle ear. Elders seldom have just one type of presbycusis, which presents another complicating factor in distinguishing between hearing impairments (DiDomenico, Ziegler, 1994; Christenson, Taira, 1990; Kinderknecht, Garner, 1993; Perlmutter, Hall, 1992).

Three types of age-related presbycusis have been identified: **sensory, neural,** and **mechanic.** Sensory presbycusis is caused by atrophy and degeneration of the hair cells at the base of the basilar membrane. It produces a loss of high-frequency sounds but does not interfere with the discrimination of speech. Neural presbycusis is caused by the loss of auditory nerve fibers. It affects the ability to distinguish speech sounds, especially in the higher frequencies, but does not affect the ability to hear pure tones. Mechanical presbycusis is characterized by degeneration of the vibrating membrane within the cochlea. This type of presbycusis leads to a gradual loss of hearing in all frequencies. In situations where several sounds in various frequencies are present at the same time, the ability to distinguish between the sounds becomes increasingly difficult. Table 18-1 lists common hearing conditions of elders.

A hearing loss related to presbycusis may be unnoticed in the early stages because the high-frequency tones that are initially lost are above the functional range used in most environments. As the condition progresses, elders may notice that they cannot hear the ringing of the telephone, the buzz of the doorbell, the ticking of a clock, or the water dripping from a faucet. With further progression, the sounds of certain consonants such as s, z, t, f, and g become increasingly difficult to distinguish. Eventually, elders may strain to hear and understand conversations and one-syllable words (Ellis, 1991).

Losses associated with presbycusis can have serious consequences in both social and therapeutic settings. For example, an elder who is asked to hand the COTA a "dime" may respond with the correct "time." In such a situation, the COTA should seek assistance to rule out the presence of presbycusis before questioning the elder's orientation or ability to follow directions. In addition, because women's voices are usually higher pitched than men's, female OT practitioners must understand that their voices can contribute to decreased comprehension by elders (Perlmutter, Hall, 1992).

A second hearing condition, **conductive hearing loss,** results in an inability of the external ear to conduct sound waves to the inner ear. Conductive hearing losses may be related to the buildup of cerumen (earwax), fluid accumulation in the middle ear from eustachian tube dysfunction, or an upper respiratory infection. These conductive problems can often be corrected by cleaning the ear, adminis-

TABLE **18-1**

Common Hearing Conditions of Elders

Condition	Cause	Symptoms
Sensory presbycusis	Atrophy and degeneration of the hair cells at the base of the basilar membrane	Loss of high frequency sounds; condition does not interfere with speech discrimination
Neural presbycusis	Loss of auditory nerve fibers	Condition affects ability to distinguish speech sounds in higher frequencies; does not affect ability to hear pure tones
Mechanical presbycusis	Degeneration of the vibrating membrane within the cochlea	Condition leads to gradual loss of hearing in all frequencies, ability to distinguish sounds becomes increasingly difficult
Conductive hearing loss	Inability of the external ear to conduct sound waves to the inner ear; may be related to buildup of ear wax, fluid accumulation in the middle ear, or upper respiratory infection	Condition can often be corrected by cleaning the ear, medications, or surgery; hearing aids or cochlear implants may be considered
Tinnitus	May be related to conductive or sensorineural loss, Ménière's disease, otosclerosis, presbycusis, earwax buildup, lesions, or fluid in middle ear	Buzzing, ringing, whistle, roar in ears, most noticeable at night; may be necessary to rule out underlying conditions before implementing treatments designed to mask symptoms

tering medications, or performing surgery. Hearing aids may be prescribed for persons who have untreatable or residual conductive hearing loss. **Cochlear implants** may be considered for persons whose residual hearing is greatly limited or who are severely deaf (Hooper, 1994).

Tinnitus is a subjective auditory problem consisting of a ringing, whistling, buzzing, or roaring noise in the ears. Tinnitus may occur as part of a conductive or sensorineural hearing loss. It may also be associated with Ménière's disease, otosclerosis, presbycusis, an accumulation of cerumen pressing on the ear drum, tympanic membrane lesions, and fluid in the middle ear. Medications such as the doses of aspirin prescribed for arthritis or other medical conditions can be additional contributing factors (Hooper, 1994; Perlmutter, Hall, 1992; Saxton, Etten, 1978). Before planning interventions to mask the symptoms of tinnitus, possible underlying conditions such as cardiovascular disease, anemia, and hypothyroidism should be ruled out by a physician.

Tinnitus is often most noticeable at night when other noises are reduced. A radio, tape recording, or appropriate hearing aid may mask the tinnitus so the individual can fall asleep. Other therapeutic interventions may include relaxation techniques and biofeedback (Corso, 1990).

PSYCHOSOCIAL ASPECTS OF HEARING IMPAIRMENTS

Even though much information about the environment is learned through the sense of hearing, the importance of hearing in work, personal, and social lives often goes unnoticed. Some researchers suggest that when hearing loss is the only loss elders experience, they can adjust well (Thomas et al, 1983). Others suggest that a hearing loss may lead to isolation and even paranoia (Corso, 1990; Ohta, Carlin, Harmon, 1981). Unfortunately, many elders experience other losses or lifestyle changes at the same time a hearing loss occurs. Retirement may lead to a loss of role identity, income, and social contacts. Adjusting to the death of a spouse or undergoing changes in vision or mobility may take priority over a loss of hearing. Elders who are predisposed to loneliness or have difficulty in initiating or maintaining relationships may become more isolated or avoid interpersonal relationships if they experience a hearing loss. This can result in an increased sense of loneliness or isolation, especially if the hearing impairment is associated with other losses (Perlmutter, Hall, 1992). Early assessment of a perceived hearing loss and recommendations for adaptations may help reduce an elder's sense of loneliness.

The elder with a hearing loss often guesses at or misses the content of conversations, is reluctant to ask for clarification, or is embarrassed when mistakes are made because of a misunderstanding. Consequently, communication can be exhausting for these elders. For example, an 85-year-old man registering for OT treatments at a rehabilitation clinic will likely be very embarrassed if he misinterprets the receptionist's request for his address as a request to undress. He may also experience isolation if his accompanying family member interrupts and answers all remaining questions. Repeated frustrating and embarrassing experiences can contribute to feelings of vulnerability, insecurity, and doubts related to self-esteem that can lead to withdrawal from social, cultural, and family contacts.

BOX 18-1

Observable Behaviors That May Indicate Hearing Loss

- Inappropriate volume increase when speaking; for example, appearing to shout while talking to a person nearby
- Turning the television or radio volume inordinately high when there is no one else in the room and no noises in the background
- Turning in a chair or turning the head to get a better hearing position when being addressed
- Consistently asking for statements to be repeated
- Not responding to verbal questions or conversation
- Responding to verbal questions only when there is accompanying visual cueing
- Looking disoriented or confused or giving inappropriate responses to questions; for example, answering "yes" to a multiple choice question
- Answering questions addressed to another person when there are several persons conversing simultaneously in the same room
- Withdrawing from social situations
- Exhibiting short attention span, which is especially apparent when two persons are talking simultaneously

Adapted from Kane, Ouslander, Abrass: Sensory impairment. In *Essentials of clinical geriatrics*, ed 2, New York, 1989, McGraw-Hill.

Some elders with hearing impairments may hear well at home and only struggle to hear in social settings. Others may be isolated not only from family and friends but also from the broader world because they cannot get information from television, radio, movies, and even telephone conversations. Elders may become increasingly frustrated as family, friends, and even health care workers begin to make decisions for them.

An age-related hearing loss may only further complicate the effects of illnesses and mental health conditions such as Alzheimer's disease. Hearing loss in elders can lead to or exacerbate paranoid ideas, suspicions, loss of contact with reality, and related tendencies (Perlmutter, Hall, 1992). Corso (1990) stated that a hearing loss can magnify previously existing paranoid personality attributes. Continued expression of suspicions, hostilities, and accusations of lying may result in friends and family members avoiding the hearing-impaired elder.

REHABILITATION AND THE HEARING-IMPAIRED ELDER

Rehabilitation is often an overlooked option for elders with hearing impairments and is seldom considered for those who are in the old-old age range (Commission on Education of the Deaf, 1989). The contributions of OT

practitioners in the areas of functional communication, socialization, and environmental assessment of home, work, and institutions is an integral part of enabling elders to live independent and productive lives (Mann et al, 1994). Without rehabilitation, elders may be at risk for increased frequency of falls, functional dependence, loss of self-esteem, and institutionalization.

The effectiveness of rehabilitation for maximizing functional independence is based on many factors. Those related to hearing loss may include age-related situational changes at the time of onset of the hearing impairment, such as vision and mobility losses, retirement, death of a spouse, and loss of clearly defined life roles. Other factors include the severity and rapidity of the loss, the degree of residual hearing, the presence of other medical conditions, and the involvement of the individual and family members in the rehabilitative process. COTA and OTR teams may work together to identify elders who have hearing impairments through observation of behaviors (Box 18-1). The Self-Rating Hearing Inventory can also be an effective tool for assessing the effects of a hearing impairment on perceived functional performance (Janken, Cullinan, 1990). The American Academy of Otolaryngology–Head and Neck Surgery has developed a 5-minute hearing test to determine the need for referral to a hearing specialist (Figure 18-1). For more profound hearing losses, a consultation and referral regarding use of a **hearing aid,** individual or computerized training in speech reading (lip reading), and instruction regarding the use of an **assisted listening device (ALD)** may be needed. In addition, referrals for accessing both formal and informal support services through public and community agencies may be beneficial.

COTAs may be involved in direct treatment interventions; adapting the environment for individuals, groups, or institutional facilities; and consultation and referrals. The skills and experience of COTAs may be directed toward designing and implementing individual or institutional activities. These recommendations, intended to promote successful adaptation for hearing-impaired elders, can also assist families, friends, and institutional personnel.

RECOMMENDATIONS FOR IMPROVING ELDER COMMUNICATIONS

Psychosocial issues associated with hearing impairments often affect family members and friends as well as the hearing-impaired elder. Information and education about the various types of age-related hearing losses and conditions may assist COTAs in developing coping strategies (Kinderknecht, Garner, 1993). The COTA should encourage family members and friends to be involved in the education and consultation process so that conversational and environmental adaptations that encourage inclusion of the elder can be promoted.

Five-Minute Hearing Test

	Almost always	Half of the time	Occasionally	Never
1. I have a problem hearing over the telephone.				
2. I have trouble following the conversation when two or more people are talking at the same time.				
3. People complain when I turn the TV volume too high.				
4. I have to strain to understand conversations.				
5. I miss hearing some common sounds like the phone or doorbell ringing.				
6. I have trouble hearing conversations in a noisy background such as a party.				
7. I get confused about where sounds come from.				
8. I misunderstand some words in a sentence and need to ask people to repeat themselves.				
9. I especially have trouble understanding the speech of women and children.				
10. I have worked in noisy environments (jackhammers, assembly lines, jet engines).				
11. Many people I talk to seem to mumble (or don't talk clearly).				
12. People get annoyed because I misunderstand what they say.				
13. I misunderstand what others are saying and make inappropriate responses.				
14. I avoid social activities because I cannot hear well and fear I'll reply improperly.				
To be answered by a family member or friend: 15. Do you think this person has a hearing loss?				

Scoring
To calculate your score, give yourself 3 points for every time you checked the "Almost always" column, 2 for every "Half of the time," 1 for every "Occasionally" and 0 for every "Never." If you have a blood relative who has a hearing loss, add another 3 points. Then total your points. The American Academy of Otolaryngology-Head and Neck Surgery recommends the following:
- 0 to 5: Your hearing is fine. No action is required.
- 6 to 9: Suggest you see an ear-nose-and-throat (ENT) specialist.
- 10 and above: Strongly recommend you see an ear physician.

FIGURE 18-1 5-minute hearing test. (Copyright 1993 by the American Academy of Otolaryngology–Head and Neck Surgery, Alexandria, Va.)

Hearing-impaired elders may need to gain confidence in requesting adaptations that help them adjust to their hearing losses. Having elders role play situations in which they request specific needs or adaptations may increase self-confidence for reentering social situations that they may have been avoiding.

Environmental adaptations should first center on identifying and minimizing the influence of background noises. Background noises greatly limit enjoyment of

conversations and often contribute to avoidance of social gatherings (Christenson, Taira, 1990). Common sources of background noise include music, conversations on television or of persons in the room, dishes being clanked, fans in use, outside traffic, overhead intercoms in use, and ice machines in use. Personnel shift changes in institutions may also create background noise.

COTAs can recommend environments that reduce background noise. Examples include going to restaurants during times that they are less crowded, requesting to sit in less crowded areas, or sitting away from distracting background noises such as kitchen traffic or music. Using theaters and church communities that offer ALDs that amplify specific sounds are other ways to reduce interference from background noises in public spaces.

Personal environmental modifications for reducing background noise include adding carpet to floors and acoustical tiles to ceilings, hanging drapes on windows, hanging banners from high ceilings, and replacing wood or metal furniture with upholstered furniture. Although these recommendations are intended to help absorb sound, they can also add aesthetic appeal to a home or institution (Christenson, Taira, 1990).

Additional interior modifications to reduce background noise within institutions include adding insulated sheetrock around noisy areas such as kitchens, maintenance, and mechanical areas, and tightening window weather seals. COTAs can assist individuals, families, and facility administrators in weighing the benefits of certain recommendations against the expenses. COTAs can also point out that, in some situations, background noises may provide helpful cues to locations of activity rooms, lounges, and beauty shops.

Environmental safety issues and concerns may center on the difficulties that hearing-impaired elders may have in locating the source of sounds in their home. Inability to locate sounds may contribute to a sense of insecurity in an individual's own environment and to the possibility of auditory illusions. Fire and smoke alarms tend to have high-pitched sounds that are difficult for persons with presbycusis to hear (Hooper, 1994). Adding visual cues such as flashing lights is recommended for alarms. Flashing lights, lower-pitched rings, or low-toned musical chimes are also available options for telephones and doorbells. COTAs should recommend adapting telephones with volume and tone controls for persons who need these modifications. Portable telephones, although convenient for some individuals, may add to confusion and frustration for persons with hearing impairments. The ring of a portable telephone may not be heard or the telephones may be difficult to locate if needed for an emergency.

Tobias et al (1990) reported a greater incidence of falls in hearing-impaired individuals than in those who are not hearing impaired. Studies indicate that instruction in ways to substitute visual cues for hearing cues reduces the incidence of falls. COTAs should also make family members and health care providers aware that approaching hearing-impaired elders from the back and talking to and touching them may startle them and possibly cause them to lose balance. COTAs should recommend that hearing-impaired persons be approached from the front, where visual contact can be made before beginning a conversation or expecting a response to a question.

To enhance conversations in areas where groups gather, COTAs should recommend that hearing-impaired individuals stay away from windows and plaster walls. Standing or sitting near soft materials that absorb sound, such as draperies, bookshelves, and upholstered furniture, is also recommended. Sitting in high-backed, upholstered chairs can help shield background noise. Focusing on the speaker's lips during conversation can help to increase comprehension. If an individual has more impairment in one ear than the other, the individual can find the position that maximizes hearing with the unaffected ear (Perlmutter, Hall, 1992; Christenson, Taira, 1990).

For family members and friends who want to improve communication with hearing-impaired elders, COTAs should recommend that they position themselves in the elder's field of vision and get the elder's attention before speaking. While conversing, they should look directly at the elder, reduce the rate of speech, and speak distinctly with a low tone. Additional recommendations include asking the elder to repeat what was said and providing written instructions to reinforce verbal directions. COTAs should stress that a hearing impairment does not lower an individual's intelligence. Accommodations for the hearing impairment should not be overly exaggerated or simplified to the point where elders with hearing loss feel that their intelligence or judgment is in question.

Because presbycusis and its corresponding reduction in the ability to hear high-pitched sounds is the most common hearing disorder in elders, lowering the voice is especially important for women who address hearing-impaired elders. Increasing volume only increases tone and contributes to personal and social embarrassment (Christenson, Taira, 1990).

In restaurants and institutional and private dining rooms, the social aspects derived from conversations during meals can be enhanced by seating no more than four persons at a table so eye contact can be easily made. In larger dining rooms, padded room dividers between tables can absorb sounds from surrounding tables. General recommendations regarding reduction of background noises should also be considered.

The effects of glare on the visual and nonverbal cues that enhance auditory communication should be considered when speaking with a hearing-impaired elder. Sources of glare may include windows, lights, and glass surfaces either from behind the person speaking or reflected from eyeglasses. Before beginning a conversation, the COTA, family member, or friend should adjust blinds or shades, adjust lighting, and reposition seating arrangements as needed.

TABLE **18-2**

Environmental Adaptations for the Hearing-Impaired Elder

Problem	Intervention
Background noises (institutional and home)	Add carpeting to floors, acoustical tiles to ceilings, and drapes on windows, and replace wood and metal furniture with upholstered furniture.
Background noises (institutional)	Hang banners from ceilings; add insulating sheetrock around kitchens, maintenance, and mechanical areas; tighten window weather seals. In dining rooms seat no more than four persons at a table and add padded room dividers between tables to absorb sound. On special care units, eliminate ringing telephones, televisions, and intercoms; serve meals in small groups; pass medications at times other than meal times.
Background noises (public places)	Go to restaurants at less crowded times; request to sit in areas away from music and kitchen. Seek out theaters and churches that offer listening devices to amplify specific sounds.
Safety (home)	Add flashing lights or lower-pitched rings to smoke detectors, doorbells, and telephones. Add volume controls to telephones. Learn to substitute visual cues for hearing cues to reduce incidence of falls.
Communication (conversation)	Focus on lips, get visual attention before speaking, look directly at person, speak clearly, lower voice tone, reduce glare.
Communication (television, radio, music)	Position to reduce glare, add closed captioning, use ALDs. Use remote controls to select programming, and alternate between music, television, and radio.

Entertainment via television, music, and radio offers opportunities for stimulation that are not dependent on other people. When elders control the times and selections for television and radio programs and music, the cognitive stimulation can be rewarding. When televisions and radios are on constantly or programs selected are not those the elder would choose, they become an additional source of background noise rather than a source of stimulation (Hooper, 1994; Christenson, Taira, 1990; Perlmutter, Hall, 1992). Closed captioned television is an additional option to suggest. COTAs should identify and reduce sources of glare on the screen when positioning elders for television viewing. ALDs offer a means of controlling the volume for the hearing-impaired elder without disturbing others. Adjusting the volume and sound for music for those individuals with presbycusis requires increasing the bass and decreasing the treble. Although this type of adjustment requires newer technology, the cost of this technology is quite reasonable when the potential benefits are considered (Christenson, Taira, 1990). (Table 18-2 summarizes environmental adaptations.)

PROVIDING ASSISTANCE WITH HEARING DEVICES

One of the most common assistive devices for persons with a hearing impairment is a hearing aid. An **audiologist** assists in determining if a hearing aid would be appropriate. The audiologist also determines whether other factors associated with aging, lifestyle, and personality are compatible with a hearing aid. COTAs may refer

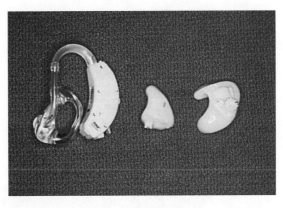

FIGURE **18-2** Hearing aids. (From Bingham BJG, Hawke M, Kwok P: *Atlas of clinical otolaryngology*, St. Louis, 1992, Mosby. Courtesy Dr. Julian Nedzelski.)

elders to a physician or audiologist for assessment and evaluation.

Recent improvements in hearing aid technology have made hearing aids more acceptable. The improved devices are smaller and fit in the ear and therefore are more cosmetically appealing (Figure 18-2). In addition they dampen certain frequencies. Some evidence indicates that younger persons report more satisfaction than elders do with hearing aids (Stoneham, 1994; Kane, Ouslander, Abrass, 1989; Rieske, Hostege, 1996). This increased satisfaction may result from several factors. The onset of age-related hearing loss is often gradual, and elders may have accommodated to their hearing loss over

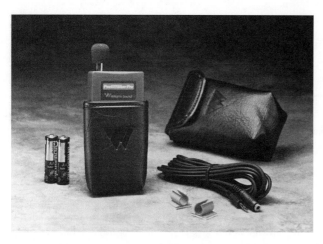

FIGURE 18-3   COTAs may need to instruct elders on maintenance of ALDs such as cleaning and battery changing. (Courtesy Williams Sound Corporation, Eden Prairie, Minn.)

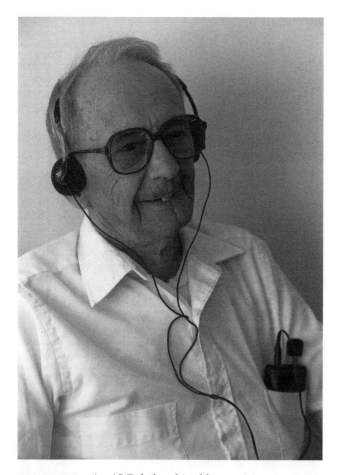

FIGURE 18-4   An ALD helps this elder participate more fully in social interactions.

an extended period, eventually finding the sudden amplification of all sound to be invasive and disturbing. In addition, the fine finger and hand dexterity required to manipulate volume and frequency controls and change batteries makes the hearing aid difficult to operate. Possible cognitive changes and short-term memory loss may affect the elder's ability to remember to turn the device on and off. The cost of replacement batteries, and the elder's acceptance of new technologies are other factors to consider when determining the appropriateness of a hearing aid (Stoneham, 1994; Christenson, Taira, 1990). Goals for an elder who uses a hearing aid may include identifying alternative ways of operating it, building handles for tools used with the controls, changing or testing batteries with less difficulty, and learning the proper way to insert the device. (The Appendix contains additional information on hearing aids.)

Even with improved technology, hearing aids may not be effective for some individuals. For others, sound distortions may be louder with a hearing aid. When hearing aids are not effective, ALDs may be used. ALDs consist of a microphone to capture spoken sounds, an amplifier to increase sound volume, and a headset worn by the hearing-impaired person (Figures 18-3 and Figure 18-4). Because the amplified sound from an ALD reaches the ear directly, background noises are reduced. ALDs can augment hearing in a noisy clinic or hospital room. When an ALD is plugged into a television, the sound is amplified only for the hearing-impaired person. Use of an ALD should also be considered when visual impairment does not allow the elder to lip-read or to supplement hearing loss by responding to other nonverbal cues.

CONCLUSION

As the numbers of elders with hearing impairments increase, the challenges and opportunities for COTAs continue to grow. The functional performance and psychosocial and environmental issues that surround a hearing impairment demand that COTAs be informed and able to recommend appropriate interventions. COTAs can assist elders in attaining both performance and quality of life expectations by identifying limitations in hearing, referring elders for additional evaluation and treatment, and providing appropriate therapeutic interventions.

CASE STUDY

Susan, a COTA who is employed by a home health agency, has been working with Mrs. Smith, a 78-year-old woman who has a hearing impairment. During a session, one of Mrs. Smith's daughters told Susan that the family has lately been struggling during their weekly Sunday dinners. Mrs. Smith's children have traditionally invited her for dinner on Sundays; however, the weekly interactions have been less than ideal and have been complicated by the poor quality of Mrs. Smith's vision and hearing abilities. During the last few weeks, Mrs. Smith has nearly fallen while moving around grandchildren, who sit in front of the television in the living room. Because she is totally deaf in her right ear and has only partial hearing in her left ear, Mrs. Smith has difficulty hearing conversations during dinner.

During these dinners, the children usually argue. The television is usually on in the adjacent living room. Mrs. Smith's daughter stated that she frequently finds her mother not paying attention to conversation or sitting silently at the dinner table. Also, when her mother does respond, her responses are often unrelated to the conversation and are sometimes totally strange. The daughter interprets Mrs. Smith's silence and preoccupation as disinterest. Susan was asked her opinion of what she thinks about the mother's behavior.

▮ CHAPTER REVIEW QUESTIONS

1 Referring to Mrs. Smith's case, list her strengths.
2 List the OT problems and needs of Mrs Smith and her family.
3 List possible OT recommendations for improving communication in Mrs. Smith's family.
4 List possible environmental modifications that may assist Mrs Smith and her family.
5 List possible referrals and resources that might be considered.
6 Referring to the whole chapter, what are some age-related hearing changes in elders?
7 How do age-related hearing impairments in elders affect their communication and socialization skills as well as their safety?
8 How can COTAs contribute to improving communication and socialization skills in hearing-impaired elders?
9 What environmental modifications can COTAs suggest to reduce background noises in an elder's home?
10 What environmental modifications in an institution might be used to reduce confusion caused by hearing impairments?
11 Why might an elder prefer not to use a hearing aid?
12 How might a COTA use an ALD to help an elder in a clinic setting?

REFERENCES

Christenson MA, Taira E, editors: *Aging in the designed environment*, New York, 1990, Halworth Press.

Commission on Education of the Deaf: *Toward equity: education of the deaf*, Washington, DC, 1989, US Government Printing Office.

Corso JF: Sensory-perceptual processes and aging. In Schaie KW, Eisdorfer C, editors: *Annual review of gerontology*, ed 2, New York, 1990, Springer.

DiDomenico RL, Ziegler WZ: Sensitivity training. In *Practical rehabilitation techniques for geriatric aides*, Gaithersberg, Md, 1994, Aspen.

Ellis NB: Aging, functional change and adaptation. In Kiernat JM, editor: *Occupational therapy and the older adult: a clinical manual*, Gaithersberg, Md, 1991, Aspen.

Hooper CR: Sensory and sensory integrative development. In Bonder BR, Wagner MB, editors: *Functional performance in older adults*, Philadelphia, 1994, FA Davis.

Janken JK, Cullinan CL: Auditory, sensory and perceptual alteration: suggested revision of defining characteristics, *Nurs Diag* 1(4):147, 1990.

Kane RL, Ouslander JG, Abrass IB: Sensory impairment. In *Essentials of clinical geriatrics*, ed 2, New York, 1989, McGraw-Hill.

Kinderknecht CH, Garner JD: Living productively with sensory loss. In Garner JD, Young AA, editors: *Women and healthy aging: living productively in spite of it all*, New York, 1993, Halworth.

Luey HS: Sensory loss: a neglected issue in social work, *J Gerontol Soc Work* 21(3/4):213, 1994.

Mann WC et al: Environmental problems in homes of elders with disabilities. *Occup Ther J Res* 14(3), 191, 1994.

Ohta RJ, Carlin ME, Harmon BM: Auditory acuity and performance on the mental status questionnaire in the elderly, *J Am Geriatr Soc* 10:476, 1981.

Perlmutter M, Hall E, editors: Sensation and perception across adulthood. In *Adult development and aging*, ed 2, New York, 1992, John Wiley & Sons.

Rieske RJ, Hostege H: *Growing older in America*, New York, 1996, McGraw-Hill.

Saxton SV, Etten MJ: *Physical change and aging: a guide for helping professions*, ed 2, New York, 1978, Tierisas Press.

Stoneham MA: Technology and disability, *Andover Medica* 13(1):47, 1994.

Thomas PD et al: Hearing acuity in a healthy elderly population: effects on emotional, cognitive, and social status, *J Gerontol* 38:321, 1983.

Tobias JAS et al: Falling among the sensorially impaired elderly *Arch Phys Med Rehabil* 71(2):144, 1990.

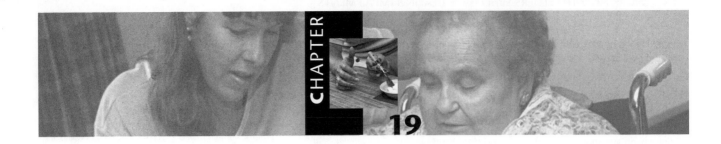

Strategies to Maintain Continence in Elders

KRIS R. BROWN

KEY TERMS

urinary incontinence, fecal incontinence, behavioral techniques, environmental modifications

CHAPTER OBJECTIVES

1. Determine the prevalence and cost associated with incontinence.
2. Indicate common causes of incontinence.
3. Review the normal anatomy and physiology of urination and defecation.
4. Identify the different types of urinary and fecal incontinence.
5. Explain the effect of the Omnibus Budget Reconciliation Act (OBRA) in dealing with the problem of incontinence in nursing homes.
6. Specify the role of each team member, emphasizing the importance of an interdisciplinary approach.
7. Identify the COTAs role in the management of incontinence.
8. List suggestions for the management of incontinence.

Incontinence of urine and stool is a common problem many elders face. Incontinence is often considered part of the normal aging process and is therefore accepted but not treated. Society's acceptance of this condition is manifested by the availability of absorbent products and high-fiber foods found in local stores. Some elders afflicted with this problem may feel ashamed and embarrassed, which may lead to psychological conditions such as depression and avoidance of social relations or activities. Other elders may think the problem will correct itself, or they may fear that it will lead to a surgical procedure. Prolonged hospitalizations are common when incontinence is left untreated. Incontinence may even be a primary reason caregivers decide to place elders in long-term care facilities.

During the normal aging process, bladder capacity and the ability to delay urination and defecation decrease. These changes can increase the risk of incontinence, especially with medical conditions such as pneumonia and chronic heart failure. Often, fecal incontinence results from changes in sphincter musculature and hormonal imbalances.

URINARY AND FECAL INCONTINENCE
Prevalence

The prevalence of **urinary incontinence** in the nursing home setting can range as high as 45% to 50% (Turpie, Skelly, 1989). For noninstitutionalized older adults, the range is 15% to 30% (US Department of Health and Human Services [DHHS], 1992). Women are twice as likely as men to experience this problem.

Cost

The total annual cost of health care in nursing homes for elders with urinary incontinence is estimated at 3.3 billion dollars (DHHS, 1992). This cost can be itemized to include routine care such as labor, supplies, and laundry, diagnostic and medical evaluation; treatment such as surgery and pharmacy and drug costs; incontinent consequences such as skin erosion, urinary tract infection (UTI), and falls; and added admissions resulting from incontinence (Hu, 1990). The total cost of managing urinary incontinence for those living in the community is 7 billion dollars (Hu, 1990).

Private insurance companies and government programs will usually only pay for urodynamic evaluation, surgical procedures, and catherization (Hu, 1990). Consequently management of incontinence is routine care. Elders and their families may feel financially strained if incontinence is the only reason for institutionalization. Therefore poor reimbursement encourages management of incontinence rather than determination of the underlying problem and provision of the most effective treatment.

ANATOMY AND PHYSIOLOGY

The anatomical structures of the male lower urinary tract primarily responsible for normal urination include the bladder neck, prostate gland, pelvic floor musculature, and urethra. In women, the structures include the bladder neck, proximal urethra (internal sphincter), and the pelvic floor muscles that provide the strength needed to maintain the pelvic floor tone and urethra resistance.

The bladder fills and empties. As the bladder fills to an average of 400 m, the pelvic floor and sphincter sense the increased pressure and the individual feels the urge to void (Doughty, 1991). The urethra then relaxes, allowing the bladder to empty.

The anatomic structures involved with normal defecation include the pelvic floor muscles, anal sphincter mechanisms (internal and external), colon, rectum, and anal canal.

A stool of an appropriate consistency is delivered to the rectum and anal sphincter via the gastrointestinal tract and colon. The normal sensory system acknowledges that the rectum is filling and alerts the structures of the type of rectal content (that is, solid, liquid, or gas). Once the stool passes the rectum, the internal sphincter relaxes, allowing the stool to pass.

Etiology

Causes of urinary and stool incontinence may be pathological, anatomical, or physiological. The most common potential causes of urinary incontinence are transient, or reversible. These include delirium, infec-

tion such as symptomatic UTI or vaginitis, and psychological factors such as depression. Excessive urine production, hypercalcemia, hyperglycemia, diabetes insipidus, chronic heart failure, lower extremity venous insufficiency, and drug-induced ankle edema are other causes of transient incontinence (DHHS, 1992).

Pharmaceutical causes of transient incontinence are sedative hypnotics (that is, benzodiazepines); diuretics, leading to polyuria; calcium channel blockers; anticholinergic agents (that is, antihistamines, antidepressants, antipsychotics, antiparkinsonian agents, and alphaadrenergic agents); sympathomimetics; and sympatholytics. Potential causes of **fecal incontinence** include abnormal delivery of feces to rectum, which may be drug-induced, metabolic, or caused by infection; sphincter dysfunction from trauma, diabetes mellitus, or inflammation; reduced rectal compliance such as rectal ischemia or fecal impaction; and anatomic derangement such as from a tumor or from third-degree hemorrhoids or injury. Other causes of fecal incontinence include muscular and neuromuscular disorders such as congenital or hereditary myopathy, behavioral and developmental dysfunction such as mental retardation or psychiatric disorders, and neurological impairment such as with the central nervous system, spinal system, or peripheral nervous system (Doughty, 1991).

TYPES OF URINARY INCONTINENCE
Urge Incontinence

Elders commonly have a combination of types of urinary incontinence. Urge incontinence is defined as the inability to hold urine for a time long enough to reach the bathroom (Newman et al, 1991). Elders may experience a massive and sudden loss of urine without warning and often strain to empty the bladder. This type of urge incontinence is common at night and is referred to as *nocturnal incontinence*. Urge incontinence may also occur when elders hear water trickling or when they drink small amounts of water. Uncontrolled contraction of the detrusor (bladder muscle), a condition that is also referred to as *detrusor hyperflexia*, may be part of the problem (Newman et al, 1991).

Stress Incontinence

Stress incontinence is considered more prevalent in women than in men. Elders with stress incontinence experience uncontrolled loss of urine when intraabdominal pressure is placed on the bladder. This type of incontinence can occur while coughing, laughing, sneezing, exercising, bending, lifting a heavy object, and arising from a chair. A child sitting on an elder's lap may place sufficient pressure on the elder's bladder, which can lead to incontinence. Stress incontinence is usually caused by weakened pelvic floor musculature as a result of the childbirth process in women, or a weakened or damaged sphincter mechanism.

Overflow Incontinence

An individual with overflow incontinence suffers from frequent or constant dribbling of urine, voiding only small amounts at a time. The bladder is always full, and the elder is never able to completely empty it. The elder cannot sense its fullness. The cause is often an underactive detrusor muscle. In men this type of incontinence is common when there is a blockage in the bladder.

Mixed Incontinence

Mixed incontinence is a combination of urge and stress incontinence. Most cases of urinary incontinence are in this category.

Functional Incontinence and Other Types

Functional incontinence is related to impaired cognitive functioning and mobility. This type of incontinence often warrants OT intervention to help with environmental and other adaptations. Other types of incontinence, which are not as common, include reflex incontinence and detrusor instability. Reflex incontinence is a storage and emptying problem resulting from a spinal cord lesion. Detrusor instability is common in individuals diagnosed with dementia. With this type of incontinence, the bladder contracts before it is full.

FECAL INCONTINENCE

Fecal incontinence is often a result of problems with the gastrointestinal (GI) tract and colon. GI problems cause changes in the consistency and volume of stools, leading to problems such as diarrhea and constipation (Doughty, 1991). Diarrhea is defined as "the frequent passage of loose, watery stools" (Anderson, Anderson, Glanze, 1994). Associated symptoms are abdominal pain and cramping. Diarrhea can be a symptom of problems such as dietary intolerance, malabsorption syndromes, inflammatory bowel disease, fecal impaction, gastroenteritis, and GI tumors.

An individual suffering from constipation will complain of abdominal pain and fullness in the rectum. Defecation usually occurs infrequently, and consistency of the stool is hard and dry. Constipation can result from intestinal obstruction, diverticulitis, tumors, dehydration, lack of exercise, and poor diet.

OBRA AND RELATED RESEARCH

The Agency for Health Care Policy and Research (AHCPR) was created as a result of the Omnibus Budget Reconciliation Act (OBRA) to conduct research on diseases and disorders. Following are the initial guidelines for information on urinary incontinence developed as a result of the studies conducted by the AHCPR panel:

1. Improve education and dissemination of urinary incontinence diagnosis and treatment alternatives to the public and to health care professionals.
2. Educate the consumer to report incontinence problems once they occur.
3. Improve the detection and documentation of urinary incontinence through better history taking and health care record keeping.
4. Establish appropriate basic evaluation and further evaluations.
5. Reduce variance among health care professionals.
6. Encourage further biomedical, clinical, and cost research on prevention, diagnosis, and treatment of urinary incontinence in the adult (DHHS, 1992).

This special panel concluded that most elders were improperly diagnosed for urinary incontinence and ineffectively treated. Both urinary and fecal incontinence are areas that surveyors look at closely during their annual inspections because of the secondary complications such as skin erosion and falls associated with these problems (Figure 19-1). (See Chapter 6 for a review of the MDS.) According to OBRA guidelines, the goal is to encourage the nursing home staff to use a rehabilitative model in the care of incontinence (NovaCare, 1993).

INTERDISCIPLINARY TEAM STRATEGIES

Only half the elders residing in the community actually relate their incontinence problems to their physicians to receive treatment (Mitteness, 1990; National Institutes of Health Consensus Development Conference, 1990). When the problem is reported, many health care professionals treat incontinence as a disease rather than determine the underlying cause.

Health care providers involved in the treatment of incontinence in elders include urologists, gynecologists, psychiatrists, nurses, psychologists, social workers, dietitians, pharmacists, and enterostomal therapists (ET nurses). Other health professionals include OT practitioners and physical and speech therapists. All members of this team work together to determine the most effective plan of care, and each provides a unique role in the interdisciplinary team.

Physicians begin care of elders with incontinence by taking a thorough medical history, performing a physical examination, and scheduling laboratory tests. They may refer the client to a specialist such as a urologist or gynecologist if the problem is recurrent. However, a conservative approach is usually initiated. The primary preference is the use of **behavioral techniques** followed by pharmacologic approaches. Because of potential complications, surgery is considered the last resort. Surgery for stress incontinence in women, which requires repositioning the bladder neck, has a success rate of 78% to 92%. The success rate of surgery in men with overflow incontinence, which requires removal of the cause of blockage, is similar (DHHS, 1992). Surgery for fecal

SECTION H. CONTINENCE IN LAST 14 DAYS

1.	CONTINENCE SELF-CONTROL CATEGORIES ***(Code for resident's PERFORMANCE OVER ALL SHIFTS)*** **0. CONTINENT** — Complete control (includes use of indwelling urinary catheter or ostomy device that does not leak urine or stool) **1. USUALLY CONTINENT** — BLADDER, incontinent episodes once a week or less; BOWEL, less than weekly **2. OCCASIONALLY INCONTINENT** — BLADDER, 2 or more times a week but not daily; BOWEL, once a week **3. FREQUENTLY INCONTINENT** — BLADDER, tended to be incontinent daily, but some control present (e.g., on day shift); BOWEL, 2–3 times a week **4. INCONTINENT** — Had inadequate control. BLADDER, multiple daily episodes; BOWEL, all (or almost all) of the time				
a.	**BOWEL CONTINENCE**	Control of bowel movement, with appliance or bowel continence programs, if employed 1, 2, 3 or 4 = **16**			
b.	**BLADDER CONTINENCE**	Control of urinary bladder function (if dribbles, volume insufficient to soak through underpants), with appliances (e.g., foley catheter) or continence programs, if employed			
2.	**BOWEL ELIMINATION PATTERN**	Bowel elimination pattern regular – at least one movement every 3 days	a.	Diarrhea	c.
				Fecal impaction **17•**	d.
		Constipation **17•**	b.	*NONE OF ABOVE*	e.
3.	**APPLIANCES AND PROGRAMS**	Any scheduled toileting plan	a.	Did not use toilet room/commode/urinal	f.
		Bladder retraining program	b.	Pads/briefs used **6**	g.
		External (condom) catheter **6**	c.	Enemas/irrigation	h.
		Indwelling catheter **6**	d.	Ostomy present	i.
		Intermittent catheter **6**	e.	*NONE OF ABOVE*	j.
4.	**CHANGE IN URINARY CONTINENCE**	Resident's urinary continence has changed as compared with status of **90 days ago** (or since last assessment if less than 90 days) **0.** No change **1.** Improved **2.** Deteriorated			

FIGURE **19-1**   MDS (2.0) form section H. Form is used by nursing staffs to rate incontinence. (From Briggs' Health Care Products, Des Moines, Iowa, 1995.)

incontinence is indicated for traumatic, idiopathic, neurogenic, congenital, and medical problems. Surgery may consist of a bowel resection, sphincter repair, or gracilis muscle transfer (Doughty, 1991).

Medications are often prescribed to improve incontinence by treating infection, replacing hormones (estrogen), decreasing abnormal bladder contractions, and tightening sphincter muscles. This type of treatment is effective primarily with urge incontinence resulting from detrusor hyperactivity. Anticholinergics such as atropine, antispasmodics, tricyclic antidepressants, and calcium channel blockers are the drugs commonly prescribed. Antidiarrheal agents such as loperamide and fecal softeners and lubricants are common medications used to treat problems with defecation (Doughty, 1991).

The dietitian can determine hydration or nutrition patterns in the elder's diet that may be contributing to both urinary and stool incontinence. Recommendations such as a high-fiber diet and liquid intake of 48 to 64 oz per day help to maintain proper functioning of bowel and bladder. (Newman et al, 1991) Caffeine intake should be limited because it acts as a diuretic.

A nurse should complete a bowel and bladder profile indicating the length of time that incontinence has been present, and the frequency and timing of episodes (Figures 19-2, 19-3). The nurse usually initiates behavioral approaches.

Social service specialists and psychologists are important in determining the family dynamics and support available to elders. They may help determine the effect that incontinence has on the involvement of elders in social activities and relationships. They may also provide counseling to assist elders in expressing feelings about their incontinence problems.

Name_____ Date _____

Time toilet is offered	Leakage (yes or no)	Was client aware of urge? (yes or no)	Did client void? (yes or no)	Comments
0800				
1000				
1200				
1400				
1600				
1800				
2000				

(2200 and so forth)

FIGURE 19-2　Bladder record. (From Doughty DB: *Urinary and fecal incontinence nursing management*, St. Louis, 1991, Mosby.)

Date and Time	Stimulus to evacuation (digital, suppository, or none)	Response (amount and consistency of stool)	Incontinent episodes (time, amount, and type of leakage)

FIGURE 19-3　Simple diary of bowel function. (From Doughty DB: *Urinary and fecal incontinence nursing management*, St. Louis, 1991, Mosby.)

Speech and language therapists are involved in evaluating elders' abilities to communicate either verbally or nonverbally to make their needs known in a timely and effective manner. These professionals assist elders in compensating for impaired communication by providing instruction in the use of gestures and communication aids.

Specific training is also provided to the caregiver to ensure proper carryover.

Physical therapists (RPTs) are involved in completing a comprehensive musculoskeletal and functional mobility assessment to ascertain range of motion, muscle strength, bed mobility, sitting balance, and gait. The treatment provided by RPTs may also include teaching and instruction on the use of an assistive device such as a walker, cane, or brace to improve the elders' abilities to ambulate to the bathroom. Caregiver training by RPTs may include the proper use of a hoyer lift or sliding board with transfers or encouraging elders to carry over a program involving range of motion and strengthening exercises. Electrical stimulation to strengthen the muscles in stress incontinence, biofeedback, and Kegel exercises may all be part of the physical therapy (PT). These approaches can also be applied by OT with demonstrated competency.

COTAs work closely with the other disciplines to determine the cause of incontinence and develop an effective treatment plan. The following treatment techniques can be provided by members of the treatment team, including COTAs, to help increase voiding.

Timed Voiding and Habit Training

Timed voiding and habit training consist of establishing a fixed schedule that requires the client to void every 2 hours. Toileting is adjusted according to the client's normal pattern and is determined after approximately 2 weeks of monitoring. Attempts are made to increase the intervals between voiding. This habit training is often used in the nursing home setting and is successful with neurologically impaired residents.

Prompted Voiding

Prompted voiding is commonly used in the nursing facility and is recommended for frail or cognitively impaired individuals. Caregivers are responsible for documenting whether the client is wet or dry on a regular basis, usually every 1 to 2 hours. Caregivers are encouraged to ask whether elders have a need to void.

Bladder Training

Bladder training is recommended with stress and urge incontinence. Studies have shown a 10% to 15% improvement rate in urinary continence using bladder training (National Institutes of Health Consensus Development Conference, 1990). The goal is to decrease the frequency of voiding and lengthen the intervals between voiding. Caregivers instruct elders to resist the urge to urinate and to follow a planned time schedule rather than responding immediately to the urge.

Biofeedback

Biofeedback offers elders visual and auditory information to teach voluntary control of certain functions. Most elders are taught to relax the detrusor and abdominal muscles while contracting the sphincter muscle. An improvement rate of 20% to 25% in urinary incontinence has been noted for individuals using this technique (National Institutes of Health Consensus Development Conference, 1990). A 70% to 90% success rate is reported with fecal incontinence (Doughty, 1991).

Pelvic Floor Exercise

Pelvic floor exercises are also known as *Kegel*, or *childbirth*, exercises. Kegel exercises are commonly used and have a 30% to 90% success rate in women with stress incontinence (National Institutes of Health Consensus Development Conference, 1990). Elders are taught to relax the abdominal muscles while contracting the pelvic floor muscles. After assistance is given to identify the correct muscles, elders are told to complete 40 to 80 contractions of the pelvic floor muscles per day (Wells et al, 1991). This technique is commonly used to improve fecal incontinence and increase muscle tone in the pelvic floor to prevent stool leakage (Doughty, 1991). PTRs and OTRs can initiate these exercises.

ENVIRONMENTAL ADAPTATIONS

When considering problems with functional mobility, COTAs are encouraged to look at the elder's environment to determine whether modifications are necessary to facilitate independence and ensure safety while toileting (Box 19-1). COTAs should make recommendations for improvement where required (Table 19-1). (Refer to Chapter 16 for more information on fall prevention.)

BOX 19-1

Considerations for Environmental Adaptations to Help with Incontinence

1. Does the client need or use side rails to assist with bed mobility?
2. Is the call light easily accessible to the client?
3. Is the height of the bed appropriate for safe transfers?
4. Is the client restrained in bed or in the wheelchair, which would limit mobility to the bathroom?
5. Is there adequate lighting to and from the bathroom? (60-year-old elders require 3× more lighting than a 20-year-old adult.)
6. Are there any obstacles or clutter that would interfere with safe mobility?
7. Is the client able to manage the door leading into the bathroom?
8. Are the floors highly waxed, which could cause a fall?
9. Is the doorway leading into the bathroom wide enough to allow proper clearance for a wheelchair or walker?
10. Is the height of the toilet appropriate?
11. Are there any grab bars or support to assist with a transfer to the toilet?

Many **environmental modifications** can be made in the bathroom. For example, grab bars can be mounted either in a 45-degree horizontal fashion to assist in pushing up or in a vertical position to facilitate pulling up. The length of the bars should be between 24 and 36 inches on the back wall and 42 inches on the side wall (Schmitz, 1994).

Physical restraints can be used by caregivers in the nursing facility to prevent an individual from falling out of bed or the wheelchair. COTAs may be involved in assisting with restraint reduction. Because of the OBRA law, the use of restraints is carefully monitored. Restraints are only recommended to encourage more functional independence, to decrease the risk of a life-threatening medical problem, or to promote a better anatomical seating position that is minimally restrictive (OBRA, 1995). The use of a restraint may cause increased agitation because the elder will be unable to take care of bathroom needs if call lights are not answered in a timely manner to prevent incontinence. OBRA protects the rights of elders to freedom of movement and access to the body. COTAs must work closely with other staff members in deciding on a restraint program that allows the client to remain continent while minimizing the use of restraints.

TABLE 19-1

Environmental Adaptations to Help With Incontinence

Room	Adaptations
Bedroom, nursing home room, or hospital room	Place a commode near the bed
	Make a urinal or bed pan available
	Adjust the height of the bed
	Add side rail to the bed for ease with transfers
Bathrooms	Add a night light to increase visibility with mobility
	Add any combination of a toilet safety frame, elevated toilet seat, and grab bars to facilitate independence and ensure safety with transfers and clothing management
	Eliminate throw rugs or bath mats
	Add a nonskid material (dycem) in front of the toilet or commode

CLOTHING ADAPTATIONS AND MANAGEMENT

Clothing management before and after toileting is a functional independence measure (FIM). This measure is often used to evaluate toileting and bowel and bladder management at admission to and on discharge from inpatient facilities (Uniform Data System For Medical Rehabilitation, 1993). COTAs can help elders improve clothing management by providing activities that use fine motor coordination, such as increasing dexterity with manipulation of zippers or buttons. Range-of-motion and strengthening exercises may facilitate pulling pants over the feet and hips.

ADAPTATIONS FOR CLIENTS WITH FUNCTIONAL INCONTINENCE

An increased incidence of incontinence is often seen in elders with dementia. In addition to an inability to manage their clothing, these elders also have difficulty locating the bathroom and toilet. Some may have problems with their strength, coordination, range of motion, and sense of balance, which affect their abilities to toilet in a timely and safe manner. They may be seen

urinating and defecating in inappropriate places. Allen, Earhart, and Blue (1992) described this level of functioning as the *Allen Cognitive Level 3*. (See Chapter 7 for more information on this theory.) Elders with dementia might perform part of the toileting task but become confused at some point and require verbal or physical assistance or both to continue. COTAs can encourage maximal functioning by determining what tasks the client can do and by training caregivers to assist with only those tasks that become difficult.

Impaired functional mobility of elders can be addressed by COTAs in conjunction with physical therapy. The goal is to improve functional mobility skills and train caregivers to provide the proper physical and verbal cues needed for elders to become successful with safe mobility.

PREVENTION OF SKIN EROSION

One of the secondary effects of incontinence as previously mentioned was skin erosion. Caregivers must be educated on a bowel and bladder program, a repositioning schedule, and proper wound care. Skin integrity may be improved by placing a special mattress on the bed or an incontinence cushion on the sitting surface.

Nutrition is extremely important in wound healing. COTAs must consider elders' abilities to feed themselves. Elders may need to learn how to use adaptive equipment to aid this procedure. Elders must be able to obtain and drink fluids to maintain hydration.

CASE STUDY

Bertha is a 94-year-old elder who was admitted to a skilled nursing facility after falling in an assisted living apartment. She was hospitalized with a fracture of the right hip and received a total hip replacement. Past medical history includes right wrist fracture, chronic heart failure, and venous insufficiency. Current medications include pentoxifylline (Trental), diltiazem (Cardizem), diguxin (Lanoxin), furosemide (Lasix), potassium, nitroglycerine (Nitro-Bid), and magnesium hydroxide (Milk of Magnesia). OT and PT receive orders to treat 5× per week. Bertha's goals are to regain abilities with ADL functions and return home. The initial nursing assessment revealed that Bertha had poor nutritional status, frequent urinary incontinence (stress) and hard stools. Stage 1 pressure sores were noted in the perineal area and in the heels bilaterally.

The OTR and the COTA completed the evaluation. Following were the significant findings:

1. Difficulty noted in orientation and memory.
2. Able to follow a two-step command and attend to a task for 2 minutes.
3. Maximal assistance needed with bathing, dressing, transfers, and grooming.
4. Setup required for feeding.
5. Normal active range of motion in the upper extremities bilaterally.
6. Slight weakness in the upper extremities.
7. Functional and fine gross motor coordination.
8. Sensation and perception intact.

9. Fair dynamic and poor standing balance.
10. Touch weight bearing.

■ CHAPTER REVIEW QUESTIONS

1 List the different types of bladder training techniques that may be appropriate for Bertha.

2 What are some recommendations that a dietitian may make with regard to Bertha's diet to improve urinary incontinence?

3 List any medications that may be contributing to Bertha's incontinence problem. With whom would the COTA consult to obtain this information?

4 What are the treatment strategies that the OTR and COTA may establish to facilitate Bertha's independence?

5 With reference to the whole chapter, list the members of any incontinence team.

6 Describe how OBRA has affected the management of incontinence in the nursing facility.

7 Discuss whether urinary and fecal incontinence are part of the normal aging process.

8 What type of incontinence is more prevalent in women?

9 Describe the effect of incontinence on nursing home placement.

10 Which behavioral technique is commonly used for incontinence training with the client who has dementia?

11 What are some of the secondary complications associated with incontinence?

12 What is the role of the COTA in the management of incontinence?

13 What are some environmental modifications that can improve continence?

REFERENCES

Allen C, Earhart C, Blue T: *Occupational therapy treatment goals for the physically and cognitively disabled*, Rockville, Md, 1992, American Occupational Therapy Association.

Anderson KN, Anderson LE, Glanze WD, editors: *Mosby's medical, nursing, and allied health dictionary*, ed 4, St. Louis, 1994, Mosby.

Doughty D: *Urinary and fecal incontinence*, St. Louis, 1991, Mosby.

Hu The-wei: Impact of urinary incontinence on health-care costs, *J Am Geriatr Soc* 38(3):292, 1990.

Mitteness L: Knowledge and beliefs about urinary incontinence in adulthood and old age, *J Am Geriatr Soc* 38(3):3374, 1990.

National Institute on Aging: Age Page, Urinary incontinence, Bethesda, Md, 1991.

National Institutes of Health Consensus Development Conference: Urinary incontinence in adults, Bethesda, Md, 1990.

Newman D et al: Restoring urinary continence, *Am J Nur* 28, 1991.

NovaCare Inc: *OBRA guidelines for occupational therapy and physical therapy clinicians*, 1993 (handout).

Omnibus Budget Reconciliation Act: Baltimore, Md, 1995, Health Care Financing Administration.

Schmitz T: Environmental assessment. In O'Sullivan SB, editor: *Physical rehabilitation: assessment and treatment*, ed 3, Philadelphia, 1994, FA Davis.

Turpie I, Skelly J: Urinary incontinence: current overview of a prevalent problem, *Geriatrics* 44(9):32, 1989.

Uniform Data System for Medical Rehabilitation *Guide for the uniform data set for medical rehabilitation (Adult FIM)*, Buffalo, NY, 1993.

US Department of Health and Human Services: *Urinary incontinence in adults*, Rockville, Md, 1992.

Wells T et al: Pelvic muscle exercise for stress urinary incontinence in elderly women, *J Am Geriatr Soc* 39(8):785, 1991.

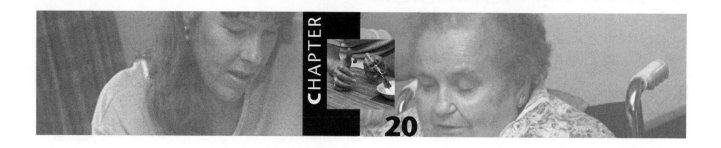

CHAPTER 20

Dysphagia and Other Eating and Nutritional Concerns With Elders

DEBORAH MORAWSKI AND TERRYN DAVIS

KEY TERMS

oral intake, undernourishment, malnutrition, dehydration, institutionalized, chronic care setting, hydration, bolus, compensations, dysphagia, positioning, aspiration pneumonia, alternative means, nutrition, contraindicated

CHAPTER OBJECTIVES *

1. Discuss the increased incidence of swallowing, eating, and nutritional problems occurring with elders.
2. Identify the basic anatomical structures related to swallowing and the swallow sequence.
3. Relate the physiological changes and the onset of increased age-related medical conditions with the increased incidence of swallowing problems.
4. Identify treatment strategies and precautions for improving oral intake and nutrition.
5. Discuss the roles of the team members and the importance of teamwork in addressing swallowing and nutritional concerns.
6. Relate ideas for managing different types of feeding problems.
7. Discuss the psychological and ethical concerns that are present when swallowing problems develop.

Eating is basic to survival and is an activity of daily living (ADL). As the elder population continues to increase, the incidence of swallowing, eating, and nutritional problems is expected to rise. Death and illness resulting from impaired **oral intake** is now considered a major health problem of elders (Feinberg et al, 1990).

Most noninstitutionalized elders have at least one chronic medical condition; many have multiple ailments. These conditions include arthritis, hypertension, heart disease, hearing impairments, orthopaedic impairments, sinusitis, diabetes, ringing in the ears, and vision impairments. These chronic conditions can influence elders' abilities to effectively and independently perform ADL functions such as eating, self-care, transfers, going outside and instrumental ADL functions such as meal preparation, shopping, money management, and housework. The need for individuals to receive help increases with age (American Association of Retired Persons [AARP], 1995).

When such help is unavailable, this lack of assistance can lead elders to social isolation and depression, which may lead to decreased oral intake. This decrease can result in **undernourishment, malnutrition,** and **dehydration.**

Among **institutionalized** elders, the prevalence of malnutrition may be as high as 70%. This high prevalence may be explained by the increased numbers of elders who need assistance with feeding and the lack of sufficient staff to assist them. In **chronic-care settings,** 19% to 24% of residents are reported to need total feeding assistance and 50% to 66% require some feeding assistance. In these settings, the staff provided assistance with eating on an average of 18 minutes per day to elders with severe dementia, and 14 minutes per day to elders with mild-to-moderate dementia (Musson et al, 1990).

These statistics clearly reflect the growing need for OT involvement with elders to help them maintain optimal independence in a home, hospital, or nursing home setting. OT assistance may include training in self-feeding, safe swallowing, positioning, mobility, meal preparation and cleanup, shopping; money management; provision of adaptive equipment; and caregiver and nursing instruction. All these activities are essential for elders to adequately maintain nutrition and **hydration.**

THE ROLE OF THE COTA

The COTA works in partnership with an OTR to collect data to identify the strengths and weaknesses of elders and establish and implement treatment plans to attain their goals. Ongoing assessment and communication between the COTA and the OTR is necessary for program and goal changes. The COTA is involved in individual and group treatment and in staff and caregiver instruction. Providing quality care is the function of the entire health care team. The amount of involvement of the COTA with elders with swallowing problems depends on the COTA's level of experience. An entry level COTA may work on activities that reinforce good nutrition and hydration such as meal preparation, money management, shopping, oral-facial exercises, instruction in adaptive devices, and energy conservation during activities. An experienced COTA, who has demonstrated competence in this area, may participate in videofluoroscopic swallow studies and assist tracheostomized and ventilator-dependent elders with self-feeding and swallowing.

THE NORMAL SWALLOW

The swallow response requires a rapid interplay between the brain, 6 cranial nerves, 48 pairs of muscles, the salivary glands, and cartilaginous structures (Figure 20-1). The COTA working with elders who have dysphagia must clearly understand the anatomy and physiology of swallowing (Nelson, 1995).

Four phases of swallowing have been defined: oral

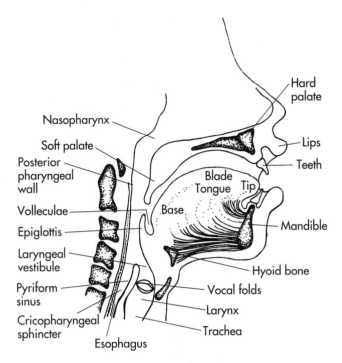

FIGURE 20-1 Oral structures and mechanisms at rest.

preparatory, oral, pharyngeal, and esophageal (Logeman, 1983) (Figure 20-2, *A-E*).

1. *Oral preparatory phase.* The oral preparatory phase includes seeing, smelling, reaching for the item, bringing it to the mouth, and putting it in the mouth. Once the item is placed in the mouth, the lips close to maintain a seal, and the tongue and cheek muscles move the **bolus** (that is, the food or liquid) around the mouth in preparation for swallowing. Saliva mixes with the bolus to aid in swallowing. Taste, temperature, and texture receptors of the tongue also play a part in preparing for the action of swallowing.
2. *Oral phase.* The oral phase occurs once the bolus is prepared and formed by the tongue. The bolus is then propelled by the tongue to the back of the mouth.
3. *Pharyngeal phase.* The pharyngeal phase occurs when the bolus passes over the base of the tongue and enters the pharynx. At this time, the soft palate elevates to seal the entrance to the nose, the hyoid bone and larynx elevate upward and anteriorly, the vocal folds close, the epiglottis tilts downward, and the cricopharyngeal sphincter opens to allow the bolus to enter the esophagus.
4. *Esophageal phase.* The esophageal phase occurs when the bolus passes into the esophagus and is propelled to the stomach.

Changes of Swallowing Structures

When individuals eat and swallow, the oral and pharyngeal structures adapt easily to different liquid and food

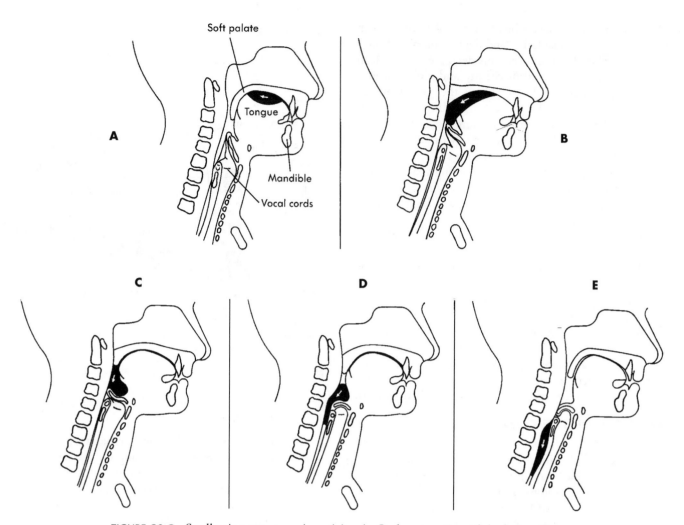

FIGURE 20-2 Swallowing structures in activity. **A,** Oral preparation of the bolus. **B,** Bolus moves from oral cavity to pharynx; swallow response initiated. **C,** Bolus passes through the pharynx; the airway is protected. **D,** Bolus enters upper esophagus. **E,** Bolus passes through the esophagus to the stomach. (From Logeman J: *Evaluation and treatment of swallowing disorders,* San Diego, 1983, Pro-Ed.)

consistencies and to the texture, temperature, and volume of the bolus. These structures also adapt to the different positions that the head and body may assume while swallowing. As individuals age, changes in these swallowing structures occur naturally (Sheth, Diner, 1988). Individuals develop **compensations** to these changes spontaneously and often unknowingly. These compensations allow them to eat safely and efficiently, such as with smaller bites, longer chewing time, and softer food (Buccholz, 1985). However, if individuals also develop a medical or neurological disorder, these compensations may no longer be effective and may result in increased swallowing problems (Table 20-1) (Cherney, 1994; Jaradeh, 1994). In addition to understanding the physical changes that occur, COTAs must also be aware of the psychological effect of swallowing problems on individuals who can no longer eat as they once did. COTAs should acknowledge elders' and care-givers' feelings about certain types of liquids or favorite foods being eliminated from their daily diet.

ETIOLOGY OF DYSPHAGIA

Dysphagia is the inability to swallow. This condition is often seen in elders and may have a variety of causes. These may be neurological such as from a cerebrovascular accident, brain tumor, and head injury, neuromuscular such as from Parkinson's disease, multiple sclerosis, and amyotrophic lateral sclerosis, dementia such as with Alzheimer's disease and multiinfarct, structural such as from cancer, and systemic such as from diabetes, rheumatoid arthritis, and scleroderma. Dysphagia may also result from prolonged illnesses or from the side effects of medications. If swallowing problems are not identified, they can result in **aspiration pneumonia,** malnutrition, dehydration, and death (Cherney, 1994; Logeman, 1983; Nelson, 1995).

TABLE 20-1

Age-Related Swallowing Changes

Swallowing phase	Healthy elder	Frail elder
Oral preparatory	Vision may be declining. Sense of smell and taste decrease and may result in decreased intake. Elder may be missing teeth and need to wear full or partial dentures and require more time to chew food.	Cognitive impairment (that is, poor memory and decreased attention may exaggerate influence of normal aging changes). Isolation and depression result in decreased food intake and weight loss. Decreased endurance may interfere with chewing and result in slow eating and low intake. Missing teeth and poor-fitting dentures may result in slow eating and poor intake.
Oral	Tongue and lip muscles atrophy, and elder may take smaller bites and softer food. Elder may require longer time to form bolus in mouth.	Decreased strength in lips and tongue and jaw muscles may result in drooling, decreased chewing, and problems moving the bolus in the mouth.
Pharyngeal	Phase becomes mildly prolonged. Muscle tone decreases and may delay clearing of food residuals. Bolus moves more slowly through the pharynx. Upward movement of hyoid and larynx become delayed. Epiglottis may become smaller and move more slowly. Cricopharyngeal sphincter remains open for shorter time.	Time of passage of bolus increases. Structures move more slowly and may put person at higher risk for aspiration.
Esophageal	Decreased strength of muscles results in increased time for passage of bolus to stomach.	Increased time needed for bolus to reach stomach. Food contents may escape from stomach and reenter esophagus and pharynx.

Adapted from Cherney L: *Clinical management of dysphagia for adults and children*, Rockville, Md, 1994, Aspen.

INTERVENTION STRATEGIES

Elders achieve a sense of empowerment, control, and motivation when they are successful at self-feeding and swallowing. To achieve this success, COTAs should implement individually planned interventions to resolve swallowing problems and promote functional self-feeding. The COTA must first establish a therapeutic relationship with the elder. This will enhance the interventions affecting empowerment and quality of life during mealtime. Treatment of swallowing disorders entails focusing attention on every aspect of the mealtime experience, including preparation, the dining environment, **positioning** of the elder, adaptive devices, direct intervention, dietary concerns, precautions, and caregiver training (Box 20-1).

Environmental Concerns

In American society people usually eat three meals each day, or about 1092 meals each year, excluding snacks. Eating is a vital part of socialization and greatly adds to the quality of an individual's life. To promote an enjoyable dining experience, pleasant surroundings and personal comfort should be provided to elders during meals. Aesthetics of the dining area should include tablecloths, centerpieces, flowers, and cleanliness. If elders are institutionalized, food items should be taken off serving trays and put directly on the table to help establish a homelike atmosphere. Deficits in visual acuity, light sensitivity, and color perception are common in elders. Poor lighting can greatly exaggerate these problems, so insufficient light and glare should be avoided. Natural light without glare, or soft, diffused overhead lighting is best. A quiet, calm environment excludes television, but may allow for age-appropriate dining music. Television may be distracting and detract from social interaction. Compatible table mates in small groups around a table can add to a positive dining experience (Figure 20-3). COTAs and other service providers should maintain a therapeutic attitude by allowing elders plenty of time to eat a meal. Lengthy waiting periods before being served may decrease the elder's interest in food and may increase fatigue. The table height should be between 28 and 30 inches to accommodate both regular chairs and wheelchairs. The distance between the table surface and an elder's mouth

BOX 20-1

Preparation Checklist for Dysphagia and Self-feeding Interventions

1. Collect information
- Evaluate dysphagia
- Review medical chart
- Consult nursing
- Assess changes in medical status
- Assess changes in diet
2. Inform elder
- Give evaluation results
- Recommend treatment
- Discuss treatment goals with client
- Provide input
3. Create environment
- Ensure that environment is positive and appropriate
- Ensure that environment is conducive to eating
4. Ensure proper fit
- Eyeglasses
- Hearing aides
- Partial and full dentures

5. Assess
- Arousal and alertness
- Safety for eating
6. Position safely
- Trunk
- Lower extremities
- Upper extremities
- Head
- Height of table surface
7. Complete oral preparation as prescribed by OTR
- Have client perform oral exercises
- Have client perform sensory stimulation
- Have client perform tone reduction techniques
8. Check food tray
- Correct diet consistency
- Provide needed adaptive equipment

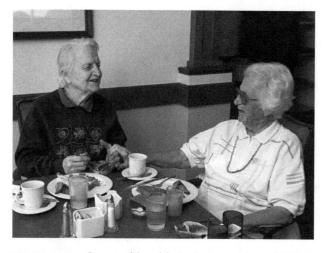

FIGURE 20-3   Compatible table mates can make dining a pleasurable experience.

should be between 10 and 15 inches (Hotaling, 1990). Adopting these suggested environmental factors can help provide a pleasurable experience during mealtime and possibly assist elders to increase their food and fluid intake.

Positioning Techniques

COTAs must have knowledge of proper positioning techniques with elders who have dysphagia. Proper positioning is important for effective and safe swallowing, correcting mechanical problems with swallowing, and increasing dining pleasure. The trachea, or airway, is next

to the esophagus, which is the food pipe. Safe positioning can prevent food from going into the trachea, causing aspiration. Proper positioning of elders also increases alertness, normalizes muscle tone, provides comfort, and helps with digestion, while allowing dynamic movement for self-feeding.

The preferred seating position for mealtime is sitting in a dining room chair with armrests rather than sitting in a wheelchair. A wheelchair, however, is preferable to a geriatric chair, which is preferable to sitting up in bed. COTAs should transfer an elder to a regular chair if the elder can possibly sit in one. If optimal posture cannot be obtained in a regular chair, use of a wheelchair may be necessary. (Figure 20-4). The elder's head, neck, trunk, and hips should be aligned. First, the pelvis should be positioned in neutral with a slight anterior tilt. The elder should have an erect posture and sit symmetrically with weight distributed equally on each hip. Second, the elder's head should be positioned in midline with the chin slightly tucked. Both upper extremities should be fully supported on a table or lap tray of appropriate height. Finally, the lower extremities should be in a weight-bearing position. Hips and knees should be flexed 80° to 90° with ankles in neutral position under the knees and the feet flat on the floor. If the feet do not reach the floor, a stool or wheelchair footrests should be used to provide a secure base of support.

If feeding in bed is essential, elders should be as close to the headboard as possible before the head of the bed is elevated to 45° or more (Figure 20-5). A pillow may be placed behind the elder's back to increase upright trunk

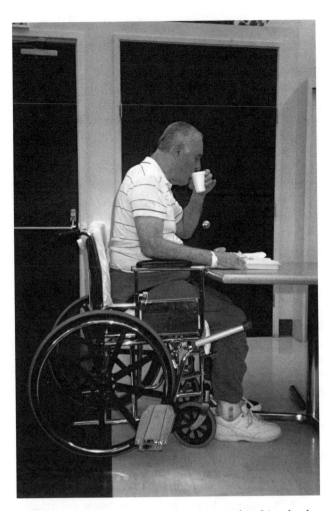

FIGURE **20-4**   Mr. S. is correctly positioned in his wheel-chair for self-feeding. This position promotes dynamic trunk movement (From Community Hospital of Los Gatos, Calif, 1996).

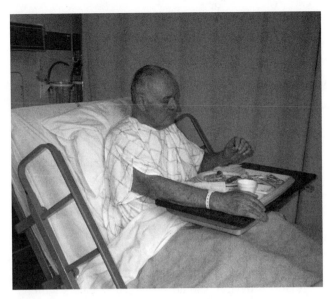

FIGURE **20-5**   Mr. S. is correctly positioned in bed for self-feeding (From Community Hospital of Los Gatos, Calif, 1996).

posture and hip flexion. To prevent elders from sliding down in the bed, the knees should be flexed and supported from underneath with pillows if necessary (Hotaling, 1990). As with sitting in a chair, elders should be upright and aligned symmetrically for optimal safety while eating and drinking.

Positioning devices are often required to aid elders in maintaining a straight midline for a dynamic, upright posture. Padded solid back and solid seat inserts provide better postural support that offsets the slinging seats and backs of wheelchairs. Lumbar and thoracic support can facilitate increased scapulohumeral control for self-feeding. Elders with low muscular tone may benefit from high-back wheelchairs. Wedges, lateral and forward trunk supports, head rests, pelvic belts, pillows, and towel rolls are often used to obtain proper positioning. Seating systems must be designed to correct or accommodate postural problems while preventing skin erosion, main-

taining comfort, promoting self-feeding, and providing the right position for safe swallowing.

Many variables affect elders' positioning. If an elder is sitting in a kyphotic posture, the COTA should have the elder lean back slightly so the chin is parallel to the floor. Special considerations are also needed for elders with scoliosis, depending on the curve of the spine. Elders with hemiplegic arms should always have the arms placed on the table. The arms should be incorporated as gross stabilizers during meals. Those elders who have recently had a lower extremity amputation may also have special positioning needs. COTAs must also consider poor sitting tolerance. Elders with back pain or low endurance need to complete their meal within the time limitations of their upright tolerance. The lower extremities may need to be elevated when sitting up in a chair if edema is present, which often occurs as a result of congestive heart failure. Hearing and visual deficits should also be considered when positioning elders to increase their awareness of their surroundings and to maximize social interaction. The COTA is responsible for following through with the OTR's instructions for positioning while considering the elder's individual needs.

Adaptive Devices

An abundance of options for adaptive devices is available to assist elders in maintaining independence in self-feeding and safe swallowing. Some devices are prefabricated, whereas others are designed by the creative minds of the COTAs. A hole punched in the plastic lid of a cup can hold a straw and will prevent spilling for elders who have tremors or ataxia. Built-up handles can be used for joint protection or a weak grasp. A universal cuff is available for elders who have no grasp. A swivel spoon or a long-handled spoon is available to assist elders with limited range of motion. Nonslip mats or plates with suction cups can keep items from sliding on the table. Plate guards and plates with lips prevent food from spilling off the plate. Cut-out-cups and straws can reduce the need for the elder to tilt the head back while drinking, thus protecting against aspiration while swallowing. Straws and cups with spouted lids also can limit the amount of each sip and are helpful for elders with severe dementia who only have a sucking reflex. Small rubber-coated spoons can help control bite size and prevent elders from hurting themselves when biting down on utensils. Rocker knives can be used for one-handed cutting. Mobile arm supports can provide stabilization and assist in hand-to-mouth movement.

Adaptive devices should be issued if elders suffer a decrease in function. However, elders should be encouraged toward further independence rather than to continue using adaptive devices. Before adaptive equipment is issued, the COTA should consult with the OTR regarding the available options.

Direct Intervention

Various feeding strategies may be used to help elders with dysphagia to feed themselves and swallow safely. To ensure that mealtime is a pleasurable experience, the COTA should avoid making parental comments or giving parental cues (for example use the word *napkin* rather than *bib*). A method of communication must be established with nonverbal elders so they can indicate when they are ready for another bite or drink. All team members, including family and other caregivers, should use this method consistently. Examples may be nodding of the head or raising a finger. In addition, the COTA should sit next to the elders rather than standing over them during meals.

As noted in the preparation checklist in Box 20-1, oral exercises, sensory stimulation, and muscle tone reduction techniques are often needed before eating. Slow, deep pressure on facial and jaw muscles in the opposite direction to the pull of increased muscle tone may help to reduce it. Tongue and facial exercises can increase strength for bolus manipulation. Sensory stimulation may include brushing teeth and icing the cheeks and tongue to increase oral tone and sensation. Brushing teeth also stimulates the salivary glands and helps elders with dry mouths manipulate the bolus easier. After using these necessary strategies, elders are ready to begin eating.

These and many other general strategies help elders with eating and should be enacted before food enters the mouth. Hand-over-hand guiding can provide tactile cueing while bringing food to the mouth and is especially helpful for elders with perceptual difficulties. Proximal upper extremity stabilization techniques can compensate

for tremors, ataxia, and weakness. To help with weakness, elders may also use the opposite hand to assist in the movement of the dominant hand when bringing food to the mouth. The "clock method" is helpful for blind elders or those with other visual deficits to orient them to the position of the plate, cup, eating utensils, and food in front of them. Items should be positioned consistently for this method to be most effective. Elders who are impulsive may require cues for both bite size and pacing of bites. Elders can be guided or instructed to put the eating utensil down between bites to pace the amount of food entering the mouth. Presenting elders with one food item at a time may also be helpful. Large food items should be cut into bite-sized portions. Using a spoon for liquids is often helpful. COTAs should coordinate eating with breathing for elders on ventilators or those with other breathing difficulties. Energy conservation may also be indicated, including limiting conversation during mealtime. For elders with low endurance, alternating food textures during the meal, ordering foods that are easy to chew, and/or having six small meals available during the day may be helpful.

Several strategies may be helpful to use with elders who have severe dementia. Frequent small feedings and finger foods are useful for elders with low attention spans or who pace constantly and cannot sit still long enough to complete a meal. Decreasing environmental stimulation, maintaining consistency in feeding-helpers, and reducing verbal communication during the meal may help decrease distractions and permit elders with dementia to focus longer on eating. When such elders refuse a particular food item, a helpful strategy is to place that food item on a plate of a different color, reheat it, and serve it again. With this particular elder population, COTAs should be careful that elders do not eat nonedible items placed on the table such as plants and napkins. Removing the knife from the place setting of such elders may also be necessary for safety (Hall, 1994).

Several interventions may be used during the oral phase. Tongue sweeps prevent oral pocketing of food. Alternating solids and liquids helps to clean the mouth and to wash down any food residue but may be contraindicated when dysphagia is present. Food should be placed in the center of the tongue. Varying food temperatures with each bite may promote a safer swallow by stimulating the mouth and increasing awareness of the bolus. Occasionally, elders with hypertonicity need food to remain at a consistent temperature to avoid increasing muscle tone. Asking elders to increase the number of times they chew a bite of food helps to break down the bolus and reduce the pace of eating. Elders may need to be cued to close the lips to prevent spillage. The oral cavity should be checked for any residue after each meal. Dentures must fit well and should be thoroughly cleaned after each meal to prevent ulcers from developing in the mouth and to prevent chipping of the dentures from hardened food (Good Samaritan Medical Center, 1995).

Problems during the pharyngeal phase of swallowing may require many treatment strategies. Elders should be given sufficient time to swallow between bites. COTAs should learn to observe and palpate swallowing and be able to recognize delays in the swallow response. These skills help in the ongoing assessment of elders. Individuals with hemiplegia may benefit from turning the head toward the hemiplegic side or tilting the head toward the nonhemiplegic side to protect the airway while swallowing (O'Sullivan, 1990). Elders should be checked for voice clarity after a swallow to make sure that there is no food or liquid residual on the vocal folds. Coughing or clearing the throat followed by a dry swallow may help eliminate a wet-sounding voice after a swallow. Multiple swallows after each bite may also be encouraged. The COTA should work closely with the OTR when feeding elders with tracheostomies. If approved by the physician, the tracheostomy may or may not be plugged and the cuff can be deflated during feeding to increase air pressure for a stronger swallow.

Several advanced techniques, including the supraglottic swallow, Valsalva's maneuver, and Mendelsohn's maneuver, may be required, for which close instruction and supervision from the OTR is essential (Logeman, 1983). Because of the wide range of individual dysphagia problems, the strategies presented here can be modified as necessary. When interventions are planned and carried out with the elder's quality of life in mind as well as their safety while swallowing, elders' motivation for food intake and their sense of empowerment prevail.

Dietary Concerns

Research into the nutritional needs of elders has recently gained momentum, but at this time, only limited knowledge exists. COTAs should understand elders' nutritional requirements. Elders often prefer to eat softer, sweeter, and easy-to-prepare foods, and also often drink less fluids. These habits may result in the elder becoming under nourished or malnourished. If elders become ill and are institutionalized, undernourishment or malnutrition can lead to other health problems and delay recovery.

Diet modifications are frequently used for elders with dysphagia. These modifications may include different consistencies of liquids (for example, thin like water, semithick like nectar, and thick like honey) and different methods of preparing solid foods (for example, pureed, minced, chopped, and soft). If oral intake is limited or impossible, elders with dysphagia may receive nutrition and hydration through **alternative means** (such as a nasogastric tube, a gastrostomy, a jejunostomy, or parenteral nutrition). The entire treatment team is responsible to monitor intake and ensure that elders consume the appropriate amounts of protein, fiber,

vitamins, minerals, and fluids (Axen, Schou, 1995; Kerstetter, Holthausen, Fitz, 1993; Howarth, 1991). Misinterpretations regarding intake may occur when intake is being monitored if food sources are not also recorded together with calories consumed.

Food preferences, food allergies, and any diet restrictions resulting from medical conditions such as diabetes and congestive heart failure should be considered when food and liquid selections are being made with elders and their families. Cultural issues regarding food must also be considered when planning for an elder's care. Increased discussion has occurred regarding the ethical and legal issues associated with permitting elders to consume unsafe liquid or solid food consistencies or imposing alternative means for feeding. Ultimately, the physician is responsible for finalizing a decision regarding this issue with elders and their families. This issue, however, requires much input from the team regarding the benefits, risks, alternatives, and prognoses. If the decision is made to allow elders to consume unsafe food items, OT intervention is recommended to be discontinued (Groher, 1990).

Precautions

When working with elders with feeding and swallowing problems, COTAs should consider many factors concerning the safety of oral intake. Some of these factors include level of alertness, orientation and cognitive status, positioning, general endurance, and the ability to self feed. The presence of a delayed swallow, food pocketing, effortful chewing, coughing, choking, a runny nose, and a wet-sounding voice all indicate swallowing difficulties with the food or liquid being consumed. The COTA should either discontinue the troublesome food or liquid or modify it to a safer consistency. The OTR should be informed of this as soon as possible so that the elder can be further evaluated.

Other indicators of swallowing and nutritional problems may include an increased temperature, lung congestion, and poor intake. Increased temperature and lung congestion may be a sign that the elder has aspirated food or liquid and is developing pneumonia. Poor intake may indicate an inability to swallow rather than a poor appetite. All personnel working with elders with possible swallowing problems must be aware of these indications and be trained in the Heimlich maneuver and CPR in case an elder chokes.

Many elders receive medications for various conditions. Medications must be taken with the correct liquid or semisolid consistency. More than one ounce (30 ml) should be taken after each pill to ensure adequate transport to the stomach. Elders should be sitting up and should be prevented from reclining for 20 minutes after a meal or after taking medication to ensure the safe passage of the food or pill to the stomach. Pills should be taken as specified by the physician. COTAs should consult with the physician or pharmacist to check if the pills can be halved or crushed because some pills are time released, and crushing them may result in too much medication being absorbed at once. Nursing staff should be present while the medications are taken to ensure swallowing has actually occurred.

Many elders are at higher risk of aspiration when using straws and taking serial swallows with liquids. The OTR should alert the COTA if an elder is safe to drink fluids in these ways. Many elders who are impulsive require close supervision to prevent overfilling the mouth or eating too fast, activities that may result in choking. The COTA should gain extensive knowledge and experience with the swallowing process before attempting to work with elders who have tracheostomies or are on ventilators.

Nursing/Caregiver Instruction

COTAs have a vital role in training caregivers to assist elders with self-feeding and dysphagia management. Caregivers may include spouses, partners, family members, friends, hired attendants, and other health care workers such as nurses and nurse's aides. COTAs must consider the caregiver's culture and lifestyle when making decisions about the most beneficial type of teaching technique to use. Some individuals learn best through observing the COTA. Others may learn best by doing it themselves under the direction of the COTA, and others may perform best with verbal instruction. Written information and instructions should be provided to elders and caregivers whenever possible. In general, all these techniques should be used with each caregiver to assure the best follow-through. COTAs must be aware of their verbal tone when teaching the caregiver, taking care not to sound condescending.

The education of caregivers must include training in many aspects of self-feeding and swallowing. First, caregivers should understand the feeding strengths and weaknesses of elders. The need for quality time during the meal and for presentation of a positive attitude to promote elder motivation and independence should be stressed. Thorough instruction should be given on proper body mechanics required by caregivers when assisting elders with feeding. Additional instruction should be provided regarding safe positioning, environmental concerns, use and care of adaptive equipment, specific intervention techniques, appropriate verbal and nonverbal cueing, dietary modifications, and signs of possible food or liquid aspiration. Caregivers may take some time to develop good observation and problem-solving skills. Caregivers must understand the importance of communicating any problems or changes in an elder's status to the appropriate team member. Caregivers should also be familiar with the Heimlich maneuver and emergency suctioning procedures. Problem solving together with caregivers is useful when dealing with elders that have difficult feeding behaviors. COTAs may share with caregivers their anecdotal successful experiences in cueing and obtaining desirable behaviors and eliminating undesirable ones with a particular elder.

An integral part of caregiver training is monitoring the food and fluid intake of elders while considering nutritional value and maintaining a modified diet. Family and friends may occasionally present a problem by not complying with the dietary restrictions of their loved one. The possible negative consequences of not following through with the prescribed feeding program should be stressed. COTAs should work with dietitians and caregivers in helping families plan meals. COTAs may also ask the caregivers of institutionalized elders to bring a meal from home and modify it with the assistance of a COTA.

Instructing caregivers on the swallowing and self-feeding protocols set up for elders helps COTAs promote continuity and quality of care. Caregivers should be integrated as soon as possible in the treatment and care of elders. Training several family members and nursing staff helps spread the responsibility of assisting elders during the meal. As with any intervention given to elders, all training of caregivers should be thoroughly documented.

IDEAS FOR MANAGING A FEEDING PROGRAM

Residents of skilled nursing facilities who are fed in their rooms are frequently positioned poorly, spend most of their day in bed, are often rushed, and often cannot finish their meals. Consequently, their intake, nutrition, and body weight decrease (Axen, Schou, 1995). A well-organized facility-wide feeding program helps get elders out of bed, changes their environment, provides social stimulation, ensures good nutrition and hydration, and increases safety. This type of program also helps maximize their functional abilities and enhances the quality of the mealtime for institutionalized elders. Although many feeding program formats designed for a variety of settings are available, the following is a generic program that requires adjustments to fit the needs of particular elders and particular facilities.

An interdisciplinary approach is the most beneficial in a feeding program. Usually the elder, the occupational therapist, COTA, speech and language pathologist (SLP), dietician, kitchen staff, physician, nursing staff, and family are involved. The RPT may also be included to assist with positioning, and the respiratory therapist may be included to assist with issues of pulmonary hygiene or coordination of tracheostomy or ventilator equipment. Elders with self-feeding and dysphagia difficulties are evaluated and referred to the dining group by the OTR and/or the SLP. These elders then are placed in one of several groups organized by the amount of assistance they require. The ratio of elders to COTAs varies depending on the needs of the group. COTAs should always have a group size that can be safely managed. A written protocol should exist that includes information on the purpose of the program and the format, staffing, size, and site of the group. There should also be criteria for referral to, continuation in, and discharge from the program. Timelines, goals, and responsibilities of the COTA or other leader should be made explicit, and documentation and equipment protocols should be explained. There should also be an established system to maintain communication with the entire team to ensure a successful program.

The feeding program should address all meals. In some settings, COTAs are unable to be present at each meal. In other settings a COTA may not be needed to assist higher-level groups that require minimal assistance or supervision. In these situations, nursing aides, restorative aides, family members, and volunteers may be best used. However, before volunteers are used in this capacity, the guidelines from regulatory agencies should be consulted. For all individuals to perform effectively and safely, they must receive formal training on leading groups, on therapeutic interventions, and on safety.

CASE STUDY

Eric is a 68-year-old, right-hand dominant man who suffered a left cerebrovascular accident (CVA) and now has right hemiplegia. He has impaired movement and sensation on the right side. In addition, he has apraxia, aphasia, right hemianopsia, and right neglect. One week after his stroke Eric was transferred to a skilled nursing facility's rehabilitation unit.

A dysphagia evaluation and videofluoroscopy were done and the following observations were noted: decreased muscle tone with impaired movement and sensation of the face, tongue, and soft palate on the right side, resulting in facial droop, poor lip seal, minimal drooling and food spillage, slurred speech, and a nasal quality to the speech. The videofluoroscopy revealed impaired oral control of the bolus and spillage of food and liquid into the pharynx before the swallow was initiated. Initiation of the swallow was delayed up to 5 seconds. Residual pooling was observed in the valleculae and pyriform sinuses after the swallow. Spontaneous clearing of the throat with additional swallows was impaired. Eric required verbal cueing to initiate clearing swallows. Aspiration into the trachea was observed while Eric swallowed thin and semithick liquids by spoon and thick liquids by cup, and a mixed consistency bolus (liquid and solid combination, such as soup). Eric did cough spontaneously when aspiration occurred. He had difficulty chewing dry, hard solids and did better with moist, soft solids and semisolids, although oral pocketing and spillage from the mouth was observed with these consistencies. When Eric used the compensation method of turning his head to the right, decreased pooling in the right valleculae and pyriform sinus resulted.

Therapeutic recommendations included one on one assistance at meals for self-feeding and a modified diet of thick liquids by spoon. Semisolids and minced, soft solids with no mixed consistencies were also recommended. Further suggestions were to provide verbal and tactile cues for Eric to turn his head to the right side during the initial swallow and

to follow up the initial swallow with two dry swallows. In addition, Eric's caloric and fluid intake were to be closely monitored.

Before the meal, the COTA reviewed the chart for any recent orders and nursing and therapy progress notes to understand how the elder's day had gone thus far. The COTA arranged to meet Eric's family in the dining room for them to observe this meal. When Eric arrived in the dining room, the COTA observed that he was not sitting erectly in his wheelchair and that he needed to be repositioned. When Eric was sitting erect, the COTA brought him to the table, locked the wheelchair, positioned Eric's feet on the floor, and placed his hemiplegic arm forward on the table.

Before the meal the COTA directed Eric through several oral-facial exercises. Icing was also used to increase tone and sensation in his right cheek and throat. The COTA iced the outside of Eric's mouth with ice wrapped in a washcloth and then iced the inside of his cheeks with a cold metal spoon that was dipped in a cup of ice. Icing would also be done on the cheek and the anterior part of the neck during the meal.

When the tray with Eric's meal arrived, the COTA checked to ensure that the consistencies of both solids and liquids were correct. The liquid on the tray was semithick, so the COTA thickened it with a thickening agent. No other modifications were needed. A plate guard was put on the plate to prevent food from spilling.

Because Eric requires assistance with tray setup and self-feeding, the COTA guided Eric's left hand (nonhemiplegic) using the hand-over-hand method to remove the container lids, butter the bread, cut the food with the rocker knife, and bring the food to his mouth. When Eric was able to integrate the movement and its rhythm and was able to feed himself independently, the COTA stopped providing hand-over-hand guiding. However, when Eric moved too quickly and took too large a bite, the COTA resumed the guiding. When Eric drooled, the COTA guided him to wipe his face with a napkin. With each bite the COTA directed Eric to double swallow and felt Eric's throat for the swallow. The COTA asked Eric to speak occasionally to check his vocal quality, and when it was wet-sounding, the COTA asked Eric to clear his throat. Whenever Eric was unable to clear his throat, the COTA asked him to dry swallow. Finally, the COTA periodically checked Eric's mouth for food pocketing and directed him to clear residuals in his right cheek by using his tongue or left index finger.

After the meal the COTA guided Eric to use a toothette to clean his oral cavity of the food residue. The COTA instructed Eric to remain upright for at least 20 more minutes. A nurse then arrived with medications, which were crushed and mixed with the thick liquid and given to Eric with a spoon. After he swallowed the medication, Eric was given additional thick liquid by spoon to ensure that the medication passed to the stomach.

The COTA then asked the family if they had any questions and provided them with additional instructions. Finally, the COTA documented what and how much Eric ate; the level of assistance that was required; how long it took to complete the meal; the presence of any coughing, wet-sounding voice, or choking; and the food consistency given him when these events occurred. In addition, the COTA documented all instructions given to the family.

As Eric progressed during meals, he needed less and less hand-over-hand guiding and verbal instruction from the

COTA. The COTA began supervising family members as they assisted Eric with meals. Eric progressed to a group dining situation, and when Eric seemed to have a little problem with a wet-sounding voice, food pocketing, follow through with compensatory techniques, duration of the meal, caloric intake, and spiking temperatures, the COTA requested that the OTR reevaluate him. A followup videofluoroscopy was done to rule out aspiration of thin liquids and mixed consistencies, and it showed that Eric had improved but still had impaired oral control of the bolus and pooling in the pharynx. However, Eric now clears this pooling spontaneously, no aspiration is noted, and these items were added to his diet.

Because Eric can now set up his tray with minimal assistance, cut the food with a rocker knife, bring the food to his mouth, eat slowly, and check for pocketing independently, he no longer requires OT supervision at meals.

CHAPTER REVIEW QUESTIONS

1 What is the definition of *dysphagia?*

2 What are the four phases of swallowing?

3 What are the three liquid consistencies?

4 Name four signs that may indicate the presence of swallowing problems.

5 Name three common changes that occur during the phases of swallowing as an individual ages.

6 Identify at least two psychological issues that may have an effect on oral intake.

7 Explain why the COTA should be concerned about nutritional balance and amount of oral intake.

8 Why is the dining environment important for nutritional intake?

9 What should the COTA do if an elder coughs continuously during a meal?

10 Describe how an individual's body should ideally be positioned during a meal.

REFERENCES

American Association of Retired Persons: *A profile of older Americans,* Washington, DC, 1995, The Association.

Axen K, Schou R: Nutritional issues in the frail older person, *Top Geriatr Rehabil* 11(2):1, 1995.

Buccholz D: Adaptation, compensation and decompensation of the pharyngeal swallow, *Gastroenterol Radiol* 10:235, 1985.

Cherney L: *Clinical management of dysphagia for adults and children,* Rockville, Md, 1994, Aspen.

Feinberg et al: Aspiration and the elderly, *Dysphagia* 5:61, 1990.

Good Samaritan Medical Center: About dysphagia. In *The stroke and rehabilitation manual,* Gaithersburg, Md, 1995, Aspen.

Groher M: Ethical dilemmas in providing nutrition, *Dysphagia* 5:102, 1990.

Hall G: Chronic dementia challenges in feeding a patient, *J Gerontol Nurs* 20(4):21, 1994.

Howarth C: Nutritional goals for older adults: a review, *Gerontologist* 31:811, 1991.

Hotaling D: Adapting the mealtime environment: setting the stage for eating, *Dysphagia* 5:77, 1990.

Jaradeh S: Neurophysiology of swallowing in the aged, *Dysphagia* 9:218, 1994.

Kerstetter J, Holthausen B, Fitz J: Nutrition and nutritional requirements for the older adult, *Dysphagia* 8:51, 1993.

Logeman G: *Evaluation and treatment of swallowing disorders,* Austin, Tex, 1983, Pro-Ed.

Musson N et al: Nature, nurture, nutrition: interdisciplinary programs to address the prevention of malnutrition and dehydration, *Dysphagia* 5:96, 1990.

Nelson K: Dysphagia: evaluation and treatment. In Pedretti L, editor: *Occupational therapy: practice skills for physical dysfunction,* St. Louis, 1995, Mosby.

Sheth N, Diner W: Swallowing problems in the elderly, *Dysphagia* 2:209, 1988.

Working With Elders Who Have Had Cerebrovascular Accidents

RENÉ L. PADILLA

KEY TERMS

cerebrovascular accident (CVA), aphasia, midline alignment, muscle tone, shoulder-hand syndrome, hemiplegia, transfers, weight bearing, functional activities

CHAPTER OBJECTIVES

1. Discuss cerebrovascular accidents by describing the major features of strokes affecting the main arteries of the brain.
2. Discuss at least three considerations in the OT evaluation of elders who have had a stroke.
3. Describe the sequence of facilitating midline alignment while elders are supine, sitting, and standing, and ex-

plain the steps to follow when transferring elders from a supine position to the edge of the bed or from a sitting to a standing position.
4. Explain precautions for handling an elder's hemiplegic upper extremity.

Virtually every human endeavor is the result of the brain's unceasing activity. The brain is the organ of behavior, cognition, language, learning, and movement. The sophistication of the brain's circuitry is remarkable, if not baffling. Billions of neurons interact with each other to do the brain's work. To appreciate the aging process, COTAs must have an understanding of the way the brain works (Umphred, 1995; DeArmond, Fusco, Dewey, 1989; Pansky, Allen, Budd, 1988). Implications of neuropathological disorders for OT intervention with elders are described in this chapter. The many biological and behavioral changes that accompany normal aging are explained elsewhere in this chapter.

Effects of normal age-related changes in the nervous

system vary greatly among individuals and are not generally associated with specific diseases. These changes clearly have little detrimental effect on many elders. Senility is not an inevitable aspect of aging. However, a number of conditions can be devastating to elders because they present serious obstacles to the process of normal, healthy aging. Some of these conditions are related to **cerebrovascular accidents (CVAs).** (Chapter 22 presents the issues related to Alzheimer's disease, another disorder affecting the brain.)

CEREBROVASCULAR ACCIDENTS

Cerebrovascular accidents (CVAs), or strokes, are lesions in the brain that result from a thrombus, embolus,

TABLE 21-1

Incidence of Neurological Deficits Following Stroke	
Neurological impairment	**Incidence (%)***
Sensory deficits	53
Dysarthria	48
Right hemiparesis	44
Left hemiparesis	37
Cognitive deficits	36
Visual-perceptual deficits	32
Aphasia	30
Bladder control	29
Hemianopsia	26
Ataxia	20
Dysphagia	12

*Adapted from US Department of Health and Human Services: *Post stroke rehabilitation: practice guideline no. 16*, Rockville, Md, 1995.

or hemorrhage that compromises the blood supply to the brain. This inadequate supply results in brain swelling and ultimately in the death of neurons in the stroke area.

Strokes are the third leading cause of death in the United States and the leading cause of disability among adults. Approximately 550,000 individuals suffer strokes each year, and nearly 150,000 die as a result, while 3 million individuals live with varying degrees of neurological impairment following strokes (US Department of Health and Human Services [DHHS], 1995). Strokes frequently increase dramatically with increasing age, doubling with every decade after 55 years of age (Dyken et al, 1984). Men experience strokes more frequently than women (Harmsen, Tsipioganni, Wilhelmsen, 1992) and African-Americans more frequently than Caucasians (Gillum, 1988). Recurrent strokes account for 25% of yearly reported strokes (Terent, 1993). Thrombotic strokes occur more often than embolic strokes and occur more frequently in men (Sacco, Wolf, Kannel, McNamara, 1982).

Ischemic strokes, caused by both thrombus and embolus, account for about 71% of strokes, with thrombotic strokes being the most prevalent. Intracerebral and subarachnoid hemorrhagic strokes account for about 24% of strokes, and other or uncertain causes account for the remaining 5%. Mortality rates have been declining steadily since the 1950s and are reported to be between 17% and 34% during the first 30 days after a stroke, 25% and 40% within the first year, and 32% and 60% during the first 3 years. Consequently, about half the individuals with first strokes live for 3 or more years, and more than one third live for 10 years (DHHS, 1995).

Risk factors for stroke can be separated into modifiable and nonmodifiable. Modifiable factors are those that can be altered by changes in lifestyle and/or medications.

They include hypertension, carotid artery stenosis, coronary artery disease, atrial fibrillation, congestive heart failure, cigarette smoking, alcohol and other drug consumption, obesity, diabetes mellitus, and high serum cholesterol, among others. The most preventable of these risk factors is hypertension. Nonmodifiable or fixed risk factors include prior stroke, age, race, gender, and family history of stroke. Among these nonmodifiable factors, increasing age is by far the greatest, because 72% of strokes occur in people age 65 years and older (Gillum, 1988).

In elders, stroke can result in various neurological deficits (Table 21-1). Neurological and functional recovery occurs most rapidly in the first 3 months following a stroke; most elders continue to progress after that time but at a slower rate (Bear, Connors, Paradiso, 1996). For this reason, predicting functional recovery after stroke as well as which elders will benefit from rehabilitation is difficult. The World Health Organization (1989) proposes that prognosis for recovery and successful rehabilitation should be indicated in the following order: (1) clients who spontaneously make good recovery without rehabilitation; (2) clients who can make satisfactory recovery only through intensive rehabilitation; and (3) clients with poor recovery of function regardless of the type of rehabilitation. Other factors that complicate prediction of recovery include co-morbidity and depression.

The outcome of a stroke depends greatly on which artery supplying the brain is involved (Table 21-2). Medical treatment of a stroke depends on the type, location, and severity of the vascular lesion. In the acute stages, medical intervention is focused on maintaining an airway, rehydration, and management of hypertension. Measures are often taken to prevent the development of deep venous thrombosis (DVT); that is, blood clots that form in the veins of the lower extremities after prolonged periods of bedrest or immobility. If such clots are released, they can become lodged in the lungs and cause death. The COTA must be alert to any sign of DVT and should request and carefully follow mobilization and activity guidelines set by the physician. Localized signs in the lower extremity that suggest the presence of DVT include abnormal temperature, change in color and circumference, and tenderness. In addition to the use of medications, elders can prevent DVTs by wearing elastic stockings and intermittent compression garments, and through early mobilization. Because of DVT and other potential complications of stroke, the COTA should check the elder's medical record and communicate with other team members before initiating each treatment session. By doing this, all team members are fully informed and can modify the interventions with the elder to best serve the elder's needs.

Bowel and bladder dysfunction is common during the initial phases of recovery from a stroke. Usually a specific

TABLE 21-2

Impairments Resulting from Cerebrovascular Accidents of Specific Arteries	
Artery	**Impairment**
Middle cerebral artery	• Contralateral hemiplegia • Contralateral sensory deficits • Contralateral hemianopsia • Aphasia • Deviation of head and neck toward side of lesion (if lesion is located in dominant hemisphere) • Perceptual deficits including anosognosia unilateral neglect, visual spatial deficits, and perseveration (if lesion is located in nondominant hemisphere)
Internal carotid artery	• Contralateral hemiplegia • Contralateral hemianesthesia • Homonomous hemianopsia • Aphasia, agraphia, acalculia, right/left confusion, and finger agnosia (if lesion is located in dominant hemisphere) • Visual perceptual dysfunction, unilateral neglect, constructional dressing apraxia, attention deficits, topographical disorientation, and anosognosia (if lesion is located in nondominant hemisphere)
Anterior cerebral artery	• Contralateral hemiplegia • Apraxia • Bowel and bladder incontinence • Cortical sensory loss of the lower extremity • Contralateral weakness of face and tongue • Perseveration and amnesia • Sucking reflex
Posterior cerebral artery	• Homonomous hemianopsia • Paresis of eye musculature • Contralateral hemiplegia • Topographic disorientation • Involuntary movement disorders • Sensory deficits
Cerebellar artery	• Ipsilateral ataxia • Nystagmus, nausea, and vomiting • Decreased touch, vibration, and position sense • Decreased contralateral pain and thermal sensation • Ipsilateral facial paralysis
Vertebral artery	• Decreased contralateral pain, temperature, touch, and proprioceptive sense • Hemiparesis • Facial weakness and numbness • Ataxia • Paralysis of tongue and weakness of vocal folds

bowel and bladder program that includes fluid intake, stool softeners, and other remedies is ordered by the physician. The COTA may be involved in structuring a scheduled toileting program for the elders, which is essential for success. (Chapter 19 presents a more detailed discussion about bowel and bladder training programs.) Other complications during the early phases of recovery from a stroke may include respiratory difficulties and pneumonia caused by the decreased efficiency of the muscles involved in respiration and swallowing. Good pulmonary hygiene, use of antibiotics, and early mobilization are effective prevention measures. Dysphagia, or problems with swallowing, must also be addressed to prevent aspiration pneumonia (refer to Chapter 20).

OT EVALUATION

Research evidence and expert opinion suggest that stroke rehabilitation should begin in the acute stage (DHHS, 1995). OT is an essential component in this rehabilitation process. The COTA is an active participant in the evaluation process under the supervision of the OTR (American Occupational Therapy Association

[AOTA], 1993). As with any client, OT evaluation is an ongoing process that occurs during each treatment session. This is particularly true for elders who have had a stroke, because they may experience many changes during the first few months of recovery. These changes may be noted especially during treatment. Although motor, perceptual, sensory, and cognitive deficits may all contribute to functional impairments, the psychosocial skills and performance of elders and the environment in which they live and perform are critical components of any OT assessment. In addition, assessment should always consider elders' abilities, not just their deficits.

Assessment of motor, sensory, perceptual, and cognitive functions is done simultaneously during performance of an activity. Although the evaluation of each discrete area may be conducted separately, the interaction of these functions and their effects on meaningful activity are of primary importance to OT. Typical impairments are discussed in the section on treatment, but areas of necessary assessment for COTAs are discussed in the following paragraphs.

In the context of motor assessment, the COTA must have an understanding of the elder's ability to maintain the body in an upright position and in the midline against gravity (postural reactions). To do this, the COTA must observe the elder's degree of hypertonicity and the presence of abnormal movement patterns, primitive reflexes, righting and protective reactions, equilibrium, coordination, and range of motion. The COTA should remember that all these performance components may be, and often are, affected by posture and endurance, and that the optimal assessment will occur when elders are upright and not too fatigued. Alignment of the trunk and pelvis and shoulder girdle, and any voluntary motor control should be noted. Assessment of strength has limited benefit in the presence of hypertonicity and can possibly worsen this condition.

The sensory assessment should include evaluation of light touch, pressure, pain, temperature, stereognosis, and proprioception. Perceptual functioning to be evaluated includes body scheme, motor planning, and visual perceptual-motor skills. Cognitive skills often assessed include attention, initiation, memory, planning, organization, problem solving, insight, and judgment. The ability to do calculations and make abstractions may also be tested. COTAs should remember that posture can have a significant effect on sensory, perceptual, and cognitive functioning, and assessment of these areas should occur when elders are upright.

Assessment of swallowing ability and safety is crucial for all elders who have experienced a stroke. Swallowing is a complex behavior that results from the simultaneous performance of motor, sensory, perceptual, and cognitive skills, and deficits in any of these areas may result in elders being at a higher risk of aspirating food into the lungs and developing pneumonia (Chapter 20 reviews this topic).

Depending on the elder's ability to communicate, evaluation of psychosocial skills of elders may need to be completed by interviewing the family or other significant people. Knowledge of the occupations or pursuits the elder was involved in before the stroke and of the elder's values and interests is crucial in the selection of treatment strategies. Occupational task considerations should be made at every stage of OT intervention.

OT INTERVENTION

The long-range goal of OT intervention for dysfunction caused by stroke is to facilitate maximal independence in all the life contexts of the elder. To reach this goal, intervention is focused on restoration of neuromuscular, perceptual-cognitive, and psychosocial skills that support the elder's ability to perform self-care and engage in productive and leisure occupations. The degree to which each of these areas is emphasized is determined by the previous physical and social environments of elders and their plans after hospitalization. Because each elder's context is unique, the OT intervention plan is tailored specifically to that individual.

CASE STUDY

The need for tailored intervention programs is illustrated by the cases of Rose and Maria. Both women are in their late seventies and suffered strokes that left them with a hemiplegic right side and mild slurring of speech, or **aphasia**. Their levels of cognitive function appear to be intact. Rose is a widow and lives in a senior community that provides one meal a day and assists her with laundry and cleaning. Her two sons live in other states. Maria lives at home with her husband and two of her eight adult daughters. Ten grandchildren, whose ages range from 3 to 18 years, also live in her home. Both Rose and Maria want to return to their previous living environments. The OT program for both women will address all their needs, but the emphasis in Rose's program will be on self-care, because she must be independent in this area to maintain her apartment at the senior community. Maria, on the other hand, is counting on family assistance for her self-care, and is more interested in cooking again for her extended family, so her program will focus more on home maintenance and social skills. The OT programs for both women will address their neuromuscular, perceptual-cognitive, and psychosocial skills, but the activities chosen as therapeutic media should reflect their life contexts.

The cases of Rose and Maria illustrate another important principle in stroke rehabilitation. The more familiar the individual is with the activities selected for intervention, the more spontaneous and unconscious are the motor, perceptual, cognitive, and psychosocial reorganization. Consequently, changes will last longer. (Warren, 1991). Conscious, attention-focused learning is often necessary in rehabilitation, especially when the likelihood of recovery is low and compensation strategies are more viable. However, these strategies may also slow the rehabilitation process because of the mental effort they require. To illustrate this, COTAs should do the following exercise with partners. Have your partner time determine the length of time required to write your full name on a piece of paper using your dominant hand. Have your partner time you writing your name again, but this time write with your nondominant hand. Focus carefully on your body while you write your name and on the amount of mental control this task requires. The experience of rehabilitation after a stroke is similar to your experience of writing with your nondominant hand. Although clients who are recovering from stroke may not be learning to use their nondominant hand, they are relearning task accomplishment with a different body. The more these clients must concentrate on the task they are attempting, the longer it may take them to complete it. Engagement in automatic activities may take less time and reinforce the automatic postural adjustments that support all actions. Consequently, whenever possible the COTA should approach the intervention for stroke impairments with strategies designed to restore lost function in ways that use the learning and work experiences of elders before they experienced the stroke. Compensation strategies, particularly those related to the use of adaptive equipment or alternative motor patterns, should be evaluated carefully because they require conscious attention and may create habits that may be difficult to break later.

Motor Deficits

Several sensorimotor approaches exist for the treatment of motor dysfunction resulting from stroke. Some of these include Brunnstrom (1970), Bobath's neurodevelopmental therapy (NDT) and proprioceptive neuromuscular facilitation (PNF) (Davies, 1985; Voss, Ionta, Meyers, 1985). Regardless of approach, the goal of intervention is to facilitate normal voluntary movement and use of the affected side of the body. Thus normal postural mechanisms must also be developed, and abnormal reflexes and movements must be inhibited.

Although hypertonicity is often the most visible sign that a person has a motor dysfunction, this problem is best addressed in the context of postural control rather than in isolation. Abnormal tone in any extremity may drastically change depending on whether the individual is lying, sitting, or standing. Therefore motor dysfunction should be treated when the individual is in alignment. Alignment means that the individual's pelvis is in a neutral position with no anterior or posterior tilt, that the spine is in **midline alignment,** and that the upper and lower extremities are in a neutral position.

The correct positioning while the elder is reclining can have a dramatic effect on **muscle tone** and pain, especially in the presence of **shoulder-hand syndrome.** Specific issues with the **hemiplegic** upper extremity are discussed later in this chapter. Having elders lie on the more affected side is most helpful in inhibiting abnormal tone and pain because of the heavy pressure exerted on that side (Figure 21-1). However, caution must be taken

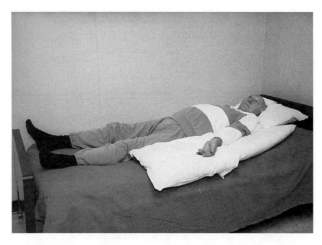

FIGURE **21-1** In the supine position, the trunk and upper extremities should be aligned. The hemiplegic upper extremity should be supported on pillows with the palm facing up.

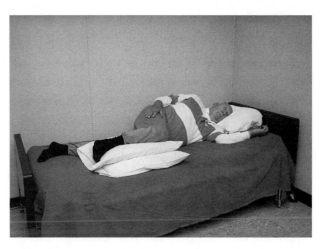

FIGURE **21-2** Lying on the hemiplegic upper extremity frees the less involved arm for functional use.

to determine that the shoulder girdle is correctly aligned, the scapula is slightly abducted, and the humerus is in external rotation. The position of the bed should be rearranged (unless the elder finds the change too disorganizing) so the elder can lie on the affected side and face the side of the bed from which **transfers** will occur. An added advantage of lying on the affected side is that it frees the less-involved upper extremity for functional use while they are in this position (Figure 21-2).

Body alignment should also be maintained during transitional movements such as changing from a side lying position to sitting at the edge of the bed and back; transferring to and from a chair, wheelchair, toilet, or car; changing from a sitting to a standing position and back; and while walking. COTAs should follow established sequential procedures when assisting elders to change from a supine position to sitting at the edge of the bed or

BOX 21-1

Sequential Procedures for Changing from a Supine Position to Sitting at Edge of Bed

1. Plan to have elder exit bed toward hemiplegic side.
2. Gently provide passive abduction to hemiplegic scapula and extend hemiplegic arm at side of body so that humerus is in external rotation and palm is facing up; an alternative is to have elder clasp hands and hold arms in 90 degree flexion with straight elbows and roll toward side of bed.
3. Have elder hook less affected leg under hemiplegic ankle and slide both legs toward edge of bed.
4. Have elder roll on to hemiplegic side, facing side of bed.
5. Have elder cross less affected upper extremity in front of body and place on bed at a level slightly below chest.
6. As the elder lowers legs at the side of the bed, have elder push up with less affected hand and hemiplegic elbow (if able).
7. Once sitting at edge of bed, have elder scoot forward by alternating **weight bearing** on each thigh and scooting the free thigh forward until both feet are flat on floor.

BOX 21-2

Sequential Procedures for Transfers

1. If transferring from wheelchair to another chair, toilet, or bed, place wheelchair at no more than 45 degrees (perpendicular) from surface going to; elder should transfer toward hemiplegic side whenever possible.
2. Make sure wheelchair is locked and footrests and armrests are out of the way.
3. Place both feet flat on floor.
4. Have elder sit upright so back is not against back rest.
5. Have elder scoot forward to front edge of chair by alternatively shifting weight on to one thigh and scooting other thigh forward; do not permit elder to push off back of chair using back extension, because this will increase abnormal muscle tone throughout body.
6. Position elder's feet so tips of toes are directly below knees; make sure feet remain flat on floor; if ankle dorsiflexion is limited, toes may be placed somewhat anterior to knees.
7. Have elder lean forward until shoulders are directly above knees.
8. Have elder push off from knees with both hands if elder is able.
9. As elder leans forward, have elder stand up; if unable to stand up fully, guide elder's body toward target chair, toilet, or bed while elder is partially weight bearing on both feet.

when doing transfers (Boxes 21-1, 21-2). In all these circumstances, COTAs must remember *not* to pull on the affected upper extremity to assist elders. COTAs should assist by holding the elder from the shoulder with the COTA's hand on the elder's scapula. Pulling the arm or supporting the elder from the axilla can easily cause or worsen glenohumeral subluxation. Glenohumeral subluxation may be painful and may discourage the elder from using that arm. This can lead to other complications such as hypertonicity, swelling, contractures, and shoulder-hand syndrome.

COTAs must pay constant attention to the elder's body alignment during sitting because this is often the elder's position during most activities, especially during the initial stages of rehabilitation. If the elder must sit fairly still for long periods, the therapist must ensure that the elder's pelvis is in a neutral position and is as far back in the chair as possible. Hips should be flexed at no more than 90 degrees. Greater hip flexion will cause posterior pelvic tilt and lumbar and thoracic spine flexion, inhibiting breathing and active upper extremity control and requiring greater cervical spine extension for the person to look straight ahead. Placing a folded towel or thin pillow in the small of the back to maintain alignment may be helpful. Too thick a pillow or support can push the lumbar spine into hyperextension, causing anterior pelvic

tilt and encouraging the elder to use back extension as the primary means of posture control. When back hyperextension is the base from which the elder begins movement in the extremities, hypertonicity throughout the body is likely to increase.

Another concern when the elder is in the sitting position is lateral pelvic tilt, or lateral flexion of the spine. Because of sensory and tone changes, half of the trunk muscles may not be working well, and consequently, the other side may be overworking. The resulting misalignment causes the spine to flex toward one side. Because of this lateral flexion, the spine is no longer in midline, and weight bearing on the elder's thighs is unequal. Pelvic tilt upward toward one side results in shortening of the trunk on the same side and elongation of the trunk on the opposite side. Weight bearing occurs primarily on the side of the elongated trunk. The COTA must help to actively or passively align the spine toward the midline, rather than to simply build up one side of the sitting surface.

When pelvic and spine alignment are achieved, the COTA can focus on placing the feet flat on the floor or on footrests so that knee flexion and ankle dorsiflexion of no more than 90 degrees is present. The COTA should take care that the femurs are in neutral rotation (that is, there is no external or internal rotation) and that there is little or no hip abduction or adduction. Thus the heels will be resting directly below the knees, and the knees will be aligned with the hips. Unless the elder is being pushed in a wheelchair, both feet should be placed on the floor so that they bear weight more evenly. Consequently, hemi-wheelchairs, the seats of which are slightly lower than standard chairs, are recommended so that the elders' feet can comfortably reach the floor.

After attending to the pelvis, spine, and lower extremities, the COTA can align the elder's hemiplegic upper extremity. The strategies for positioning are similar for both hypotonic and hypertonic arms. The elder should be placed in front of a table or be outfitted with a lap board so the hand can be placed facedown on a flat surface to benefit from the normalizing effects of weight bearing. To accomplish this, the COTA should ensure that the elder's scapula is slightly abducted, the shoulder is flexed so the elbow is anterior to the shoulder, the humerus is in neutral or slight external rotation, and the forearm is pronated. The elbow should not be resting on the lap board, and the hand should be lower than the elbow. This permits the hand to bear weight normally. The normal weight-bearing surface of the hand includes the lateral external surface of the thumb, fingertips, lateral border of the hand, and thenar and hypothenar eminencies. The COTA should maintain the arch formed by the metacarpophalangeal joints so the hand is not flattened. The hand should not be fastened in any way to the lap board except in extreme cases in which clear evidence indicates that the elder may be hurt otherwise. Restricting normal, spontaneous weight bearing inhibits normalization of muscle tone. In cases of extreme hypertonicity in the hand, the COTA can place a soup bowl face down on a square of nonslip material on the lap board, thus permitting some weight bearing against a hard surface (Figure 21-3). However, the elder's hand should never be placed on nonslip material. Such material can contribute to shoulder subluxation because the hand cannot move toward the body when the shoulder is pulled backward.

During intervention sessions that do not require sitting still for long periods, the elder should sit at the edge of the chair or mat. The concerns with alignment in this position are similar to those described above for long periods of sitting, but the focus of intervention will be on the elder moving into and out of alignment while participating in activities. Sitting at the edge of the mat forces active trunk control because there are no back or arm rests for support and the base of support under the thighs is reduced. Concerns regarding lower-extremity placement are the same as described previously. However, as the elder's ability to control the trunk increases, the

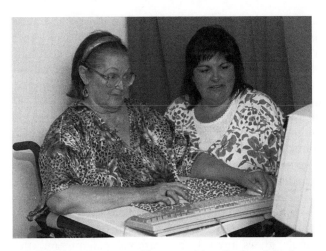

FIGURE 21-3 In cases of hypertonicity, the hemiplegic hand can be placed on an inverted soup bowl to bear weight more comfortably.

height of the mat can be increased, thus gradually increasing and challenging the amount of active weight bearing on the lower extremities. This gradation prepares the elder for the trunk and postural control required during standing activities. If the elder has little or no active control of the hemiplegic upper extremity, the elder should lay on a table, following similar guidelines as those described previously. As the height of the mat increases, so should the height of the table or surface that supports the hand.

Although ambulation training does not traditionally fall in the realm of OT, it should be considered a transitional movement that permits elders to maneuver from one task or occupation to another. For example, elders may need to ambulate from the bed to the bathroom to complete toileting tasks or from the sink to the stove to the refrigerator to complete a meal preparation task. Consequently, COTAs should assist in maintaining alignment in the same way as described previously. During ambulation, the person's shift of the midline toward the less affected side is most obvious. This often is accentuated when elders are taught to walk using a broad-based cane and they establish the habit of maintaining the midline in the middle of the less affected side rather then in the middle of the body. Because there is less control, or less sensory feedback, elders may hesitate to bear weight equally on each leg as they step. The COTA should coordinate intervention with the RPT to understand what ambulation pattern to reinforce with elders during OT intervention.

Special attention should be given to the hemiplegic upper extremity. This extremity should be purposefully included in any activity early during the course of intervention, even if little or no active motor control is present, because this will keep the elder's attention on the extremity and reduce its neglect. Before any active or passive motion is expected of the elder, the COTA must first passively mobilize the elder's scapula to ensure that it glides when the arm is moved. The scapula may not glide sufficiently or may stop altogether because of muscle paralysis or hypertonus. Consequently, the COTA should never flex or abduct the shoulder of elders more than 90 degrees unless the COTA can be sure that the scapula is gliding properly. If elders do not have active scapular control, the COTA can passively move the scapula while ranging the shoulder. When the shoulder is flexed more than 90 degrees, the scapula glides downward on the posterior wall of the rib cage. In addition, the inferior border, or angle, of the scapula rotates slightly upward. When the shoulder is abducted more than 90 degrees, the scapula glides toward the vertebral column and the inferior border rotates slightly downward.

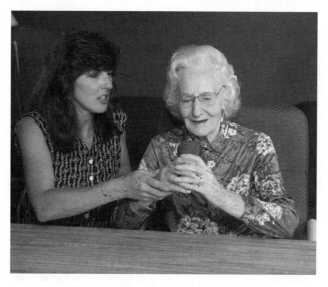

FIGURE 21-4 When clasping hands, the thumb of the hemiplegic hand should be on top.

If elders have no active movement in the hemiplegic upper extremity, they should be instructed to move it by clasping hands with the thumb of the hemiplegic hand on top (Figure 21-4). While clasping the hands in this manner, elders should be instructed to extend the elbows and hold the shoulders flexed at approximately 90 degrees. With the arms in this position, elders can go from a supine to a side-lying position and from a sitting to a standing position, or they can hold on to the knee of the hemiplegic lower extremity during dressing or other **functional activities.** The COTA's imagination and creativity are essential in assisting elders to use this clasped-hands technique to perform numerous functional activities such as picking up a mug to drink and mixing a cake. In addition, elders can flex or abduct the hemiplegic shoulder themselves by guiding the arm with clasped hands. This bilateral integration assists with normalizing tone and encourages elders to actively care for the hemiplegic upper extremity (Davies, 1985).

Elders may develop shoulder-hand syndrome if the hemiplegic upper extremity is not managed appropriately. This syndrome is characterized by swelling, tenderness, loss of range of motion, and vasomotor degradation. Pain and subluxation of the glenohumeral joint may not necessarily be present. The COTA should address all these problems immediately to avoid irreversible atrophy of bones, skin, and muscles (Davis, 1990). The swelling is best decreased by filling a bucket or pail two-thirds full with crushed ice and adding cold water to the level of the ice. Elders should sit, while maintaining good alignment, in front of the bucket, which is placed on the floor, and should lean forward to place the hemiplegic hand and wrist in the water. The edematous hand should be kept in the water for 3 to 5 seconds. The COTA should dry it gently with a towel. The COTA should ask the elder to flex the fingers if possible, or the COTA should provide gentle passive ranging of the fingers and hand. This

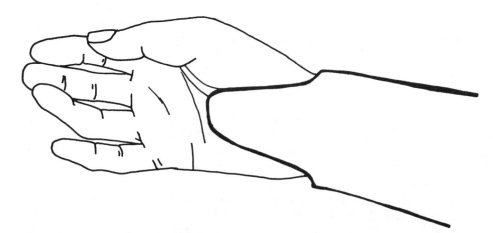

FIGURE 21-5 A modified cock-up splint holds the wrist in slight extension and helps reduce fluid build-up in the hand.

procedure is then repeated 3 or 4 times in a session. The whole procedure should be done 3 to 4 times daily until swelling subsides. While the COTA is providing the range of motion exercise, retrograde massage can also be done, and a simple cock-up splint can be used to hold the wrist in extension (no more than 30 degrees) to help reduce the buildup of fluid in the hand when elders are not receiving therapy (Figure 21-5).

COTAs can use graded activities to facilitate voluntary control of an elder's hemiplegic upper extremity. Such activities should be geared toward developing control in a progression from shoulder to elbow to hand. Elders may develop control in the hand before the more proximal parts of the arm, but this result is often caused by misalignment of the rest of the body. This is an associated reaction to effort in the opposite arm, or learned control of hypertonicity. In spite of apparent control in the hand, the COTA should first facilitate active movement in the shoulder by engaging elders in activities that emphasize the body moving on the arm while the hand is maintained in weight bearing. The weight-bearing surface of the hand is limited to the lateral surface of the thumb, the thenar eminencies, and the fingertips. In this position the palm of the hand is free and not in contact with the weight-bearing surface. Weight bearing on the hand does not need to be forceful, and elders should *never* have the hand completely flattened. Placing weight on a flat hand can lead to loss of the normal and functional arches of the hand and, consequently, can interfere with elders' abilities to develop grasp later. Placing weight on the hand can be done in both sitting and standing positions. In a sitting position, for example, an elder's affected hand can be placed in a weight-bearing position on the table or on a stool placed next to the elder. In a standing position, the elder should be taught to place the affected hand on a weight bearing surface such as a table or countertop while performing functional tasks such as putting away dishes or groceries or folding laundry (Figure 21-6). As control of the shoulder increases, activities should be introduced that emphasize free movement of the hemiplegic extremity on the more stable part of the body. During all these activities, the COTA should continue to ensure that good body alignment is maintained and that elders are not using abnormal movements in one part of the body to obtain control in another.

COTAs should instruct elders in proper one-handed dressing techniques to protect the hemiplegic upper extremity and to avoid falling. Dressing should be done while sitting in a chair and, in general, the hemiplegic extremity should be dressed first and undressed last to avoid pulling on it or twisting it unnecessarily. Front-buttoned shirts or blouses are easiest to don by dressing the hemiplegic arm first and then draping the shirt over

the shoulders by holding on to the shirt collar with the other arm. When the shirt is draped over the opposite shoulder, the elder can reach into the sleeve with the unaffected arm. This procedure is reversed when taking the shirt off. The process is similar when putting on pants with the exception that the elder should cross the hemiplegic leg over the opposite leg to dress the hemiplegic leg first. If the elder is able to stand to pull up the pants, the elder may do so when both legs are clothed. If standing is not possible, the elder can shift weight to each side while sitting in the chair and gradually can pull the pants up over the buttocks.

All the principles mentioned previously should be considered when training elders in functional activities or selecting adaptive equipment. Although progress may seem slower at the beginning, following these principles

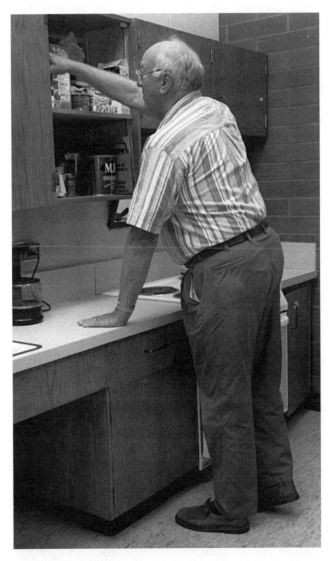

FIGURE 21-6　Bearing weight on the hemiplegic hand can be done while standing at a counter.

can make a marked difference in the quality of movement elders develop. When tasks are too difficult, elders are more likely to use abnormal movement patterns, become fatigued quickly, and become discouraged. The COTA must use good observation and clinical reasoning skills in selecting activities that challenge elders at the appropriate levels.

Perceptual-Cognitive Deficits

Although the motor deficits resulting from a stroke are the most easily observed, many less visible problems can severely hinder the rehabilitation process if not appropriately addressed. Depending on the type of brain lesion, the individual may have sensory disturbances that range from a total absence of sensation to a heightened perception of pain and other distorted sensations. These problems are accentuated when the individual has a body scheme disorder or difficulties planning motor actions, which is known as *apraxia*. Consequently, the individual has difficulty integrating and using any perceptual input from the hemiplegic side. Visual deficits common in strokes include hemianopsia, poor figure ground perceptions, and difficulty with spatial relationships. Unilateral neglect results from a unique constellation of these symptoms when elders have no sense that the hemiplegic side of the body even exists, and they fail to visually scan toward that side. All these disorders should be addressed simultaneously during intervention, using bilateral functional activities that encourage the use of the hemiplegic side of the body. The more normal movement is likely to provide a more normal and repeated sensory stimulation to the hemiplegic side, which is more likely to be processed correctly in the brain and used as feedback in determining where each body part is and what it is doing. Consequently, the COTA should grade a variety of motor and sensory activities so that they maximize the elders' abilities to control movement independently and provide increased sensory input. However, the activities should not be so overwhelming that they cause withdrawal reactions or increases in abnormal tone. Various textures, smells, colors, distances, and depths can be graded during most functional activities. In addition to these remedial approaches, the COTA should teach elders to compensate for deficits by providing repeated practice in establishing habits of visually scanning the hemiplegic side and methodically protecting and integrating the hemiplegic extremities in whatever activity they may be involved. (Additional information on issues that involve the visual system are covered in Chapter 17.)

Other areas of concern for the COTA include elders' abilities to comprehend and produce language and to plan and safely perform activities. As a result of stroke, elders may not be able to understand what others are saying, a condition known as *receptive aphasia*, may not be able to produce the words they intend to utter, a condition known as *expressive aphasia*, or both disorders may be present, which is known as *global aphasia*. These disorders may also extend to nonverbal language, and as elders may be unable to interpret or appropriately use gestures. Treatment of language deficits is generally directed by the speech-language pathologist, but strategies must be reinforced during OT intervention. When talking to elders, COTAs should keep instructions and explanations simple and concrete and should state them in an empathetic, patient way. Demonstration is usually helpful. The best way to ensure elders have understood the instructions is to observe their performance (Pedretti, Smith, Pendelton, 1995).

Cognitive dysfunction is often believed to be a major cause for failure of elders to reach rehabilitation goals and must be considered, particularly when planning for discharge (Woodson, 1995). Safety may be compromised if elders cannot plan activities, make judgments, solve problems, or express verbally their needs for emergency care. For example, limited memory may cause elders to overmedicate in a day or not turn off the stove after cooking. Being unable to remember all the steps involved in a task may mean that elders can often be surprised by the outcome. Elders may get stuck on a step and may be unable to determine what to do next or may neglect to realize that something dangerous could happen if an inappropriate action is taken. OT intervention, as mentioned earlier, should involve graded repetition of procedures until elders can routinely perform them safely. Emphasis should be placed on varying the context or situation in which the procedure is practiced to enhance learning (Toglia, 1991).

Emotional Adjustment

COTAs should consider the emotional adjustment of elders to the disability caused by the stroke. Depression, a common reaction to any catastrophic event, is one of the most underidentified and undertreated responses to stroke (Pedretti, Smith, Pendelton, 1995). Depression may be caused by not only natural grief because of the loss of function, but also in part by the result of chemical changes in the brain caused by the stroke. Depression is present between 6 months and 2 years after the stroke in up to 45% of clients (Robinson, Price, 1982). Poor frustration tolerance, denial, anger, and emotional liability are all signs that elders are struggling to deal with the reality of their condition. COTAs must listen empathetically and supportively, while sensitively maintaining the focus on areas of realistic recovery. Permitting elders to control choices in intervention as much as possible can reinforce the sense that they can affect their environments. Although a complete recovery cannot be guaranteed, neither can a lack of recovery. COTAs must honestly explain to elders that residual limitations will be present, but the best chance for recovery will be in much practice of skills. COTAs should use their creativity and ingenuity skills to help elders adapt tasks or environments that elders consider lost, and thus instill new hope and motivation in the rehabilitation process. As with any area of intervention, family and social involvement is crucial for elders to accept residual limitations and maximize their residual abilities. Ultimately, elders must see that they can continue to be effective in some measure and can still actively pursue activities and ideals they valued highly before the stroke.

CHAPTER REVIEW QUESTIONS

1 Sit at the edge of a bed or chair and lift up the left side of your pelvis. What happens with your spine and trunk when you do this? What occurs with the imaginary midline of the body when you sit in this position? Where on your thighs do you feel the most pressure while sitting in this position? Can you tell any difference in how your arms work while sitting this way? How would you feel after sitting in this position for ten or fifteen minutes?

2 Sitting on a firm chair, make sure that your pelvis is as far back in the chair as possible, and your back is well supported. From that position, without moving forward, attempt to stand. What did you do with your arms while attempting to stand? How much work did your trunk have to do to get you to a standing position? Now repeat the activity but first scoot to the edge of the chair before you stand. Did you notice any differences in the amount of work your upper trunk and arms had to do to get you upright? From which position was it easier to stand?

3 Sitting at the edge of a chair with your trunk well aligned, move your feet as far forward as you can, making sure that they are flat on the floor. From that position, attempt to stand. Were you able to do so? How much work did your upper trunk and arms have to do? Return to sitting at the edge of the chair, and now attempt to stand again, but first place your feet as far back behind your knees as possible. Was standing from this position more or less difficult than your first attempt? Did you fall forward? Now return to sitting at the edge of the chair, and this time place your feet so that your toes are directly aligned below your knees and are flat on the floor. Did this help to keep your midline where it should be, even during movement?

REFERENCES

American Occupational Therapy Association: Occupational therapy roles, *Am J Occup Ther* 47:1087, 1993.

Bear M, Connors B, Paradiso M: *Neuroscience: exploring the brain,* Baltimore, 1996, Williams & Wilkins.

Brunnstrom, S: *Movement therapy in hemiplegia,* New York, 1970, Harper & Row.

Davies, P: *Steps to follow: a guide to the treatment of adult hemiplegia,* New York, 1985, Springer-Verlag.

Davis, J: The role of the occupational therapist in the treatment of shoulder-hand syndrome, *Occup Ther Pract* 1:30, 1990.

DeArmond S, Fusco M, Dewey M: *Structure of the brain: a photographic atlas,* ed 3, New York, 1989, Oxford University Press.

Dyken ML et al: Risk factors in stroke: a statement for physicians by the Subcommittee on Risk Factors and Stroke Council, *Stroke* 15: 1105, 1984.

Gillum, RF: Strokes in blacks, *Stroke* 19:1, 1988.

Harmsen P, Tsipioganni A, Wilhelmsen L: Stroke incidence rates were unchanged while fatality rates declined during 1971-1987, *Stroke* 23:1410, 1992.

Pansky, B, Allen D, Budd, G: *Review of neuroscience,* ed 2, New York, 1988, Macmillan.

Pedretti L, Smith J, Pendelton H: Cerebral vascular accident. In Pedretti L, editor: *Occupational therapy: practice skills for physical dysfunction,* ed 4, St. Louis, 1995, Mosby.

Robinson R, Price T: Post-stroke depression disorders: a follow-up study of 103 patients, *Stroke* 13:635, 1982.

Sacco RL et al: Survival and recurrence following stroke. The Framingham Study, *Stroke* 13:290, 1982.

Terent A: Stroke morbidity. In Whisnat J, editor: *Stroke: populations, cohorts and clinical trials,* Boston, 1993, Butterworth-Heinemann.

Toglia J: Generalization of treatment: a multicontext approach to cognitive perceptual impairment in adults with brain injury, *Am J Occup Ther* 45:506, 1991.

Umphred D, editor: *Neurological rehabilitation,* ed 3, St. Louis, 1995, Mosby.

US Department of Health and Human Services: *Post stroke rehabilitation: practice guideline no. 16,* Rockville, Md, 1995.

Voss D, Ionta M, Meyers B: *Proprioceptive neuromuscular facilitation,* ed 3, New York, 1985, Harper & Row.

Warren M: Strategies for sensory and neuromotor remediation. In Christiansen C, Baum C, editors: *Occupational therapy: overcoming human performance deficits,* Thorofare, NJ, 1991, SLACK.

Woodson A: Stroke. In Trombly C, editor: *Occupational therapy for physical dysfunction,* ed 4, Baltimore, 1995, Williams & Wilkins.

World Health Organization: Recommendations on stroke prevention, diagnosis, and therapy: report of the WHO Task Force on stroke and other cerebrovascular disorders, *Stroke* 20:1460, 1989.

CHAPTER 22

Working With Elders Who Have Dementia and Alzheimer's Disease

CARLY **R**. HELLEN

KEY **T**ERMS

Alzheimer's disease (AD), activity-focused care, "therapeutic fibs," rescuing, chaining, bridging

CHAPTER **O**BJECTIVES

1. Gain awareness and sensitivity to the cognitive, physical, and psychosocial needs of elders with Alzheimer's disease (AD).
2. Describe activity-focused care.
3. Relate suggestions to promote wellness through task simplification and modification.
4. Identify caregiving techniques, approaches, and interventions that can be used to help empower elders who have Alzheimer's disease to participate in daily living tasks.
5. Suggest appropriate communication responses to elders with Alzheimer's disease.
6. Problem solve antecedents and approaches to refocus unwanted behavioral responses.

Carl is a COTA who works in a skilled nursing facility (SNF). One of his responsibilities is consulting with staff at a special care unit for people with **Alzheimer's disease (AD).** John, the charge nurse on the unit, contacts Carl. "We are having problems with Mrs. K. She is wandering in and out of other's rooms and taking their possessions, which is irritating the other residents. She is also having difficulty communicating her needs. Her performance with ADL functions seems variable. We are also having problems with increased agitation of all of our residents, especially at change of shift. Do you have any ideas?"

Chris is a COTA working on a subacute unit. Ruth, one of the elders, has been admitted after a total hip replacement. After reviewing her chart, Chris finds out that Ruth has a history of AD. Both Carl and Chris can provide practical suggestions to help these elders with AD function better. This chapter provides background information about AD and occupational therapy treatment interventions.

Dementia is a syndrome that includes confusion, forgetfulness, decreased judgment, and loss or failure of mental abilities. Depression, medications, and metabolic dysfunction may cause a reversible dementia. Causes of nonreversible dementia include small strokes (multiinfarct dementia), Parkinson's disease, Pick's disease, and Alzheimer's disease (AD). AD affects 4 million elders in

BOX 22-1

Four Stages of Alzheimer's Disease

Mild impairment/early stage
Average 1-3 years, possibly longer
Memory loss, especially with recent events
Difficulty with complex cognitive tasks
Difficulty with decision making and planning
Decreased attention span and concentration
Decreased ability to initiate activity or be spontaneous
Impaired word-finding skills
Preference for familiar settings

Mid/Moderate impairment stage
Average 5-7 years, possibly longer
Chronic recent memory loss
Difficulty with written and spoken language
Tendency to ask questions constantly
Tendency to experience visual-spatial perceptual problems
Topographical disorientation
Increasing difficulty with familiar objects and tasks
Assistance with ADL functions necessary
Ability to respond to multisensory cueing
Tendency to wander, pace, rummage

Late/severe impairment stage
Average 2-3 years
Dependence on others for ADL functions
Ability to respond to hand-over-hand activity
Decreased interest in food
Difficulty with chewing and swallowing
Incontinence
Decreased vocabulary
Misidentification of familiar objects
Impaired ambulation/gait, increased falls
Repetitious movement or sounds

Terminal stage
Average 3 months–1 year
Usually in bed or wheelchair
Limited ability to track visually
Loss of appetite, severe weight loss
Tendency to utter sounds rather than words
Total dependence on others for care
Possible development of contractions, skin breakdown
Possible reaction to music and touch, fleeting attention span

The problems start gradually and become more severe over time, leading to a total inability to perform self-care. Although the rate of change varies, the usual stages are mild, moderate, severe, and terminal (Box 22-1).

Alzheimer's disease can last 2 to 20 years. Most people die after 8 years, often from pneumonia or other systemic problems. Causes of AD are not known, but current research suggests the involvement of brain chemicals, amyloids, and genetic factors (Aronson, 1987; Alzheimer's Association, 1990). Treatment is based on medical and psychosocial support. The disease has no known cure at this time.

Aronson (1994) reported that of the 1.5 million residents of nursing homes in the United States, more than half have AD or some form of dementia. COTAs work with elders who have AD and related dementia in nursing homes as well as in homes, adult day programs, and hospitals. COTAs often provide therapy to elders with AD on special care units or as part of their regular caseload. Occupational therapy treatment for these elders usually focuses on ADL functions, communication, strengthening, and adaptations of purposeful activities.

ACTIVITY-FOCUSED CARE FOR ELDERS WITH AD

Activity-focused care for elders with AD recognizes that life consists of being and doing. The tasks of life are interconnected. The activities of responding to a question or participating in a group, for example, connect all components of life. The objectives of activity-focused care include focusing on abilities, not limitations, and promoting the purposeful use of time. Other objectives include supporting a sense of belonging, enabling verbal and nonverbal communication skills, encouraging positive behaviors, and developing interventions to refocus unwanted behaviors (Hellen, 1992).

Activity-focused care redefines interventions, especially in long-term care settings and special care units. Success is achieved through augmenting the client's strengths by reframing expectations. It involves the willingness to enter the client's world with sensitivity and flexibility and the provision of holistic support.

COMMUNICATION: UNDERSTANDING AND BEING UNDERSTOOD

Communicating with people who have AD is often challenging. As the disease progresses, verbal abilities decrease and communication continues through nonverbal gestures and sounds. Verbal and nonverbal communication have the same objectives: expressing thoughts and needs and supporting self-image and a sense of worth. Other objectives for communication include improving socialization and involvement in a supportive community, understanding others, and enhancing the environment. During the early stages of AD, changes that occur in

the United States and is projected to affect up to 6 million by 2010 (Evans et al, 1990). It is a progressive, degenerative disease of brain tissue that leads to memory loss and problems with thinking and carrying out daily life activities. Performing routine tasks, using good judgment, being aware of surroundings, communicating effectively, and coping become more difficult as the disease progresses.

language and communication include the onset of difficulty with using nouns. Substituted words are sometimes used for the noun. For example, Mary was asked to identify an object (a comb). Her response was, "Oh, honey, you know," as she ran her hand through her hair. She was unable to use the noun "comb" (Figure 22-1).

Reality orientation is usually embarrassing for elders with AD because of their inability to remember. One type of response that maintains the dignity of elders with disorientation is to refrain from confronting them with corrections, especially if the confrontation would increase agitation. Instead, caregivers should refocus elders on the task at hand by redirecting them or agreeing with them. These strategies are called **"therapeutic fibs."** For example, when Jim states "My wife is taking me home in 5 minutes," the COTA agrees with him, knowing that a discussion would increase his agitation. The COTA then redirects Jim to do a meaningful task. Elders asking for their mothers or wanting to go home may be seeking acceptance. They may also be expressing the need for safety, purposeful use of time, or the company of others. Telling them that their mother is dead or the facility is

now their home can upset them. Instead, the COTA may say, "You are safe with me and I will be here today with you. If you are like your mother, she must have been wonderful. I miss my mother too; we used to have fun folding the wash, perhaps you and I can work together."

As the disease progresses, the ability to speak and understand decreases. Some of these elders become more intuitive, often with increased awareness of people's attitudes and the environment (Hellen, 1992). Therefore caregivers should be aware of nonverbal messages. In time, elders with AD lose almost all language skills, but they may still occasionally utter a perfectly correct statement. For example, John talked a lot, but his words were just sounds that made no sense. When a caregiver impatiently spoke to him in an abrupt and firm tone, saying "John, time out; go to your room," John responded, "In the military, I was in solitary confinement and I can do that standing on my head." The family later confirmed that John had indeed been in the military and

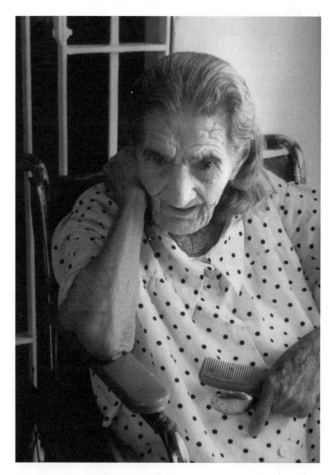

FIGURE **22-1** Elders with AD may display difficulty identifying and verbalizing the names for common objects. (Courtesy Yolanda Griffiths.)

BOX 22-2

Suggestions for Improving Communication

1. Attract the client's attention by using touch and talking at eye level.
2. Use short, simple sentences to express one thought at a time. Be willing to repeat as needed, allowing time for the elder to respond.
3. Be aware that asking questions can often be embarrassing for people with AD, who often have difficulty finding the right words for the answer. Instead, help them respond by giving as many multisensory verbal or nonverbal cues as possible.
4. Do not try to apply logic or give people long explanations.
5. State requests with positive words ("Please sit here" rather than "Don't sit there").
6. Listen carefully to all the words, gestures, and facial expressions the person uses. Validate feelings behind the words. For example, if Henry's words seem to make no sense but sound angry and upset, say, "You sound upset, Henry. I know when I feel that way I like a hug. Can I give you a hug?" However, be aware that some people are tactile defensive and become agitated when touched.
7. Realize that elders with AD often respond literally to words (because the fire alarm says "pull," Hazel pulls it).
8. Be aware that elders with AD often revert to their primary language. COTAs may have to learn appropriate key words in that language to encourage therapy.
9. Singing a familiar song is a method to encourage speech.

the story was true. The caregiver's "drill sergeant" tone and body posture triggered John's response.

People with AD need to experience acceptance and success, especially as their language skills diminish. COTAs can keep the dialogue going even when the words are few (Box 22-2).

BEHAVIOR AND PSYCHOSOCIAL ASPECTS

People with dementia are not stupid; they are forgetful. Like anyone else, they have needs and should be approached and cared for with respect. They should also have opportunities for pride and meaningful involvement. Knowledge of their client's life story often becomes the basis for COTAs to plan and carry out therapy. A Life Story book can be used for this purpose. This book can include pictures with captions, lists, favorite recipes, family traditions, schools attended, and military history. Using the book is an excellent tool for refocusing behaviors and reducing agitation (Hellen, 1992).

The behaviors of people with dementia are often attempts to communicate. For example, increased agitation may be the client's way of communicating illness. Rapid pacing might be a sign of an inability to cope with others, excessive noise, or environmental factors.

Some of the typical behaviors displayed by people with AD include wandering, pacing, and rummaging or redistribution of personal belongings (Figure 22-2). Combativeness and aggression can also occur. Catastrophic reactions are explosive responses to distress. These reactions result from the inability to understand, interpret, and cope with real or imagined situations, people, the environment, or oneself. "Sun-downing" results from a combination of increased behavioral responses in the mid-to-late afternoon. These responses often reflect physical problems such as dehydration and emotional exhaustion. Screaming, yelling, and calling often reflect fear, a need for acceptance, and a lack of active participation during the day. Other behavioral manifestations may include inappropriate sexual conduct, accusing or demanding speech, withdrawal from activities, and apathy. Elders with AD might also show perseveration in their actions by repetitious movement or sounds, such as wiping or patting the table surface, pulling on clothing, and shouting.

Difficult behaviors are not purposeful; they are part of the disease. Behaviors can often be a problem to others but not to the elder. For example, Betty, who lives in a special care unit, goes into other people's rooms. She looks through their closets and takes clothing and items from their drawers. This behavior suggests that Betty feels in control and is cleaning up the house. Whose problem is it? Bertha, the owner of these possessions, is angry and feels that her privacy has been invaded. The facility staff meet the challenge of working with both people in a supportive way by identifying acceptable places for Betty to rummage, such as the top drawer in the

family room and "busy boxes" filled with safe items. This measure addresses Betty's need to feel in control.

A respectful response exists for every behavior. In some cases, attempting to reason with people who have AD may not work, especially if they mistake others for someone they do not like. Logic also may not work with people who are having a visual or auditory hallucination. Usually, COTAs can identify the event that precipitated the unwanted behavior and make adjustments that might stop it or decrease the likelihood of recurrence. Three problem-solving tools can help refocus unwanted behavior. These are the behavioral profile, the behavioral analysis, and the Behavioral Observation Form.

The behavioral profile is a tool used to examine the situation. COTAs can ask themselves the following thought-provoking questions: WHAT exactly is happening? WHY has the behavior happened, and WHAT was the antecedent? WHO is involved, and WHERE is the behavior exhibited? WHEN does the behavior usually occur? WHAT now?

The behavioral analysis outlines the specific behavior by focusing on the client's actions, and defining the antecedent or possible causes. In addition, it outlines acceptable approaches and interventions with attention to the impact on the family, environment, and activity (Box 22-3).

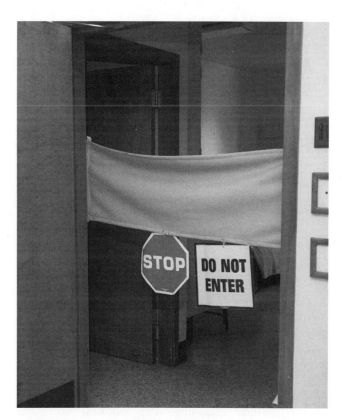

FIGURE 22-2 Environmental adaptations should help restrict elders with AD from wandering into other people's rooms but not restrict access to corridors.

BOX 22-3

Problem: Pacing and/or Wandering- Behavior Analysis Approach

Behaviors exhibited
Pacing
Trying to get a ride home
Following visitors out the door
Packing and leaving
Searching behavior for something unattainable (for example, mother)

Possible cause or antecedent
May be a stress-handling mechanism
May be escape from intolerable reality
May be search for something familiar
May be consistent with former habits (always "on the go")
May reflect need for self-stimulation
May result from hunger
May be an energy outlet
May be reflect a semiagitated state
May result from anxiety, boredom
May be the result of a habitual role pattern
May be search for security

Interventions with the resident
Ask whether the client is hungry, needs to void, feels uncomfortable, is really lost
Have elder wear Medic-Alert ID bracelet
Take photos for police
Provide alternative activities
Pin a note on clothes with address or room number
Avoid stressful situations from which the elder wants to escape
When the elder leaves, follow and gently escort back
Use sensory distraction
Walk with elder
Provide regular routine
Use restraints, when appropriate
Use a therapeutic "fib" such as notifying the elder of a phone call

Family focus
Discuss treatment approaches
Provide information on policy and procedures

Instruct them not to contradict the elder's stories; instead, they should assure the elder that everything will be all right.
Recommend not overdramatizing entrances, exits, and promises to return.
Encourage use of local support groups and discussions with other families
Encourage walks with the elder
Inform of possible risks

Facility adaptations
Remove environmental cues that suggest leaving the facility, such as coats and suitcases.
Use familiar objects in room.
Install Dutch doors
Design rooms to be close to central nursing station
Provide access to enclosed outdoor area
Develop procedure to follow for missing persons.
Provide routine orientation and escort for new admissions
Perform periodic checks for wanderers
Alert visitors to facility procedures
Employ experienced, trained staff who know the elder
Introduce the elder to all staff, especially those near the doors (for example, switchboard operator, receptionist)
Set up "safe" areas for pacing
Group elders so the wandering ones do not upset others.
Write problem/intervention on kardex

Activity
Physical exercise
Small, supervised field trips
Expressive arts
Music activities
Routine, familiar activities
Dancing
Physical fitness trail (pair elders to walk together or with trained volunteers)
Errands away from the unit (for example, picking up laundry, taking paperwork to the nursing office)

The Behavior Observational Form is used to determine a behavioral pattern involving the time of day and possible antecedents. This form can help COTAs and other health care workers make appropriate changes for reducing or refocusing difficult behaviors (Figure 22-3).

The challenge of identifying the source of the difficult or unwanted behavior and a solution to the problem also requires critical reasoning. The following are some questions that COTAs can ask themselves to help with the critical reasoning process: What is this behavior "saying?" Whose problem is it? What are some environmental factors that might be contributing to the behavior?

The story of John, an elder in an AD special care unit, illustrates the importance of critical reasoning in addressing difficult or unwanted behaviors. John tries constantly to go out the door because he thinks it is time to go to work. Possible reasons for his attempts to leave include the time of day, the fact that he sees visitors leaving with their hats and coats, and lack of involvement in meaningful activities. The staff may not be trained to redirect him when his anxiety and agitation increases, the day room may be too noisy, or he may believe that the

Name:							
Date	Time	Observed activity and behavior	Behavior				Observer
			Trigger (What started it)	Intervention (What stopped it)	Time elapsed •Before stopping •Stayed stopped		

FIGURE 22-3 Behavioral Observation Form.

intercom voice is calling him to the phone. The COTA might consider the following options: asking him to help with a project (he might forget his need to leave), painting the exit door the same color as the walls on either side so it appears less obvious, involving John in a meaningful activity, and spending some quality time with John.

Mary is another person in the same unit. She often becomes combative when performing ADL functions, especially showering. In fact, she strikes the COTA during an assessment of showering. The COTA considers possible causes for this behavior: Did Mary formerly take baths, and is she unhappy with the change in her routine? Is Mary a very private person and embarrassed that someone is helping her? Did she react to the COTA's tone of voice? Is Mary getting sick and unable to report it? Is she too tired when the shower is scheduled? Is she experiencing chronic pain such as arthritis, which may be upsetting her? Does she feel rushed? Has the showering task been simplified enough so that she can participate and feel in control? The COTA then considers the following behavioral interventions: asking Mary to help wash down the shower, singing Mary's favorite hymn with her while she showers, postponing the shower for another time, and allowing Mary to bathe with some of her clothes on or wrapping her in a bath blanket during the bathing process.

As illustrated by the preceding examples, handling the behavioral difficulties of elders who have AD can be a trial and error process until COTAs identify solutions that work. Different techniques can succeed one time and fail the next. Even when COTAs cannot ascertain the exact reason for the behaviors, they can try the following intervention techniques. Distraction is a helpful technique, especially if the person is agitated. COTAs can be creative with ideas for distraction that involve the person in a meaningful activity, such as listening to music. **Rescuing** is another distraction technique: When one caregiver is in conflict with the client, a second caregiver responds by "rescuing" that person. This technique is illustrated by the following example. Sally, a nursing assistant, says to Mary, the resident, "Don't go out the door." If Amy, the COTA, approaches Mary in the same fashion, Mary might feel outnumbered. On the other hand, if Amy says, "Sally, Mary and I want to be alone; please leave us," Mary might feel "rescued" and go with Amy.

Inappropriate timing, attempts to manipulate the elder to fit a schedule, and unrealistic performance expectations can cause negative behavior such as hitting. Consequently, caregivers must be aware of the elder's mood before approaching with a demand.

TREATMENT
Observations, Screening, and Assessment

The COTA/OTR team may collaborate in the administration of the following evaluations. The Folstein Mini-Mental State (MMS) is a short and simple quantitative measure of cognitive performance. This measure is a questionnaire in five areas of cognition, including orientation, registration (memory), attention, and calculation, as well as recall and language (following oral and written instructions) (Folstein, Folstein, McHugh, 1975). The Global Deterioration Scale measures clinical characteristics at seven levels based on the progressive stages of AD (Reisberg et al, 1982).

The Allen Cognitive Performance Tests and the Routine Task Inventory examine cognitive function through completion of tasks (Allen, 1985). The levels of function help predict behavior and effects on ADL functions. These levels range from the ability to use complex information and perform ADL functions accurately and safely to severe deficits in recognition and use of familiar objects. This assessment includes information on communication, response to tasks, and need for task simplification. It also addresses the role of the therapist during treatment. (Refer to Chapter 7 for a more detailed explanation of these tests.)

The Cognitive Performance Test (CPT) is a standardized functional assessment instrument designed for the evaluation of Allen cognitive levels (Burns, Mortimer, 1993). Six functional tasks—dressing, shopping, making toast, making phone call, doing laundry, and traveling—compose the test. This test also looks at the person's abilities to process information in relation to functional performance.

Treatment Planning

Occupational therapy for people who have AD involves attention to self-care skills, communication, mobility, and safety. Areas to address in treatment planning include decreased attention span, inability to initiate tasks, difficulty with sequencing tasks, and impaired judgment. In a special care unit, the plan of care should emphasize occupational therapy.

Treatment planning begins with establishing a cognitive and functional baseline and includes ability-based goals. These goals should identify functional capacity and needs to restore, maintain, or improve skills. The goals should focus on abilities and opportunities for participation in activities that support cognitive, physical, and psychosocial wellness. These goals should include interventions that enable caregiving and refocus difficult behaviors in a supportive and safe environment.

Treatment planning should include the use of assessment and observation to measure changes in functional status. The process of treatment planning includes providing and suggesting continuous modifications and adaptations of approaches, such as task simplification and cueing. The elder's life story may be used as the basis for treatment that focuses on past wisdom and experiences. Treatment planning also involves assessing all aspects of treatment support and factors that lead to negative responses, including environmental components. For

example, Andrew's limited attention span prohibited him from eating more than a few mouthfuls of each meal. He was seated in a large dining room with five other people at his table. Music was played on the tape deck, and the staff often talked loudly with each other. When the COTA suggested relocating Andrew to a small dining area where the tables seated two, he was able to focus on his food and complete his meal.

Treatment Intervention

Occupational therapy treatment interventions consider the effects of dementia on the elder's cognitive abilities and well-being. Success with treatment interventions entails many crucial components, including the COTA's flexibility and creativity. Success may need to be redefined, as exemplified by Susan, a resident of a special care unit. Susan liked to wear a yellow floral blouse and her favorite orange and black plaid skirt. She was proud of her ability to select and dress independently, although some disapproved of her choices.

Equally important for successful treatment intervention is the COTA's nonverbal approach. It should reflect acceptance and respect for the elder with AD. To ensure success, treatment interventions should not place elders in situations in which their inabilities may lead to failure. For example, Clara had always been a talented knitter of lovely sweaters. Her ability to do intricate stitches became impaired as her dementia progressed. The COTA set up the stitches on large needles and helped her get started knitting squares using a basic stitch. Clara was able to knit the simple squares for a baby blanket and delighted in the recognition of her success.

Applying life history and experiences to functional abilities is also meaningful. For example, Sara, age 78, a mother of five, responds to normalization activities such as washing dishes, hanging laundry, and sweeping floors. These activities provide tactile stimulation, lower and upper body range of motion, strengthening, trunk stabilization, and fine hand motor skills.

COTAs can use their skills in analyzing activities to identify steps toward task simplification. For example, Jim was able to dress himself independently when each item of clothing was placed on his bed in the appropriate sequence for dressing. Successful treatment interventions should also focus on working with elders to promote active participation and collaboration. For example, Charles had lost interest in feeding himself but accepted the COTA's suggestion to have the caregiver place a hand over his hand. That way he could continue to feed himself with assistance rather than being fed by others.

When possible, treatment interventions should be provided in appropriate and familiar settings. For example, Millie was unable to experience success with simple dressing tasks when she attempted them in the clinic. When the COTA arrived at Millie's bedside early each morning, Millie was able to use visual cues found in her bedroom, including the bureau and closet, to trigger self-dressing skills.

Activities of Daily Living (ADL)

COTAs can make a significant contribution to elders with AD and enhance their quality of life by supporting ADL functions. Understanding task breakdown, task simplification, and appropriate treatment approaches enables these elders to become involved in performing these familiar skills. This understanding can be facilitated by using one-step commands and visual cueing, including objects or gestures. The use of the Allen's stage levels can be a helpful measure of the elder's level of functioning (Allen, 1985).

Difficulties with ADL functions associated with dementia include decreased attention span, limited ability to follow directions, and increased length of time to complete tasks. Other difficulties include problems with sequencing, perception, and body awareness. Emotional responses of fear, paranoia, and reactions to excessive environmental stimulation that are real or imagined can also influence ADL functioning.

COTAs working on ADL functions will be most successful when they use creative problem solving. Therapy requires working *with* elders, not doing *to* or *for* them. COTAs should do everything possible to make ADL functions meaningful. The use of distraction techniques (for example, singing and holding items such as costume jewelry, scarves, and neckties) should be part of daily care. The COTA's attitude, approach, and direct involvement are key components in supporting the elder's quality of life.

COTAs should consider the timing when working on ADL functions. Often, these decisions are based on knowing the elder and responding to nonverbal language that suggests the best and worst times for these activities. Sometimes, COTAs must come back several times because many elders with AD are sensitive to being rushed. For example, Charles appeared agitated when the COTA wanted to work on dressing skills. After several attempts the COTA decided to return later. At that time, Charles was calmer and accepting of the activity.

Assisting with ADL functions can also provide opportunities for COTAs to monitor the elder's physical well-being and safety. Elders with AD often do not report bruises, rashes, and blisters. Decreased cognitive ability and judgment, combined with an unawareness of perceptual difficulties, may lead to unsafe situations. Elders may eat dirt or plants, walk on wet floors, put their shoes on the wrong feet, forget necessary items such as glasses, misjudge a chair seat and fall, or scald themselves in the shower because they do not know how to turn on the cold water—all these are examples of potential dangers.

When working with elders on ADL functions, COTAs should always focus on abilities by encouraging active involvement. The techniques of hand-over-hand guidance, **chaining,** and **bridging** can be used. Hand-over-hand guidance may help the elder complete the ADL task. In chaining, the caregiver begins a task by putting one hand over the elder's hand and continuing until the elder can take over and complete the task. For example, Astrid had no idea what a toothbrush was or how to use it. However, when the COTA placed it in her hand and guided it to her mouth to start the brushing action, Astrid was able to complete the task independently (Figure 22-4).

With bridging, elders who are unable to perform any part of the daily living task can focus their attention by holding the same object the caregiver is using. This technique can also help decrease anxiety. For example, Allan could not shave. The COTA demonstrated to the caregivers a bridging technique to try with Allan. She placed a turned-on electric razor in his hand so he could feel the vibration while she shaved him with another electric razor. By holding a razor, Allan was better able to focus attention on the task (Hellen, 1992).

The creativity and flexibility of COTAs can promote the remaining abilities of elders and their willingness to be actively involved in daily life tasks (Box 22-4). Knowledge of the client's past routines is helpful during ADL functions.

Using Adapted Equipment

Elders who have AD often refuse or misuse adapted equipment. Improper use may affect the elder's safety, especially if the item does not look familiar. For example,

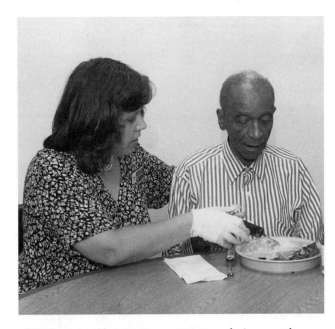

FIGURE 22-4 Chaining is a common technique used to facilitate participation in ADL functions.

BOX 22-4

Suggestions for Provision of ADL Support for Elders with Alzheimer's Disease

Bathing:
1. Know whether client prefers a bath or shower; use hand-held shower head.
2. If privacy is an issue, elder can bathe with some clothing on or with a bath blanket.
3. If needed, elder may wash one part of the body per day until they are able to accept total bathing.
4. Consider safety by using adaptations such as bath seats, grab bars, and floor mats.
5. Create a warm and homelike environment.

Shaving:
1. Use a mirror unless elders do not recognize themselves.
2. Use a bridging technique with clients incapable of actually shaving.

Oral care:
1. Use a child-sized tooth brush.
2. Pretend to be brushing your own teeth and encourage the elder to mirror the activity.
3. Use bridging technique of asking elder to hold an extra set of dentures while the caregiver is removing the elder's dentures.
4. Set up a dental chair, complete with bib, etc.

Dressing:
1. Suggest clothing one size larger for dressing ease. Keep the clothes appropriate to the elder's past lifestyle.
2. Suggest 100% cotton clothing because it does not retain the odor of urine.
3. Use verbal and visual cues to simplify each step, and always thank the elder for helping.
4. If possible, use washable shoes with Velcro closures.
5. Ask the elder to sit when dressing, especially if balance is a concern.

Toileting
1. Be aware of elder's past toileting routines and habits.
2. Use pictures of toilets on bathroom doors.
3. Determine whether the bathroom mirror prohibits elders from using the toilet because they do not recognize their image and think someone else is there.

4. Be sure the toilet seat color contrasts with the floor. Change the seat or use a washable rug around the toilet base.
5. Use key words to remind the elder about the task.
6. Offer the elder something (for example, a magazine) to hold or do while seated on the toilet.
7. Never refer to pads for incontinence as "diapers."
8. Use suspenders to keep pads in place.

Eating
1. Observe for safety problems such as overstuffing the mouth, not chewing before swallowing, and eating non-edibles (napkins, foam cups, etc.). If the elder is storing food in the mouth, check for a clear swallow. Obtain a swallowing evaluation if a problem is apparent. Refer to Chapter 20 on dysphagia.
2. Offer the meal in a quiet area to decrease distractions and improve attention span.
3. If the food needs to be set up, always do that out of the elder's sight. This prevents reinforcement of inabilities.
4. Sit with the elder.
5. Provide color contrast between the food and the plate and the plate and the table. Avoid plastic utensils, which are easily bitten and broken.
6. Obtain, if appropriate, a dietary order for variation in food textures.
7. Simplify the meal by serving one item and one utensil at a time.
8. Use finger foods, or incorporate food into a sandwich.
9. If the elder is not eating and no medical reasons prohibit it, use sugar or honey on the food to increase palatability.
10. If the elder needs to be fed, bridge the task by having the elder hold a spoon or plastic cup.
11. If the elder is disinterested in eating, alternate bites of hot and cold foods.
12. If weight loss is a problem, double the elder's breakfast.
13. Try to avoid commercial food supplements if possible by allowing time for the meal to be eaten and providing protein-enriched foods such as milk shakes.

a plate guard may appear so strange that the elder with AD might spend the mealtime trying to remove it from the plate. Sometimes, large, built-up handles on eating utensils may feel so different that clients do not use them. Reachers and other metal devices used for ADL functions can be used as weapons. Flatware with large handles and scoop dishes can be helpful because they closely resemble their ordinary counterparts. Adapting the environment by

using pictures, words, labels, and arrows are often the best ways to cue for successful involvement in ADL functions.

Using Activities to Promote Well-Being

Activities can be adapted for individuals and groups. The objectives of therapeutic activities are enhancing meaning, encouraging active participation, and ensuring success. All of life's activities can be used as treatment modalities. Suggestions for cognitive activities are adapted trivia games, crossword puzzles, rhyming games, and reminiscence. Others include spelling games, simple crafts, clothes-sorting, cards, poetry recitation, and singing. Suggestions for physical activities include parachute exercises, dancing, and tossing, hitting, and kicking balls and balloons. An exercise program may include use of hand-held wands, light weights, scarves, and fabrics. Psychosocial activities include parties, service projects, grooming tasks, celebrations of special days, field trips, and pet care. Recommendations for normalizing activities are folding and hanging up laundry, dusting and sweeping, sorting silverware, and shining shoes (Hellen, 1992).

Communication with and Teaching Caregivers

Occupational therapy treatment of elders who have AD focuses on maintaining functional abilities and preventing secondary complications. These objectives can be achieved by tailoring communication and education to caregivers. Caregivers benefit from a variety of techniques, including written instruction and demonstration. The instructional method of requiring a "return demonstration" allows COTAs to observe first-hand that caregivers follow through with activities. Afterwards the COTA can make necessary suggestions or corrections.

The COTA and OTR team can formulate a maintenance program (American Occupational Therapy Association, 1993). Contributing to a maintenance program may require COTAs to sensitize caregivers to the nature and progression of AD. An understanding of task breakdown and simplification, activity modification, behavioral interventions, supportive communications, and the need for flexibility is essential in maintenance programs.

TERMINAL STAGE ISSUES

Severe dementia, or terminal stage, is exhibited when the elder is oriented only to person and depends entirely on others for self-care. Defining the exact time of terminal, or end-stage, AD is difficult because of changes and variations in the disease process. For example, John appeared to have entered the terminal stage because he had been refusing food for 2 weeks. When offered cold and sweet foods, he suddenly started to eat again with gusto.

Many elders at the terminal stage of AD are in bed or in wheelchairs or recliners. Sometimes, they lie in bed in the fetal position. These elders are dependent on others for basic life functions and display an almost total loss of communication skills. To help make them more comfortable, COTAs may provide positioning suggestions and passive range-of-motion exercises. A caring touch, hand-over-hand movement, and various sensory activities may produce a response. Some people become ill with symptoms leading to pneumonia or other systemic

problems shortly before death. This is an important time for supporting family members and staff caregivers.

REIMBURSEMENT FOR SERVICES

A functional outcome must be meaningful, utilitarian, and sustainable over time. At present, maintenance of remaining abilities of elders with dementia is not usually covered by third-party payers such as Medicare. For elders on Medicare, Part B, the COTA/OTR team may suggest a short-range program based on continuous functional support, especially if a change in functional status has occurred. Often, elders with AD who receive Medicare reimbursement for care receive an initial evaluation from occupational therapy. A maintenance program is then developed and carried out by facility staff. The OTR evaluates the elder and establishes the plan of care. The COTA may train caregivers to carry out the plan. Medicare may reimburse the facility for time spent in evaluation and teaching. Occupational therapy practitioners may follow the elder for reevaluation when significant changes occur in functional status. (Refer to Chapter 6 for a more in-depth discussion of Medicare policy.)

CONCLUSION

COTAs can make a unique contribution to elders with AD. COTAs can treat these elders from the initial stages of forgetfulness and poor judgment by offer strategies for continuing independence. COTAs may also provide advice about late-stage care by focusing on positioning, feeding, and responses to sensory activities. Understanding the changes that occur as dementia progresses challenge elders, caregivers, and families to pursue creative and supportive solutions for daily care. The holistic programs and care of COTAs support the abilities and well-being of elders. When offered activity-focused care, elders with dementia can have meaningful lives.

CASE STUDY

Mildred is 78 years of age and has mid-stage AD. Mildred was formerly a teacher and experienced a happy family life with her husband of 58 years and their two sons. She has been widowed for the past 5 years. Mildred was brought to the special care unit (SCU) where she resides when she was found wandering outside during the cold winter months.

At the SCU the COTA helped to assess Mildred's functional status. The COTA identified the following abilities: Mildred follows one-step directions, responds to multisensory cueing, maintains strong socialization skills, and refers to her former profession by often mentioning her past role as a teacher.

Mildred functions at Allen's Cognitive Level 3. The COTA observed that she was forgetful, with limited instructional carry-over. Mildred experiences problems with sequencing ADL functions. She often becomes anxious, which leads to combativeness during ADL functions, especially bathing. Other assessment findings included the inability to toilet independently and use multiple utensils with meals. Communication challenges included receptive and expressive understanding of words, especially nouns.

The COTA instructed all staff members who work with Mildred to consider her strengths as well as her attention-span deficits and feelings of depression as she attempts to cope with the disease.

▮ CHAPTER REVIEW QUESTIONS

1 Considering Mildred's case, how can visual triggers and written phrases be used to help Mildred be as independent as possible?

2 What anxiety-reducing approaches can be explored? What specific interventions can be used during bathing?

3 How can the COTA develop a system for sequencing Mildred's clothing?

4 What environmental issues might need to be addressed, especially in the bath/shower room?

5 What suggestions can be incorporated as mealtime interventions for promoting successful dining?

6 If Mildred can find the toilet, what strategies can enable her to remain continent?

7 How can the COTA use ADL functions as therapeutic modalities for reducing feelings of depression and helplessness?

8 In reference to the entire chapter, what are the basic symptoms of AD and how do they affect elders with the disease and their caregivers?

9 Identify six ways to facilitate communication with elders who have dementia.

10 How can a functional assessment be used to develop treatment goals?

11 List three guidelines for the provision of ADL support to elders functioning at the mid-stage level of AD.

12 Outline six specific mealtime adaptations for elders with a short attention span.

13 List steps for getting dressed using task simplification.

14 What are possible antecedents and appropriate interventions for agitation?

15 Why do people with dementia wander, and how can the risk of elopement be decreased?

16 Give specific examples of ways activity-focused care supports COTAs treatment interventions.

17 Describe strategies to adapt the activity of folding laundry to address the elder's cognitive, physical, psychosocial, and normalization needs.

REFERENCES

Allen CK: *Occupational therapy for psychiatric diseases: measurement and management of cognitive disabilities*, Boston, 1985, Little Brown.

Alzheimer's Association: *The "Just The Facts" kit*, Chicago, 1990, The Association.

American Occupational Therapy Association: Occupational therapy roles, *Am J Occup Ther* 47(12):1087, 1993.

Aronson MK, editor: *Understanding Alzheimer's disease: what it is; how to cope with it; future directions*, New York, 1987, Scribners.

Aronson MK: *Reshaping dementia care*, Thousand Oaks, Calif, 1994, Sage Publications.

Burns T, Mortimer J: The cognitive performance test: a new approach to functional assessment in AD, *J Geriatr Psychiatric Neurol* 7(1):46, 1993.

Evans DA et al: Estimated prevalence of Alzheimer's disease in the United States, *Milbank Q* 68:267, 1990.

Folstein MF, Folstein SE, McHugh PR: Mini mental state: a practical method for grading the cognitive state of patients for the clinician, *J Psychiatr Res* 12:189, 1975.

Hellen CR: *Alzheimer's disease: activity focused care*, Stoneham, Mass, 1992, Butterworth-Heinemann.

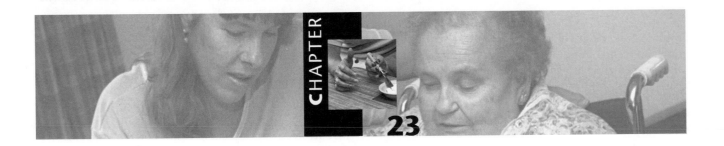

CHAPTER 23

Working With Elders Who Have Psychiatric Conditions

L. MARGARET DRAKE AND PATTY L. BARNETT

KEY TERMS

deinstitutionalization, nursing homes, mood disorders, anxiety disorders, agoraphobia, panic disorder, social phobia, post-traumatic stress disorder, acute stress disorder, schizophrenia, hypochondriasis, drug abuse, dual diagnosis, personality disorders

CHAPTER OBJECTIVES

1. Understand the prevalence of mental illness among elders.
2. Become acquainted with psychiatric diagnoses common among institutionalized elders.
3. Describe the importance of considering both mental health and medical conditions when working with elders.
4. Identify assessments commonly used by occupational therapy practitioners with elders who have mental illness.
5. Describe treatment approaches commonly used with elders who have mental illness.

In most health care settings, elders are treated for all types of medical diagnoses. Often, these diagnoses are accompanied by less obvious psychiatric conditions. For example, an elder who sustained a recent stroke and does not want to attend or participate in occupational therapy treatment may be suffering from depression. An elder with cancer who does not seem to care about her appearance may also have depression. Although mental health problems are strongly associated with disability and poor performance, few people identify mental health problems as the reason for poor functional performance (Stahl, 1996). Many researchers suspect that institution-alized elders often have untreated mental illness (Smith, et al, 1994). If COTAs are not aware of the need to monitor and address mental health conditions, they may miss treating the whole person. Elders who have mental health conditions are often found in nonmental health settings because they need additional assistance after discharge from other health care facilities. **Deinstitu-tionalization,** or the release of elders with mental illness from state hospitals, also contributes to this problem. Elders who have mental illness should be approached in the same way as any other occupational therapy client. Therefore the COTA must recognize and address mental health conditions in elders in all treatment settings, not merely in mental health facilities. This chapter considers primary mental health conditions of elders and suggests strategies for occupational therapy treatment.

CARE OF ELDERS WITH MENTAL ILLNESSES
General Facts

The deinstitutionalization movement of the 1960's and 1970's led to the closing of many state mental hospital wards that previously cared for many elders with mental illness. Before deinstitutionalization, each state received funding to pay for this care. When officials in state governments realized that this financial burden could be shifted to the federal government, they began referring these elders to **nursing homes.** A consequence of this situation is that more elders with mental illness live in nursing homes than mental hospitals (George, 1993). In addition, because of the trend toward shorter stays in acute inpatient mental health care units, many elders with mental illness end up in nursing homes for stabilization of medications. These situations have made nursing homes the major caregivers for elders with mental illness.

Consumer groups such as The National Alliance for the Mentally Ill have introduced legislation to make mental health treatment more accessible and equitable. Provider groups such as psychiatrists, mental health nurses, social workers, and occupational therapists have also lobbied for such legislation. In spite of this situation, many staff members of nursing homes have little or no training in mental health (Torrey, 1990). Failure to recognize depression is a continuing problem in nursing home care (Buckwalter, 1990). Consequently, COTAs educated in psychosocial care can be important advocates for elders and a tremendous help to other staff members at the facility.

Many medical conditions coexist with psychiatric disorders. Because this is such a common occurrence, a whole chapter is devoted to this problem in the fourth edition of the *Diagnostic and Statistical Manual of Mental Disorders* (DSM-IV) (American Psychiatric Association, 1994). This manual of mental illness categorizes and defines all known mental disorders in the United States. By using this manual, clinicians can easily find diagnoses and symptoms of each disease. The manual includes scales to measure the severity of each dysfunction as well as for disturbance of relationships. Mood, psychotic, and anxiety disorders caused by medical conditions are among the diagnostic categories discussed in this manual.

The functional performance of many elders is severely handicapped by mental disabilities (Stahl, 1996). Limitations may occur in any of the performance areas or components relevant to occupational therapy. For example, the memory deficits that occur with depression may affect the ability of elders to follow their medication schedule. The following sections discuss specific mental

health conditions of the elder population and suggested COTA treatment interventions.

DEPRESSION

The term **mood disorder** describes various kinds of depression. Two basic types of mood disorders exist: those that involve a depressed mood only and those that involve fluctuation in mood. Major depression is the most severe form of mood disorder. It involves only a depressed state. A less severe form of this disorder is known as *dysthymic disorder.* The most severe mood fluctuation disorder is bipolar disorder. A less severe form of this disorder is cyclothymic disorder (American Psychiatric Association [APA], 1994).

Researchers report varied statistics on the prevalence of depression among the elder population. Some studies show that approximately 5% of those over 65 have active, current mood disorders (Birren, Sloane, Cohen, 1992). Other studies indicate that 25% of elders experience a form of depression (Johnson, 1995). By 70 years of age, approximately 6% of elders have a mood disorder (Busse, Blazer, 1989). Depression and all other forms of mental illness are reported to be more prevalent among institutionalized elders than those in the community (George, 1993). Moreover, depression usually lasts longer in elders than in younger people. Elder females are more likely than elder males to be depressed. Even though the elder population contains many more females than males, figures on the prevalence of depression are calculated proportionally (Busse, Blazer, 1989). Since 1980 the rate of suicides among elders has increased 9%. An elder commits suicide in the United States approximately once every hour and a half. This amounts to 18 elder suicides a day, about 6500 a year. Nearly 75,000 elder Americans killed themselves between 1980 and 1995. These elders account for one out of every five suicides committed in the United States (Rosenberg, 1996).

Major Depression

The symptoms most often associated with major depression are sadness, tears, feelings of emptiness and worthlessness, changes in eating and sleeping habits, slowed movements, complaints of fatigue, decreased concentration, and suicidal thoughts. For a diagnosis of major depression, these symptoms must last at least 2 weeks. Recognizing depression among elders is often difficult because other symptoms may mask this diagnosis. Often, elders blame dysfunction on physical problems rather than depression. However, certain symptoms are common (Box 23-1). Depressed elders are more likely to neglect their personal hygiene. Because elders are more successful than other people when they attempt suicide (Busse, Blazer, 1989), COTAs should be especially aware of this risk. Major depression can occur as a result of life events, such as the loss of a mate, home, and professional role. Consequently the depression may be called *reactive* because the person is reacting to the event in an exaggerated way. If no apparent event or situation provoked the depression, it may be called *endogenous* (coming from within the person). The symptoms of reactive and endogenous depression are identical.

Mild Depression or Dysthymic Disorder

Although symptoms of major depression are the ones most commonly recognized, those associated with mild depression or dysthymic disorder can interfere with socialization and enjoyment of life. Elders with dysthymia have many symptoms associated with major depression, albeit in a less debilitating form. Symptoms of dysthymia are considered personality characteristics because they have been present for many years (APA, 1994). Depressive symptoms become part of a diagnosis only when they impair function to the extent that the elder is unable to perform necessary tasks (Busse, Blazer 1989). For example, an elder with Parkinson's disease who lacks the motivation to attempt ADL functions in treatment might be diagnosed as clinically depressed.

Bipolar Disorder

Fluctuating mood disorders are less common in elders. The mania occurring in bipolar disorder is much less common in elders than in younger people. Elders are less likely to develop bipolar disorder later in life if they did not experience their first manic episode before the age of 40 (Birren, Sloane, Cohen, 1992). The hyperactivity, impulsiveness, euphoria, and grandiosity usually associated with manic episodes of bipolar disorder in a younger person are more likely to be displayed as confusion, irritability, and increased suspiciousness in elders. Although elders with bipolar disorder may be treated with lithium like younger people, they are at increased risk of experiencing toxic effects (Busse, Blazer, 1989). Consequently, lower dosages are usually required. COTAs must recognize the symptoms of lithium toxicity to identify it early in treatment. These symptoms include nausea, cramping, vomiting, thirst, and polyuria. If symptoms are not identified early enough, elders may develop tremors, experience convulsions, or go into a coma. Very few outcome studies describe the treatment of elders with bipolar disorder (Busse, Blazer, 1989).

Cyclothymia

A less severe fluctuating disorder, cyclothymia, has symptoms that are similar to those of bipolar disorder but milder. For a diagnosis of cyclothymia, the person must have experienced these symptoms for more than 2 years. The onset of cyclothymia usually occurs early in life, and its symptoms are reflected in the person's personality; elders with cyclothymia may be described as moody or unpredictable (American Psychiatric Association, 1994).

BOX 23-1

Symptoms of Depression Among Elders

- Sad facial expression, poor posture, deep sighing, and frequent tears
- Inability to enjoy activities that previously brought pleasure
- Neglect of personal hygiene (for example, unwashed hair, unpleasant body odor, ragged fingernails)
- Weight change—usually associated with loss of appetite
- Increased preoccupation with physical problems
- Sleep difficulties such as frequent wakefulness at night and fatigue during the day
- Slowed movement in ambulation and self-care activities
- Fatigue that prevents initiation and completion of tasks
- Low self-esteem as demonstrated by self-deprecatory statements such as "I'm just not good at that anymore"
- Increased confusion as demonstrated by the tendency to get lost easily and forget dates and scheduled times
- Difficulty concentrating that interferes with ability to read and solve problems
- Indecisiveness as expressed by difficulty making simple choices between two options
- Suicidal thought as expressed by statements such as "I wish I were dead" and "Life is just too difficult. I want to end it all"

Causes of Late-Life Depression

Late-life depression, a term used by some gerontologists, may result from bereavement or a reduced activity level. Additionally, physical and chemical changes such as gradual metabolic slowing of and decreased viability of the endocrine and neurotransmitter systems may contribute to the onset of late-life depression (Busse, Blazer, 1989).

Complaints about changes in sleep patterns increase with aging. The amount of time spent sleeping decreases naturally in elders. Some theorists attribute this change to the decreased production of melatonin in the aging brain. Rapid eye movement (REM) sleep, which is associated with dreaming and completion of the sleep cycle, decreases in elders (Busse, Blazer, 1989). COTAs should recommend traditional methods known to enhance sleep such as warm baths, darkness, relaxing music before sleep, and even guided imagery. However, the short attention span of many depressed clients may make some of these activities difficult.

A medical illness can itself cause reactive depression in elders. Once the cycle of depression starts, it tends to

BOX 23-2

Medications That Contribute to Depression

Analgesics
Antianxiety drugs
Sedatives and hypnotics
Antihypertensive agents
Antipsychotics
Cancer chemotherapy agents
Cortisone

BOX 23-3

Phases of Remotivation Groups

1. Greeting phase
2. Introduction to the discussion topic (by using various objects or media)
3. Open-ended questions for discussion, such as "What is your earliest memory of . . . ?"
4. Discussion of the memories and ideas presented by the participants
5. The COTA expresses appreciation for the contributions of the group members

spiral downward. A reactive depression provoked by life events or losses may exacerbate other diseases. COTAs may be the first to recognize this secondary depression and recommend referral for psychiatric evaluation. Some medications also contribute to depression. When reviewing the medication section of the medical record, COTAs should pay particular attention to medications associated with depression (Box 23-2). If elders are taking any of these medications, the COTA should discuss this matter with the physician.

Treatment Intervention for Elders With Depression

In the assessment of elders with depression, both physical and social functioning are important considerations. Knowledge of traditional psychiatric symptoms is also important. If elders have poor social support before the diagnosis of depression, they will have this problem after discharge (Busse, Blazer, 1989).

COTAs play an important role in differentiating depression from dementia. The term *pseudodementia* is sometimes used to describe a person who exhibits cognitive symptoms associated with dementia but actually caused by depression. A clue that may help COTAs differentiate between true organic dementia and depres-

sion is that elders with depression complain of cognitive problems (such as diminished memory, problem-solving difficulties, and the ability to concentrate) whereas elders with organic dementia usually deny that they have such problems. In addition, elders with depression appear sad, whereas elders with dementia usually appear indifferent or apathetic. When asked a question, elders with depression often say, "I don't know," whereas elders with dementia may attempt to cover their cognitive deficits by manufacturing a story in response (Kaplan, Saddock, 1983).

Mental stimulation is an important part of treatment for depression. Remotivation therapy has been used successfully for a number of years to get depressed people involved again in daily activities (Lyon, 1971; Ireland, 1972). This kind of therapy is usually done in a group. The therapist uses objects, pictures, pets, and holiday symbols to stimulate discussion and memories (Box 23-3).

Some general considerations for group work include avoiding rushing, which may increase stress and lower functional performance outcomes; allowing time for elders to focus on details; reducing irrelevant noise; and speaking loudly and clearly with regular pauses for those who process information slowly. Activities such as moving to music increase oxygen in elders' blood and consequently raise their mood. Music, particularly blues, can be used to assist clients in expressing their feelings of depression (Pedersen, 1986).

Each elder who has depression reacts to the illness differently, and COTAs must interact with clients as individuals. In working with elders who have depression, COTAs obtain better results by speaking slowly and using the elder's name frequently. COTAs should be warm but not oversolicitous. In some cases, telling elders what to do may be more helpful than asking them to choose; people with depression often have difficulty making decisions. However, COTAs should permit elders to guide the intervention when they are ready to make choices. Interpersonal contacts with these clients should be frequent but short. COTAs should praise the elders' projects rather than the elders themselves, who are apt to reject personal praise. Some precautions include watching for signs of fatigue and supervision in the use of sharp tools to prevent accidents and suicide attempts. The number of therapists working with each elder should be limited. In addition, elders should be advised well in advance when a change is necessary.

Recommended activities include short-term projects that provide repetitive, structured, and well-defined routines, with few possibilities for frustration. Competitive activities and those that require high levels of concentration are best avoided until some improvement is apparent.

COTAs should be aware of community resources such as support groups, which give a voice to the elder population. The role of COTAs may involve helping elders find addresses and telephone numbers of such organizations. Support groups have been identified as strong factors in the recovery of some patients (National Alliance for the Mentally Ill, 1995). Elder females may be referred to organizations such as the Older Women's League (OWL).

ANXIETY DISORDERS

Anxiety disorders are no more prevalent in elders than in younger people. However, elders tend to experience specific types of anxiety, including the fear of being a victim of crime or elder abuse. The fear of going out after dark is one of the main phobias experienced by elders. Nursing home residents who frequently witness the deaths of other residents may develop anxiety related to the fear of death. Other common anxieties involve the fear of cognitive problems, such as memory loss, and fear of injury or sickness. These anxiety disorders manifest themselves in elders with the same symptoms as in younger people (Box 23-4). Anxiety disorders include agoraphobia, panic attacks, social phobia, and post-traumatic stress disorder (Birren, Sloane, Cohen, 1992).

Agoraphobia is a fear of specific situations from which the person cannot escape (Figure 23-1). These fears may make elders afraid to leave their houses. Other common agoraphobic fears include being in crowds of people, crossing a bridge, and using various modes of travel, such as flying or being on a boat. An elder might be unwilling to go to the laundromat for fear of not being able to put the correct coins in the washing machine and being embarrassed.

Panic disorder is characterized by recurrent panic attacks. These attacks include symptoms such as heart palpitations, shaking, excessive sweating, shortness of breath, chest pains, nausea or other digestive distress, light-headedness, feelings of unreality, fear of mental imbalance or death, and bodily sensations for which no cause is apparent. COTAs who work with these elders should involve them in activities and occupations. This involvement frequently alleviates feelings of panic. COTAs should also reassure elders that they are not dying or "going crazy."

People with **social phobia** fear that they will not be able to act appropriately in public. These people are often afraid that they will embarrass themselves by doing something socially unacceptable. A common manifestation of social phobia is the fear of being unable to talk to other people. The fear of offending others while dining in public is also common (American Psychiatric Association, 1994). For example, elders may avoid going to restaurants or become anxious when served food for fear that they will drop some on the tablecloth or their clothes. COTAs should grade involvement in anxiety-producing tasks.

BOX 23-4

Symptoms of Anxiety Among Elders

- Excessive worry about loved ones, personal health, and impending catastrophes
- Restlessness demonstrated by inability to stay seated or attentive
- Difficulty with concentration and tendency to be distracted by everything in environment
- Muscle tension that may cause pain, especially in the neck, and headache
- Irritability with those nearby (especially the health care workers) that may be expressed as a refusal to participate in treatment sessions
- Sleep disturbance that leaves elders so fatigued the following day that they decline to participate in therapy sessions
- Panic attack that may be expressed as acute fear of dying

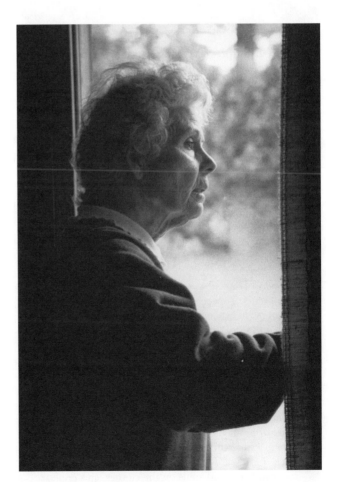

FIGURE 23-1 Elders may fear leaving home and restrict their social interactions because of mental conditions.

Post-traumatic stress disorder and **acute stress disorder** result from exposure to an event that is outside the realm of usual human experience. Examples of these types of events include a natural disaster such as a hurricane or an accident in which loved ones are hurt or exposed to danger. In the acute form of the stress disorder the symptoms occur within a month after the event. In post-traumatic stress disorder, months or years may elapse before symptoms appear. The three main symp-

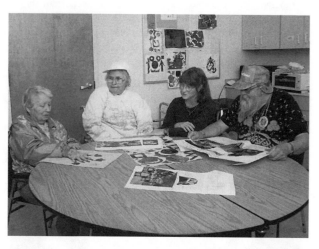

FIGURE 23-2 Expressive therapies such as drawing or making a collage can help elders deal with their feelings.

toms of these disorders are reliving the traumatic event, avoiding reminders of the event, and experiencing symptoms of anxiety similar to those of panic disorder. Encouraging elders to talk about the event, describe the experience, and express their feelings are typical strategies of COTAs. Some ways to facilitate the process include expressive arts activities, structured group interaction sessions, and video presentations that deal with similar events. After viewing such videos, COTAs can facilitate a group discussion.

Treatment Interventions for Elders With Anxiety Disorders

Some suggested interventions for elders with anxiety disorders have already been discussed. Successful occupations and activities have some additional characteristics. Although avoidance of situations causing anxiety may appear helpful, treatment of these disorders often involves exposing elders to controlled simulations of the original event and helping them gradually overcome the desire for avoidance. For COTAs, this help may involve asking elders to use expressive therapies such as movement, drawing, and making a collage to describe anxiety (Figure 23-2). Expression of these feelings may provide some relief. Some clients are soothed by repetitive motions such as those in needlework. Acceptance, reassurance, encouragement, and praise are appropriate for these elders. After elders have expressed their anxiety, COTAs can assist them in gradually confronting the anxiety-producing situation.

SCHIZOPHRENIA

The major form of psychosis in the Western world is **schizophrenia.** The first symptoms of this disabling disease usually appear before age 30 (Box 23-5). Approximately 10% of elders 60 years of age or older who are admitted to psychiatric units for psychosis developed it late in life (Birren, Sloane, Cohen, 1992). Discoveries in the dopamine receptor system have made many forms of schizophrenia treatable. Some unexplained links exist between schizophrenia and Parkinson's disease. Often, some improvement occurs with age in schizophrenic symptoms, but those of Parkinson's disease may increase (Birren, Sloane, Cohen, 1992).

People who have late onset of schizophrenia are more likely to have positive symptoms of the disease such as delusions, hallucinations, suspiciousness, and disorganized language and behavior. They are less likely to have the negative symptoms of schizophrenia such as restricted emotions, decreased speech and interaction, and limited behavior of all types. Conversely, people whose onset was at a younger age are more likely to have negative symptoms. Some people with schizophrenia who show symptoms of the disease in old age may have been considered "odd" throughout their life. Some studies

BOX 23-5

Symptoms of Schizophrenia among Elders

- Delusions—false beliefs that have no basis in reality,
- Hallucinations—most commonly auditory (in which voices direct persons to do things they would not normally consider doing, such as harming themselves or others) or tactile (in which elders might feel as if something were crawling on their skin); hallucinations involving all the senses also are possible
- Disorganized speech in which the speaker has no logical sequence or coherent theme to statements
- Lack of meaningful speech in which the elder speaks without providing information
- Disorganized behavior such as appearing to start an action but suddenly dropping it and changing to another with no apparent sense of purpose
- Lack of emotion—sometimes called *flattened affect* (voice is monotonous, and face shows no feelings)
- Lack of motivation—often demonstrated by apathetic responses to requests to participate
- Lack of self-care—often demonstrated by unruly, uncombed hair; food spills on the clothes; and unpleasant body odor

show that the majority of elders with schizophrenia have been single throughout their lives (Birren, Sloane, Cohen, 1992). This means that these elders probably have little family support.

Many people with early onset of schizophrenia commit suicide (Birren, Sloane, Cohen, 1992). However, many others live to old age and can be found in the nursing home population as well as in the geriatric wards of mental hospitals. These elders are especially vulnerable to the side effects of neuroleptic drugs. A common side effect is tardive dyskinesia, a movement disorder that includes involuntary blinking, tongue thrust, foot tapping, jerking, and twisting. Elders may also develop the "Pisa syndrome," in which they lean to one side. Elders with schizophrenia are more likely to experience faintness from neuroleptic medication than younger people (Birren, Sloane, Cohen, 1992). Because COTAs work with elders soon after these symptoms appear, they must share this important information with the team. Because COTAs see elders performing daily activities, they are able to notice any abnormal movement. Other healthcare workers may not see elders during routine activities and therefore may not recognize abnormalities. The sooner COTAs report abnormal movements resulting from neuroleptic drugs, the sooner the drug can be adjusted to prevent a potentially permanent impairment.

Treatment Interventions For Elders With Schizophrenia

COTAs can assist elders who have schizophrenia by addressing the functional areas of their lives. COTAs can make sure that elders can perform ADL functions as independently as possible. COTAs can also involve these elders in concrete projects such as simple crafts, cooking, or gardening. Projects should be structured, with clear guidelines for accomplishing the task. The project should be successfully finished in a short time. Because schizophrenia is primarily associated with sensory distortions, COTAs may first need to verify elders' feelings and perceptions. It is particularly important not to argue with elders about the reality of their hallucinatory or delusional perceptions. Unless these elders want to discuss their feelings about their symptoms or the way their illness interferes with occupational performance, COTAs should redirect them to a concrete activity that may help orient them to reality.

HYPOCHONDRIASIS

Hypochondriasis is a disorder characterized by the individual's preoccupation with personal health. The person is overly concerned about disease and usually does not realize that this concern is unreasonable. Concerns are considered unreasonable after the physician has ruled out physical illness and finds no evidence of disease. The person with hypochondriasis, however, continues to

believe that the illness is real (American Psychiatric Association, 1994). Many complaints focus on specific organ systems, particularly the digestive tract. Hypochondriasis is common in elders. Approximately half of the elders diagnosed with depression also have hypochondriasis (Birren, Sloane, Cohen, 1992). Individuals with hypochondriasis use their bodies as a way to communicate messages they are unable to express otherwise. For example, instead of directly asking someone for attention, elders with hypochondriasis may complain at length about their aches and pains. Naturally, this behavior often results in alienating elders with hypochondriasis, increasing their social isolation and their need for attention.

Healthcare workers sometimes discount reports of bodily illness among elders. However, aging often does produce physical pain as arthritis and other degenerative diseases take their toll. COTAs must know elders well enough to distinguish among physical complaints, those caused by degenerative disease, and those resulting from a mental disorder. Complaints must be believed until proved false (that is, the physician has exhausted medical tests to rule out disease).

If COTAs determine that a complaint is an attention-seeking behavior, the best response is to direct attention to positive qualities in the elder. Behavioral studies demonstrate that positive attention such as rewards changes and maintains behavior more efficiently than negative attention such as punishment and criticism (Early, 1993). Although 95% of clients blame their illnesses on physical problems, physicians find that these physical problems are often symptomatic of psychosocial problems (Stahl, 1996). For this reason, COTAs should encourage interaction and participation in group activities.

SUBSTANCE ABUSE

Historic events such as Prohibition (when alcohol was forbidden) and World War II (when many young adult women had the opportunity to smoke and drink) have affected the attitudes of elders toward these substances. The increased use of sedatives in the 1960s may also play a part in their attitudes toward drug use (Birren, Sloane, Cohen, 1992). Alcohol abuse is common among elders, and many are hospitalized for alcohol-related dysfunction after coming to the hospital for other reasons (Adams et al, 1993). For example, an elder may be admitted for a fracture that resulted from falling while intoxicated.

Any mind-altering drug may affect elders more intensely than predicted because their mechanisms of neutralizing and eliminating the drug are diminished. Therefore elders are often more sensitive to drug treatment. This sensitivity is compounded by the fact that most elders take more than one kind of medication. These medications often create unintended interactions. (Refer to Chapter 15 for a more thorough discussion of this topic.) **Drug abuse** is often part of a **dual diagnosis** in which the elder is both depressed and addicted to alcohol or drugs.

The contribution of COTAs in cases of substance abuse is to notify the physician of the problem and join the team in confronting the elder about the problem. Although elders with substance abuse problems require individual assessment to determine specific performance deficits, most need guidance in time management. COTAs can provide elders with schedule sheets and assist them in planning better use of leisure time. Many elders substitute alcohol for other entertainment when they are housebound. Drinking may also be a mechanism for coping with bereavement and loneliness. COTAs should develop plans to help elders find ways to socialize. Most communities have special transportation services available to senior citizens. Many local agencies provide programs and information on aging. Awareness of substance abuse problems is crucial if COTAs are providing home health services.

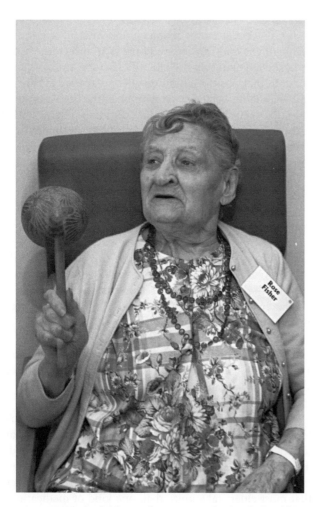

FIGURE 23-3 Activities such as group singing help elders take initiative in participation.

PERSONALITY DISORDERS

That elders do not have new **personality disorders** is a common assumption. However, some research shows the contrary (Agronin, 1994). The elder may have suppressed the behavior earlier in life, or the personality disorder may indeed be new. Elders are more likely to cover up personality traits that are undesirable. Some elders who are diagnosed as paranoid, schizoid, or schizotypal may have been considered strange even during youth. Sensory losses and changes may exacerbate elders' paranoia because the interpretation of stimuli becomes more difficult. Characteristics such as suspiciousness and inflexibility tend to remain stable throughout life.

The most common personality disorders found in elders are the dependent, avoidant, and compulsive types. People who have a primary diagnosis of depression are most likely to have a personality disorder as well (Agronin, 1994). Antisocial personality disorders are less common in later years. Elders are usually less impulsive and less likely to commit violent crimes. They are more likely to exhibit behavior such as exposing their genitals and being drunk in public (Agronin, 1994).

Because of their long- or short-term behaviors, elders with personality disorders often lack social support systems. The COTA/OTR team should therefore include building social support as part of the treatment plan (Agronin, 1994). This could mean encouraging the elder to contact old friends or attend a class or social group in the facility, adult day program, church, or other community organization. Most local newspapers publish lists of support groups and their meeting times and places.

People who are overly dependent need approval, reassurance, and support. They should be provided with opportunities to make their own decisions and gradually establish their independence in a context where the opportunities for failure are minimal. Some elders may never overcome their dependency. In such cases, COTAs can create situations in which reasonable dependence is part of an activity, such as the COTA reading the instructions while the elder assembles a project. Activities such as group singing allow elders to participate while depending on others to set the volume and rhythm of the music (Figure 23-3).

Unpredictable situations are best avoided with elders who show obsessive compulsive tendencies. Such situations sometimes provoke obsessive thoughts and compulsive behaviors in affected elders. The objective with these elders is to involve them in constructive activities that replace compulsive rituals. They should be given encouragement, praise, and approval for effort.

EVALUATION STRATEGIES

COTAs participate in the evaluation process once service competency has been established. Among the assessments commonly administered by COTAs in nursing homes and mental health settings is the Allen Cognitive Levels (ACL) test (Allen, Earhart, Blue, 1992). (Refer to Chapter 7 for details on this test and cognitive levels.) The Routine Task Inventory (RTI) is an assessment of ADL functions that COTAs may administer (Early, 1993). COTAs help clients reassess their interests and values through a variety of interview and checklist techniques. The NPI Interest Checklist (Matsutsuyu, 1969) is commonly used in assessment. Behavioral checklists are another way COTAs provide valuable assessment information. The Comprehensive Occupational Therapy Evaluation (COTE) Scale (Hemphill, 1982) is one such checklist in which 25 behaviors are scored according to a scale—0 for normal to 4 for severely impaired. This numerical score allows COTAs to identify improvement and deterioration (Early, 1993). (The reader is referred to Chapter 7 for details on other assessment tools appropriate for the aged.)

CASE STUDY

Mrs. G. is a 75-year-old woman diagnosed with depression. After being stabilized on an antidepressant at an acute care hospital, she was placed in a group home that specialized in the care of elders with mental illness. The residents are taken daily to a day treatment program, where a COTA provides the major part of the service. An OTR visits the center twice a week.

Mrs. G. is a widow and has three married daughters and eight grandchildren. Mrs. G. has sewn clothes for her daughters and grandchildren throughout her career as a parent and grandparent. She has also been a member of the same quilting club since the birth of her first child. A homemaker until age 45, she experienced the "empty-nest syndrome" after all her daughters left for college or got married. She had been depressed then, but not severely enough to require hospitalization. Her husband, a farmer, encouraged her to visit her sister, who lived in a large city. The change of scenery seemed to help her overcome the loss she felt. She returned from her visit to her home and enrolled in a technical program for office workers. From age 45 to 65 she worked as a secretary at the local high school. At 65, she retired but continued to work as a substitute. Her husband lost the farm as a result of bank foreclosure and eventually accepted a position on a corporate farm. When Mrs. G. was 68, her husband died of a sudden heart attack. She began to show symptoms of depression within a year. She began to reduce her activities, turning down jobs to fill in at the school, refusing to go out with her friends, declining to baby-sit her grandchildren, and quitting her quilting group. Her daughters did not become worried until they realized she was hoarding medication and planning suicide. They persuaded her to admit herself to the psychiatric unit of the regional hospital.

Although her medication was working at the time of her discharge from the acute care inpatient psychiatric unit, she had residual dysfunction in several self-care, socialization, and cognitive areas. Because all the daughters lived more than 3 hours away, they agreed that Mrs. G. would stay in a group home until the family felt she could adequately take care of herself again. Fortunately, they were able to place her in a local group home with 24-hour supervision.

The schedule of the group home includes chair aerobics, weekend outings to the mall, a reminiscence group, and a crafts group that makes stuffed toys for children with developmental disabilities. Mrs. G. also participates in a day treatment program 3 days a week. The family hopes that when Mrs. G. recovers sufficiently, she can resume her life in one of the assisted living units in a nearby housing development operated by her religious denomination.

Soon after Mrs. G.'s arrival in the day treatment program, the COTA asked Mrs. G. to identify activities that she missed doing. Mrs. G. began crying as she discussed her grandchildren and her quilting group. After consulting with the OTR, the COTA left a copy of the NPI Interest Checklist (Matsutsuyu, 1969) for Mrs. G. to fill out on her own. She returned a day later and gave the Allen Cognitive Levels (ACL) test. Mrs. G . scored at cognitive level 4 on the ACL, which means that although she recognized an error, she could not correct it. The COTA administered the Routine Task Inventory-2 (RTI-2) 2 days later. Mrs. G. also scored at Cognitive Level 4 on this test of ADL functions. This score means she initiated grooming tasks and completed most of them; however, she neglected the back of her hair and neglected to clean up the bathroom after she bathed herself.

Mrs. G. is able to find the mailbox in the group home when she wants to mail letters to her daughters. However, she gets lost easily when she attempts to walk unsupervised in the neighborhood. She is independent in toileting but gets anxious when she has to use any restroom other than the one in her room or the OT clinic. She usually remembers to ask the nurse for her medications. She is able to fix a sandwich in the kitchenette at the day treatment program, but she often burns the soup. The last time this happened she stated, "I can't do anything right anymore. I am just a burden to my daughters. They would be better off not having to worry about me." Although she can dress herself in the morning, she does not pay attention to whether her clothing matches or is appropriate for the weather.

After discussion with the OTR, the COTA explained her findings to Mrs. G. and one of her daughters. The OTR, COTA, daughter, and Mrs. G. then planned for Mrs. G. to participate in a daily ADL group session with the COTA to work on self-care and homemaking occupations. The plan includes the use of self-cueing devices such as timers, environmental aids such as a neighborhood map, and a medication check-off sheet. These adaptations will be useful after discharge as well. Mrs. G. will also participate in the remotivation group.

▮ CHAPTER REVIEW QUESTIONS

1 Considering the case study above, which of Mrs. G's behaviors might cause the therapist to think she was suffering from depression rather than dementia?
2 What other activities in the group home schedule might the COTA want to encourage Mrs. G. to attend?
3 What community resources could be used in guiding Mrs. G.'s recovery?

4 Identify three or more common causes of late-life depression.

5 Describe types of activities recommended for elders experiencing auditory hallucinations.

6 How should you structure occupational therapy intervention for an elder who refuses to leave home because he believes he will fall whenever he walks on cement?

REFERENCES

Adams WL et al: Alcohol-related hospitalizations of elderly people, *JAMA* 270(10): 1222, 1993.

Agronin ME: Personality disorders in the elderly: an overview, *J Geriatr Psychiatry* 27(2):151, 1994.

Allen CK, Earhart CA, Blue T: *Occupational therapy treatment goals for the physically and cognitively disabled*, Rockville, Md, 1992, American Occupational Therapy Association.

American Association of Retired Persons: *A profile of older Americans*, Washington, DC, 1994, The Association (brochure).

American Psychiatric Association: *Diagnostic and statistical manual of mental disorders*, ed 4, Washington, DC, 1994, The Association.

Birren JE, Sloane RB, Cohen GD, editors: *Handbook of mental health and aging*, San Diego, 1992, Academic Press.

Buckwalter KC: How to unmask depression, *Geriatr Nurs* 11(4):179, 1990.

Busse EW, Blazer DG: *Geriatric psychiatry*, Washington, DC, 1989, American Psychiatric Press.

Early MB: *Mental health concepts and techniques for the occupational therapy assistant*, ed 2, New York, 1993, Raven Press.

George LK: Depressive disorders and symptoms in later life, *Generations* 17(1):35, 1993.

Hemphill B: The evaluative process. In *Psychiatric occupational therapy*, Thorofare, NJ, 1982, SLACK.

Hopkins HL, Smith HD: *Willard and Spackman's occupational therapy*, ed 8, Philadelphia, 1993, JB Lippincott.

Ireland M: Starting reality orientation and remotivation, *Nurs Homes* 21(4):10, 1972.

Johnson C: *Depression workshop*, Northern Louisiana University Institute of Gerontology, (Unpublished monograph) 1995.

Kaplan HI, Saddock BJ: *Kaplan and Saddocks' synopsis of psychiatry*, ed 7, Baltimore, 1994, Williams & Wilkins.

Lyon GG: Stimulation through remotivation, *Am J Nurs* 71(5):982, 1971.

Matsutsuyu JS: The interest checklist, *Am J Occup Ther* 24(4):323, 1969.

Morency CR: Mental status change in the elderly: recognizing and treating delirium, *J Prof Nurs* 6(6):356, 1990.

National Alliance for the Mentally Ill: *NAMI families just like yours, families like yours, learning to live with severe mental illness*, Arlington, Va, Aug 1995, The Alliance.

Pedersen ID: Treatment of depression in institutionalized older persons, *Phys Occup Ther Geriatr* 5(1):77, 1986.

Rosenberg M: Elder suicide: report to the senate select committee on aging, Atlanta, 1996, National Centers for Disease Control and Prevention.

Silverman P: *The elderly as modern pioneers*, Bloomington, Ind, 1987, Indiana University Press.

Smith M et al: Evaluation of a geriatric mental health training program for nursing personnel in rural long-term care facilities, *Issues Mental Health Nurs* 15(2):149, 1994.

Stahl C: Psychosomatic illness and function, *Adv Occup Ther* 12 (4): 14, 1996.

Stancliff BL: Study shows growing older not depressing, *OT Pract* 1(3):10, 1996.

Torrey EF: Economic barriers to widespread implementation of model programs for the seriously mentally ill, *Hosp Commun Psychiatry*, 41 (5):526, 1990.

Williams AK, Schulz R: Association of pain and physical dependency with depression in physically ill middle-aged and elderly persons, *Phys Ther* 68(8): 1226, 1988.

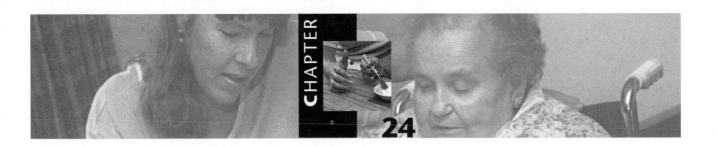

Working With Elders Who Have Orthopedic Conditions

BRENDA M. COPPARD, TYROME HIGGINS, AND KAROLINE D. HARVEY

KEY TERMS

orthopedic, fracture, osteoarthritis, compound fracture, transverse fracture, spiral fracture, comminuted fracture, closed reduction, open reduction, internal fixation, external fixation, delayed union, nonunion, malunion, hemovac, total hip replacement (THR), arthroplasty, antiembolus hosiery, rheumatoid arthritis, wrist subluxation, ulnar drift, swan neck deformity, boutonnière deformity, Nalebuff type I deformity, joint protection, work simplification, energy conservation

CHAPTER OBJECTIVES

1. Identify the causes of fractures in the elder population.
2. Identify terminology related to fractures and their management.
3. Describe the precautions required after a hip pinning and implications of such a procedure relative to occupational performance.
4. Describe the precautions required after a total hip replacement and the implications of such a procedure relative to occupational performance.
5. Identify adaptive equipment and modified methods of performance that benefit elders with hip fractures.
6. Identify the signs and symptoms of osteoarthritis and rheumatoid arthritis.
7. Describe the effects of osteoarthritis and rheumatoid arthritis on occupational performance.
8. Explain the principles of joint protection, work simplification, and energy conservation.

Orthopedic problems are prevalent among elders. The incidence of hip **fractures**, for example, account for 90% of all fractures in persons over the age of 70 years (Cummings, 1987). Orthopedic problems may result in elders being hospitalized for a surgical procedure and

rehabilitation and possibly being placed temporarily or permanently in a long-term care facility.

The role of the COTA and OTR team is to help maximize the occupational performance of elders who have orthopedic problems. Elders who would otherwise need to enter an extended care facility are often able to go home as a result of OT treatment. COTAs must be familiar with orthopedic conditions and their effects on occupational performance to ensure that appropriate evaluation and treatment are carried out. This chapter will address orthopedic problems and conditions that contribute to these problems.

CAUSES OF FRACTURES

Causes of fractures include falls, trauma from automobile accidents, **osteoarthritis,** and metastatic carcinoma. Other factors such as smoking, alcohol abuse, and decreased level of physical activity also correlate with the incidence of fractures (Jette, Harris, Cleary, 1987).

The majority of fractures in elders result from falls (Mehta, Nastasi, 1993). Factors associated with falling include poor vision, orthostatic hypotension, poor balance, diminished mobility, side effects of medication, muscle weakness, neurological diseases, reduced alertness, dementia, and environmental obstacles (Mehta, Nastasi, 1993; Tinetti, Williams, Mayewski, 1986). (an in-depth examination of the causes of falls in elders is provided in Chapter 16.)

Ninety-two percent of persons older than 65 years of age are licensed drivers. Statistics show that although elders drive less frequently than younger persons, they account for 48% of auto accidents. Trauma resulting from auto accidents accounts for a portion of the fractures seen in the elder population (U.S. Department of Transportation, 1994).

Elders are more likely to sustain fractures after a fall because of osteoporosis, osteomalacia, and diminished ability to repair microfractures (Mehta, Nastasi, 1993; Melton, Riggs, 1985). Stress fractures can also occur in elders who suddenly increase their levels of activity by jogging, walking farther than usual, or walking on a different terrain, for example (Mehta, Nastasi, 1993; Heckman, 1991).

Fractures may also be caused by cancer that has metastasized to bone. Although any cancer may metastasize to bone, metastases from carcinomas, particularly those that arise in the breast, lung, prostate, kidney, and thyroid, are most common. Metastatic lesions weaken the strength of bones and may lead to fractures (Berkow, Fletcher, 1987).

TYPES OF FRACTURES

A fracture is a break in a bone. A fracture is considered to be **"compound"** or **"open"** if bone protrudes through the soft tissue and skin. If the soft tissue and skin are undamaged, the fracture is considered to be "closed" or "simple." Different physical forces can result in certain types of fractures. A **transverse fracture** occurs as a result of a direct force, whereas a **spiral fracture**

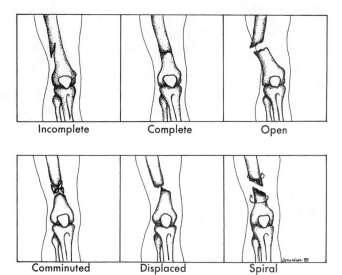

FIGURE 24-1 Types of fractures. (Modified from Garland JJ: *Fundamentals of orthopaedics,* Philadelphia, 1979, WB Saunders.)

results from a circular or twisting force. A fracture that results in more than two bone fragments is a **comminuted fracture.** Figure 24-1 shows these various types of fractures.

MEDICAL INTERVENTION FOR FRACTURES

The goals of medical management of a fracture are to reduce pain and align the fracture for proper healing. The fracture can be aligned with or without surgery. The process of manually realigning and then casting a fracture is termed **closed reduction.** The **open reduction** is a surgical procedure that is used to internally fixate the fracture site. **Internal fixation** is performed with use of orthopedic nails, screws, pins, rods, or plates. When **external fixation** is used to align a fracture, a fixator device is applied externally to maintain reduction (Figure 24-2). This device usually involves the use of screws and rods that are removed after the fracture has healed.

COTAs should also be familiar with terminology relating to the healing of fractures. Three terms used to describe fractures that do not heal well are **delayed union, nonunion,** and **malunion** (Daniel, Strickland, 1992). *Delayed union* describes a fracture that heals at an abnormally slow rate. *Nonunion* describes a fracture in which healing stops just short of a firm union. *Malunion* describes a fracture in which the bone heals in an unsatisfactory alignment.

FACTORS INFLUENCING REHABILITATION

Several factors affect the outcome of rehabilitation efforts in elders who sustain fractures. Age is a predominant factor in rehabilitation. Elders may need more time

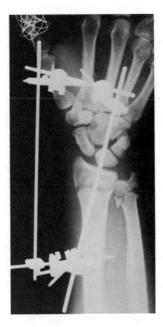

FIGURE **24-2**   External fixator in place to maintain reduction. (From Hunter J, Mackin E, Callahan A, editors: *Rehabilitation of the hand: surgery and therapy*, ed 4, St. Louis, 1995, Mosby.)

than younger persons to achieve their highest levels of independence. For example, in elders, a comminuted fracture of the proximal humerus should be immobilized for the shortest period of time possible to reduce the chances of development of adhesive capsulitis or frozen shoulder. With a younger person the threat of such a complication may not always be a concern.

The general condition of the elder also affects the course of rehabilitation. For example, elders who are in shock or are unconscious require different treatment than those who are alert and oriented. In addition, past and present medical conditions may affect the rehabilitation of elders who have fractures. For example, elders with congestive heart failure or chronic obstructive lung disease may be limited in their abilities to participate in endurance and strengthening activities. Furthermore, a large percentage of elders with fractures also have associated medical problems such as hypertension, diabetes, and stroke (American Association of Retired persons [AARP], 1995).

The presence of dementia often affects rehabilitation outcomes for elders with fractures. For example, teaching the integration of hip precautions or joint protection methods while engaging in self-care tasks to an elder with short-term memory deficits is difficult. (A detailed discussion of intervention considerations for elders who have dementia is presented in Chapter 22.)

Although hip fractures are the most common type of fracture sustained by elders, fractures of other bones also

occur. COTAs should know the common fractures and general recommended treatment techniques (Table 24-1).

HIP FRACTURES

An estimated 30% of elders fracture a hip by 90 years of age (Birge, Morrow-Howell, Proctor, 1994). Hip fractures occur more commonly in women than in men (Cooper, Barker, Morris, 1987). Fractures of the hip are classified by the type and direction of the fracture line (Morawski et al, 1996).

Hip fractures usually require an open reduction internal fixation, or pinning procedure. The open reduction internal fixation of the involved hip usually must be protected from excessive force through weight-bearing restrictions. The open reduction internal fixation site is sutured shut, and a **hemovac** may be used for about 2 days (Morawski et al, 1996). A hemovac, which is connected to a suction machine, is a device that draws and collects drainage from the site. The hemovac unit should *not* be disconnected for any activity and is usually removed by a registered nurse or a physician.

The amount of time required for a hip fracture to heal depends on the elder, fracture site, fracture type, and severity of injury. Out-of-bed therapy activities for persons with hip pinnings are usually initiated 2 to 4 days after surgery (Morawski et al, 1996). Most function returns within 6 weeks to 6 months after the fracture occurs; most persons experience little improvement in function from 6 months to 1 year after sustaining a fracture (Birge, Morrow-Howell, Proctor, 1994; Magaziner et al, 1990).

Weight-bearing Restrictions for Hip Pinnings

Depending on the type and severity of the fracture, the physician may restrict the amount of weight bearing allowed on the involved hip while the person is walking. Most weight-bearing restrictions are observed for 6 to 8 weeks, during which time the person may use crutches or a walker to ambulate (Morawski et al, 1996). COTAs must be aware of any weight-bearing precautions before initiating therapy and should know the terminology related to weight-bearing restrictions (Table 24-2).

TOTAL HIP REPLACEMENTS

Total hip replacements (THRs) are often indicated to reduce pain and restore motion for elders who have severe osteoarthritis, rheumatoid arthritis, or ankylosing spondylosis. A hip replacement, or **arthroplasty,** may be full or partial. During a full hip arthroplasty, the hip's ball and socket are replaced with metal or metal and plastic prosthetic implants (Bear-Lehman, 1995). During a partial joint replacement, which is commonly used for fractures of the femoral neck and head, the femoral neck and head are replaced with a prosthesis (Bear-Lehman,

TABLE 24-1

General Recommended Treatment Techniques for Fractures*

Fracture location	Precautions and/or contraindications	Acute injury treatment techniques	Treatment techniques after repair
Humeral	Keep elbow, wrist, finger joints mobile or per physician's order; monitor for signs of edema; position upper extremity above heart if edema occurs and not contraindicated for cardiac condition; PROM is contraindicated; discontinue immobilizer or brace with physician's order	Use shoulder immobilizer or plaster cast to immobilize; after 5 to 7 days, a humeral cuff brace can be used	Begin AROM when acute pain is subsided to prevent stiffness; PROM is contraindicated; encourage isometric exercises during and after immobilization; Codman's exercises should only be encouraged in the absence of edema
Elbow	Keep shoulder, wrist, and finger joints mobile or per physician's order; monitor for signs of edema; position upper extremity above level of heart if edema occurs and not contraindicated for cardiac condition; PROM is contraindicated; discontinue immobilizer(s) with physician's order	A plaster cast or elbow conformer can be used to immobilize the elbow in 90 to 100 degrees of flexion; a sling can also be used	Begin gentle, nonresistive AROM after removal of cast; perform AROM in a gravity eliminated plane; PROM in the early stage is not advised; person may have difficulty regaining full elbow extension, but a functional arc should be regained for ADL
Wrist (scaphoid)	Keep shoulder, elbow, and finger joints mobile or per physician's order; if an external fixator is in place, monitor sites for infection; clean pin sites with hydrogen peroxide; discontinue any splints with physician's order	A plaster cast may be worn for 2 weeks to 2 months depending on the physician; a thumb spica splint can be used after the cast is removed to position the wrist in slight flexion and radial deviation	When stabilized and cast removed, AROM should begin to all wrist motions
Colles' (distal radius)	Keep shoulder, elbow, and finger joints mobile or per physician's order; if an external fixator is in place, monitor sites for infection; clean pin sites with hydrogen peroxide; discontinue immobilizer(s) with physician's order	A volar wrist splint is used for positioning after a plaster cast or internal/external fixation is removed	Begin ROM of wrist and forearm once a bony union has occurred and cast has been removed

*Physicians may vary these protocols.
ROM, range of motion; PROM, passive range of motion; AROM, active range of motion.
Adapted from Daniel MS, Strickland LR: *Occupational therapy protocol management in adult physical dysfunction*, Gaithersburg, Md, 1992, Aspen.

1995). Hip prostheses last approximately 10 years or longer in 90% of elders (Lewis, 1989).

The two basic surgical approaches for THRs are the anterolateral approach and the posterolateral approach (Daniel, Strickland, 1992). COTAs must be aware of which type of surgical approach was used to properly carry out OT treatment (Figure 24-3). COTAs should also note the position precautions for each surgical approach.

The movement precautions are usually observed for 6 to 12 weeks as indicated in a physician's order (Morawski

et al, 1996) (Table 24-3). Cemented THRs usually have no weight-bearing restrictions. When cement is not used, bony ingrowth is used to secure the prosthesis to the elder's bone. Often 6 to 8 weeks of weight-bearing restrictions are required when this type of prosthesis is used (Morawski et al, 1996).

After THR surgery, physicians often instruct clients to wear **antiembolus hoseiery.** These thigh-high hose are worn 24 hours a day and removed only during bathing. Clients are instructed to wear this hosiery because it assists with blood circulation, prevents edema, and

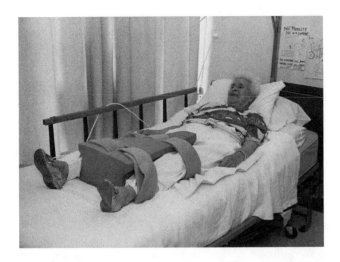

FIGURE **24-3** While the elder is supine, the elder's legs should be abducted with a wedge to prevent hip rotation and adduction.

T**ABLE 24-2**

Weightbearing Terminology	
Term	**Definition**
No weight bearing (NWB)	No body weight is borne on the involved side
Toe-touch weight bearing (TTWB)	No weight is borne on the heel; weight is borne only on the toes
Partial weight bearing (PWB)	A partial amount of the body weight can be borne on the involved side; usually a percentage of body weight (for example, 50% PWB) or pounds (PWB with 50#) is stated
Full weight bearing (FWB)	Full body weight is borne on the involved side

T**ABLE 24-3**

Motion Precautions for Clients Who Have Had a THR	
Approach	**Position precautions**
Anterolateral approach	1. Hip external rotation 2. Hip adduction 3. Hip extension
Posterolateral approach	1. Hip flexion beyond 90 degrees 2. Internal rotation 3. Hip adduction

reduces the risk of deep vein thromboses. If an elder has not been instructed to wear these hose and complains of pain or swelling in the affected leg, the physician should be consulted immediately because this could be a sign of the presence of a thrombus.

ROLE OF OCCUPATIONAL THERAPY IN TESTING ELDERS WITH HIP FRACTURES AND JOINT REPLACEMENTS

Psychosocial Issues

A number of psychosocial issues may surface during an elder's hip replacement rehabilitation. Dealing with a chronic condition such as arthritis can be very stressful and frustrating; many elders are required to deal with pain, swelling, and mobility limitations on a daily basis. Providing information on support groups may be beneficial to the elder.

After a THR some elders find it difficult to abide by the position precautions. They may view these precautions as impediments to resuming the lifestyles they had before the procedure, especially when they had no predisposing medical conditions that limited activities. COTAs should be empathetic to the elder's concerns, but they must also help elders understand the rationale for adhering to hip precautions (Figure 24-4 and 24-5). The COTA should also address the consequences of not following these precautions. COTAs may need to reassure elders that healing takes time and that involvement in activities may continue, usually with some modifications. With physician approval, elders may resume sexual activity if positioning precautions are observed.

Many elders feel guilty when they require assistance from family or friends (Morawski et al, 1996). Elders who are temporarily placed in an extended care facility while they heal may also find it difficult to accept assistance from nursing staff in the facility. Feelings of guilt are sometimes accompanied by financial worries about the cost of care. In addition, relocation to a new environment such as a hospital, extended care facility, or long-term care facility can be stressful (Morawski et al, 1996). COTAs should encourage elders to talk about their feelings. When possible, discussing the situation with elders before

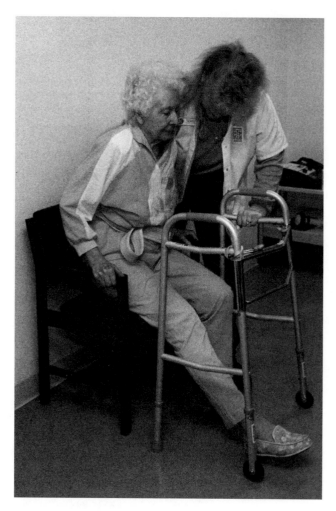

FIGURE 24-4 The elder should extend operated leg and bear weight on arms when coming into a standing position.

they are moved to a new facility is beneficial. In addition, the elder should be thoroughly oriented to the new facility.

Occupational Therapy Interventions

The specific intervention strategies and techniques used with an elder who has had a THR vary depending on whether the anterolateral or posterolateral surgical approach was used (Box 24-1, Figure 24-6).

ARTHRITIS

Arthritis affects the majority of the general population in the United States and is prevalent in nearly 100% of the elder population (Trombly, 1989). Among elders, arthritis is considered the second most prevalent cause of chronic limitation of activity, and is a major predisposing condition for fractures (AARP, 1995).

COTAs must be aware of the physical restrictions and limitations that arthritis imposes on elders' activity. Interventions by the COTA and OTR team should focus on helping elders manage their symptoms more effec-

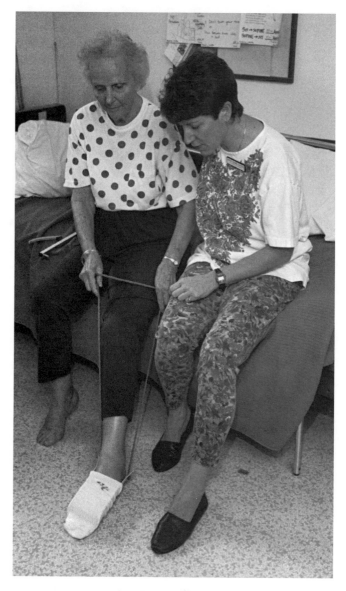

FIGURE 24-5 A sock aid is used to don socks while following hip precautions.

tively in addition to modifying occupational tasks.

More than 100 types of arthritis have been identified (Berkow, Fletcher, 1987). The two most prevalent types, osteoarthritis and **rheumatoid arthritis,** are reviewed in this chapter. Descriptions, causes, and symptoms of both of these forms of arthritis are included (Table 24-4).

Treatment for arthritis in elders can consist of any combination of therapy, medication, and surgery. Therapy may consist of the provision of PT and OT. Medications commonly prescribed to elders who have arthritis are nonsteroidal antiinflammatory drugs. Performing surgery to replace joints is often a last resort.

Occupational Therapy Intervention

The primary goal of OT intervention is to improve the quality of life of elders with arthritis. Specific goals may

BOX 24-1

Occupational Therapy Interventions for Posterolateral and Anterolateral Approaches to THR

Bed mobility
For both approaches
- Abduct legs with wedge or pillows to prevent hip rotation and adduction

Walking
For both approaches
- Avoid pivoting on the leg that has been operated on
- When approaching corners, take small steps in a circular fashion
- If possible, take 10- to 15-minute walks four times per day 6 to 8 weeks after the operation
- Walk at a slow, comfortable pace

Chair transfers
For both approaches
- Sit on chairs with firm seats, preferably with arm rests
- Avoid low, soft chairs and rocking chairs
- Extend leg that has been operated on, reach for arm rests, and bear some weight through arms when trying to sit down

Commode chair transfers
For posterolateral approach
- Use a chair with a height that accommodates for hip flexion precaution
- Wipe between legs while seated or wipe from behind while standing with caution to avoid internal rotation
- Stand and face the toilet to flush

For anterolateral approach
- An over-the-toilet commode is usually used initially in the hospital and upon discharge; elders usually have enough hip mobility to use a standard toilet seat
- Avoid external rotation while wiping
- Stand and face the toilet to flush

Shower stall transfer
For both approaches
- Use a non-skid mat to avoid slips and falls
- Use a shower chair and grab bars

Car transfer
For both approaches
- Avoid bucket seats in small cars
- Back up to passenger seat, hold onto a stable part of the car, extend the leg that has been operated on, and slowly sit in the car

- Increase the seat height with pillows if necessary
- Avoid prolonged sitting in the car

Lower extremity dressing
For both approaches
- Sit on a chair or the bed's edge when dressing
- Use assistive devices if necessary to observe precautions
- Use a reacher or dressing stick in donning and doffing pants and shoes
- Dress the leg that has been operated on first using a reacher or dressing stick to bring pants over the foot and up to the knee
- Avoid crossing the operated LE over the nonoperated LE
- Use a sock aid to don socks or knee-high nylons and a reacher or dressing stick to doff these items
- Use a reacher, elastic shoe laces, and a long-handled shoehorn if necessary

Lower extremity bathing
For both approaches
- Use a long-handled sponge or back brush to reach the lower legs and feet safety and use soap on a rope to prevent the soap from dropping
- Wrap a towel around a reacher to dry the legs
- If a bath bench is used, place a damp towel on the seat to avoid sliding off the bench

Hair shampooing
For both approaches
- Shampoo hair while seated until able to shower

Leisure interests
For both approaches
- Adapt and use long-handled tools when appropriate
- Use stools when appropriate to avoid bending, squatting, and stooping

Homemaking
For both approaches
- Avoid heavy housework (e.g., vacuuming, lifting, and bed making)
- Practice kitchen activities; keep commonly used items at countertop level
- Carry items in large pockets, a walker basket, a fanny pack, or a utility cart
- Use reachers to grasp items in low cupboards or pick up items off the floor

TABLE **24-4**

Description of Osteoarthritis and Rheumatoid Arthritis

Name	Definition	Cause	Symptoms
Osteoarthritis (degenerative joint disease)	A degenerative disease of cartilage with a secondary degeneration involving underlying bone	Possible biomechanical, inflammatory, and immunological factors; secondary factors include congenital defects, trauma, inflammation, endocrine and metabolic disease, and occupational stress	Progressively developing pain, stiffness, and enlargement with limitation of motion; crepitus with PROM; commonly affects weight-bearing joints (hips, knees, cervical and lumbar spine, PIPs, DIPs, CMCs, and MTPs); joints appear red, tender, swollen; asymmetrical presentation; deformities of joints
Rheumatoid arthritis	Chronic, systemic disease characterized by inflammation of the synovial tissue of joints; may involve the heart, lungs, blood vessels, or eyes	Unknown; seems to be of an unknown immune reaction in synovial tissue	Characterized by exacerbations and remissions; commonly affects weight-bearing joints (hips, knees, cervical and lumbar spine, PIPs, DIPs, CMCs, and MTPs); joints appear red, tender, swollen, and hot; usually a symmetrical presentation; deformities of joints

PROM, proximal range of motion; *PIP,* proximal interphalangeal; *DIP,* distal interphalangeal; *CMC,* carpometacarpal; *MTP,* metatarsalphalangeal.

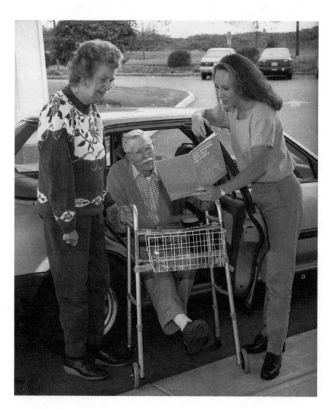

FIGURE 24-6 A COTA provides training on proper techniques for transfers.

include maintaining joint mobility, preventing joint deformity, maintaining strength, maintaining or improving functional ability, maintaining a healthy balance of rest and activity, modifying performance of activities, and improving psychosocial acceptance and coping mechanisms.

Maintenance of joint mobility. COTAs may develop an exercise program for the elder to keep arthritic joints moving. Such an exercise program should seek to minimize stress to all involved joints. Elders with arthritis often find that taking a warm bath or shower after waking up in the morning relieves joint stiffness, thereby making it easier to exercise and engage in other activities. Elders with arthritis may also find it helpful to use a paraffin bath before engaging in wrist and hand exercises.

Prevention of joint deformity. COTAs must be aware of the common types of joint deformities that may develop as a result of arthritis. Deformities include **wrist subluxation, ulnar drift** of the metacarpophalangeal joints, **swan-neck deformity, boutonnière deformity,** and **Nalebuff type I deformity** of the thumb (Figure 24-7).

Volar subluxation of the wrist frequently occurs in elders who have arthritis. A wrist cock-up splint may aid the elder in maintaining better wrist alignment, which will promote function and reduce pain (Lohman, 1996).

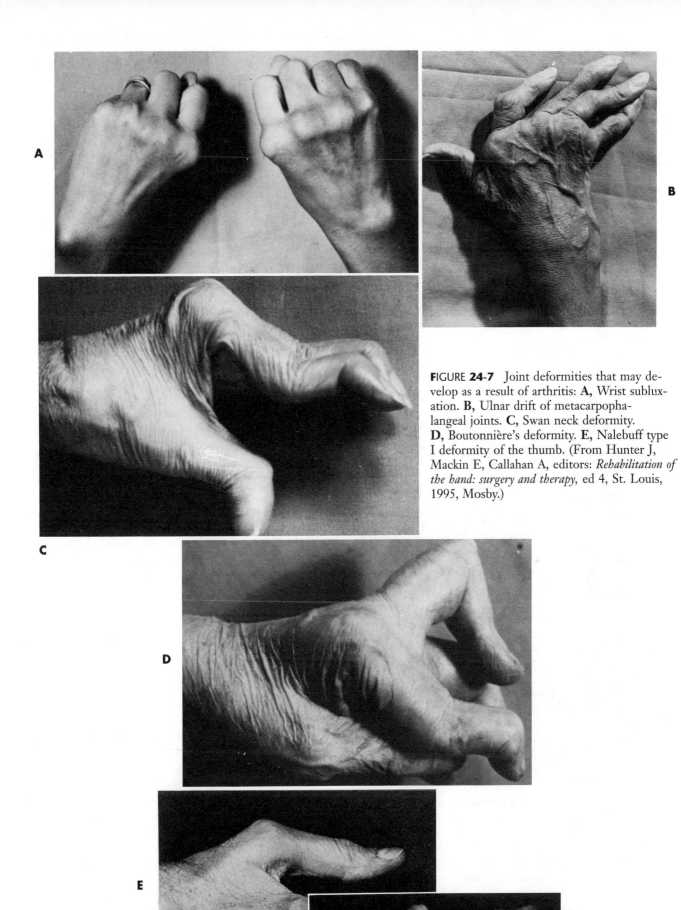

FIGURE 24-7 Joint deformities that may develop as a result of arthritis: **A,** Wrist subluxation. **B,** Ulnar drift of metacarpophalangeal joints. **C,** Swan neck deformity. **D,** Boutonnière's deformity. **E,** Nalebuff type I deformity of the thumb. (From Hunter J, Mackin E, Callahan A, editors: *Rehabilitation of the hand: surgery and therapy*, ed 4, St. Louis, 1995, Mosby.)

BOX 24-2

Joint Protection Principles

- Respect pain. Monitor activities and stop to rest when discomfort or fatigue develops. For example, if kneeling or stooping to garden causes pain and stiffness, stop and rest. Next time, try sitting on a stool.
- Reduce stresses on joints. Use the largest joint possible for activities. For example, when using hands to push up from a seated position, push up with the palms, not the back of the fingers.
- Wear splints as prescribed to protect joints. For example, wear resting-hand splints during exacerbation periods to reduce pain. Movements should be done in the opposite direction of deformity. For example, when wringing out a wash cloth, twist toward the radial side rather than the ulnar side.

- Avoid sustaining a strong, tight grasp. For example, use foam or a cloth wrap around handles to relax the grip needed to manipulate an object.
- Avoid carrying and lifting heavy objects. For example, use a cart to move heavy objects. Distribute object weight evenly over many joints. For example, use both hands to handle a carton of milk.
- Limit the amount of time spent climbing, walking, and standing. For example, take an elevator or escalators; drive or use a walking aid; sit whenever possible.
- Avoid sustained flexion of the finger joints. For example, use a large sponge for cleaning; work with the fingers extended over the sponge rather than squeezing it.
- Avoid using heavy objects. For example, cook with light-weight pots and pans rather than heavy cast-iron pots and pans.

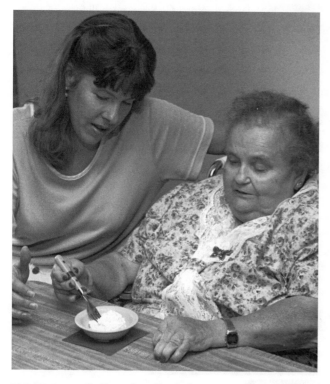

FIGURE 24-8 Built-up handles help elders with arthritis maintain independence in a variety of activities.

Ulnar drift, or ulnar deviation, of the metocarpophalangeal joints is another common deformity caused by arthritis. Ulnar drift is usually caused by destruction and loosening of the radial collateral ligaments. Some experts suggest that the use of an ulnar drift splint may prevent further deformity (Berger et al, 1996).

A swan-neck deformity of the finger results in proximal interphalangeal (PIP) hyperextension with distal interphalangeal (DIP) flexion. A boutonnière deformity results in PIP flexion with DIP hyperextension. Both these deformities can be splinted or surgically repaired with varying results. A Nalebuff type I deformity results in the metacarpal joint of the thumb flexed with hyperextension of the interphalangeal joint. A radial gutter thumb spica splint is often used for better positioning (Lohman, 1996).

To prevent further deformity, elders should be evaluated to determine if they need splints that are appropriate for the deformity and activity level. In addition, elders should be taught **joint protection** techniques (Box 24-2, Figure 24-8).

Maintenance of strength. COTAs may be asked to develop graded strengthening programs for elders who have arthritis. These programs should include the principles of joint protection previously discussed. During periods of acute exacerbation of arthritis, elders should *not* engage in strengthening programs.

Improvement of functional ability. Functional ability can be improved through careful collaboration between the COTA, OTR, and elder. This collaboration can help determine whether assistive equipment works well and is accomplishing the goal for which it was intended. For example, a rocker knife may allow the elder to continue to cut meat during meals. COTAs must observe how the elder handles the knife to ensure that the involved joints are protected as the knife is used and to ascertain that the knife actually cuts the meat.

Maintenance of life balance. Graded strengthening programs for elders who have arthritis are developed by OTRs and may be administered by COTAs. Assisting elders in achieving a balance between rest and activity is

BOX 24-3

Principles of Work Simplification and Energy Conservation

Pace

A moderate, slow pace is most productive; a slower pace is needed in a hot and humid atmosphere

Rhythm

Working in a rhythmic manner saves energy and increases efficiency

Eyes

Work in a well-lighted room, with local light for close work, and rest the eyes periodically

Rest

Plan regular rest periods that are properly spaced during the day

Body mechanics

Sit to work whenever possible; sit in a seat large enough to give full support; work with the elbows close to the body; if working at a table, the height of the table should be near the height of the elbows when they are bent at 90-degree angles

Work areas

A place should be designated for all tools, utensils, and materials; materials should be located close to the area where they will be used

Design of equipment

Handles of utensils and equipment should permit the maximum surface of the hand to come in contact with the handle; handles should be heat resistant and built up

as appropriate; handles that have impressions for the fingers should be used when possible; light-weight equipment should actually be light weight

Kitchen storage

Store supplies and utensils within each reach; arrange the cupboards so that all articles are easy to see, easy to reach, and easy to grasp; store heavy equipment (for example, stacks of plates and pans) on shelves that are easy to reach; use vertical dividers for dish storage, baking pans, trays, and lids; avoid clutter by eliminating or discarding unnecessary equipment

Cooking

Use a cart for transporting food and dishes; slide heavy pots from the sink to the stove instead of lifting them; avoid holding containers or mixing bowls when preparing food; select equipment that can be used for more than one job

Bedmaking

To avoid numerous trips around the bed, make one side completely and then the next side; if possible, keep the bed away from the wall; have the bed put on rollers if it must be moved

Cleaning

When cleaning the bathtub, use long-handled brushes and sit on the edge of the bathtub; use a dust cloth on a long-handled stick for dusting baseboards and ceilings; have cleaning equipment available both upstairs and downstairs

---

paramount. For example, elders are often tempted to schedule all activities during the morning hours with hopes of resting in the afternoon. However, a better balance is achieved when activities are scheduled throughout the day and an appropriate period of rest is incorporated after each activity. This type of schedule will help decrease the fatigue of elders, and is less likely to lead to an exacerbation of their conditions. In addition, elders will likely accomplish more during the day.

Modification of activity. **Work simplification** and **energy conservation** techniques often benefit elders who have arthritis (Box 24-3). These elders must attempt to distribute their energy output evenly over the number of tasks to be accomplished. Incorporating energy conservation and work simplification techniques into the elders' daily routines can assist them in maintaining a functional lifestyle.

Improve psychosocial well-being and coping mecha-

nisms. The combination of acute and chronic pain, coupled with joint stiffness and immobility, can result in limitations of activities of daily living (ADLs) such as dressing, and recreational and social outlets such as dancing. The population of elders who experience pain is challenged daily to use strategies that will enhance productive living. Elders who do not have coping and support systems will need assistance in developing such systems. COTAs may provide assistance by linking elders who have arthritis with community resources that can provide support and help elders developing coping mechanisms. Self-help courses sponsored by the Arthritis Foundation can provide social interaction. Alternative methods of pain control may include relaxation training, cognitive restructuring and modification, medication fading, and social assertiveness training. The process of helping elders cope with arthritis must involve a multidisciplinary approach for chronic pain management to be successful.

CASE STUDY

Mr. H. is a 76-year-old elder who sustained a right hip fracture after falling when attempting to make his way to the bathroom in the middle of the night. Mr. H. underwent an open reduction internal fixation and pinning of the right hip. He is waiting for a home health care agency to contact him about providing assistance with his home rehabilitation. Mr. H., a widower, is unable to drive because of poor vision and rheumatoid arthritis. He resides in a ranch-style home in which the kitchen, bedroom, and bathroom are located on the main level. However, laundry facilities are located in the basement.

▌ CHAPTER REVIEW QUESTIONS

1 List the precautions that Mr. H. might need to follow after his hip pinning procedure.

2 List the ADL functions that will be directly affected by Mr. H.'s hip pinning procedure.

3 Describe the problems that Mr. H. may be dealing with as a result of his rheumatoid arthritis.

4 Name the wrist and hand deformities associated with rheumatoid arthritis that may be afflicting Mr. H.

5 Describe some possible causes for Mr. H.'s fall that should be investigated.

6 Describe the ways in which Mr. H.'s performance of ADL functions and environment will need to be modified.

REFERENCES

American Association of Retired Persons: *A profile of older Americans*, Washington, DC, 1995, The Association.

Bear-Lehman J: Orthopedic conditions. In Trombly CA, editor: *Occupational therapy for physical dysfunction*, ed 4, Baltimore, Md, 1995, Williams & Wilkins.

Berger, SM et al: Geriatric splinting. In Coppard BM, Lohman H, editors: *Introduction to splinting: a critical-thinking and problem-solving approach*, St. Louis, Mo, 1996, Mosby.

Berkow R, Fletcher AJ, editors: *The Merck manual*, Rahway, NJ, 1987, Merck Sharp and Dohme Research Laboratories.

Birge SJ, Morrow-Howell N, Proctor EK: Hip fracture, *Clin Geriatr Med* 10:589, 1994.

Cooper C, Barker DPJ, Morris J: Osteoporosis, falls and age in fracture of the proximal femur, *Br Med J* 295:13, 1987.

Cummings SR: Epidemiology of osteoporotic fractures, *Osteoporosis Update* 7(3):113, 1987.

Daniel MS, Strickland LR: *Occupational therapy protocol management in adult physical dysfunction*, Gaithersburg, Md, 1992, Aspen.

Heckman JD: Stress fractures in the elderly, *Hosp Pract* 26 (Suppl 1): 36, 1991.

Jette AM et al: Functional recovery after hip fracture, *Arch Phys Med Rehabil* 68:735, 1987.

Lewis SC: *Elder care in occupational therapy*, Thorofare, NJ, 1989, SLACK.

Lohman H: Thumb spica splints. In Coppard BM, Lohman H, editors: *Introduction to splinting: a critical-thinking and problem-solving approach*, St. Louis, 1996, Mosby.

Lohman H: Wrist cock-up splints. In Coppard BM, Lohman H, editors: *Introduction to splinting: a critical-thinking and problem-solving approach*, St. Louis, 1996, Mosby.

Magaziner J et al: Predictors of functional recovery one year following hospital discharge for hip fracture: a prospective study, *J Gerontol Med Sci* 45:M101, 1990.

Mehta AF, Nastasi AE: Rehabilitation of fractures in the elderly, *Clin Geriatr Med* 9:717, 1993.

Melton LJ, Riggs BL: Risk factors for injury after a fall, *Clin Geriatr Med* 1:621, 1985.

Morawski D et al: Hip fractures and total hip replacement. In Pedretti LW, editor: *Occupational therapy: practice skills for physical dysfunction*, St. Louis, 1996, Mosby.

Tinetti ME, Williams TF, Mayewski R: Fall risk index for elderly patients based on number of chronic disabilities, *Am J Med* 80:429, 1986.

Trombly CA: Arthritis. In Trombly CA, editor: *Occupational therapy for physical dysfunction*, ed 3, Baltimore, 1989, Williams & Wilkins.

U.S. Department of Transportation, 1994.

CHAPTER 25

Working With Elders Who Have Cardiovascular Conditions

JANA K. CRAGG, JEAN T. HAYS, AND CLAIRE PEEL

KEY TERMS

cardiac rehabilitation, cardiovascular diseases, heart rate (HR), blood pressure (BP),
maximum heart rate, metabolic equivalents, energy conservation, work simplification

CHAPTER OBJECTIVES

1. Identify the signs and symptoms of cardiac dysfunction.
2. Describe the phases of cardiac rehabilitation.
3. Recognize the role of OT in cardiac rehabilitation.
4. Describe assessments, treatment techniques, and precautions used with elders who have cardiac conditions.
5. Describe treatment approaches for elders with cardiac conditions in various treatment settings.

Some COTAs may specialize in cardiac rehabilitation, and others may work in settings with elders who have cardiac conditions as primary diagnoses or that accompany other diagnoses. Joan is a COTA who specializes in **cardiac rehabilitation.** She works closely with the cardiac team as she provides OT treatment. Mark is a COTA employed by a skilled nursing facility. He treats elders with a variety of conditions. Many of the elders are admitted for specific reasons such as rehabilitation after a total hip replacement or stroke. Most have accompanying chronic illnesses, including cardiac conditions. Mark often informally consults with Joan when he has a treatment question about cardiac conditions because he does not have the same specialty experience that she has and values her expertise. This

chapter primarily focuses on COTAs' roles in cardiac rehabilitation settings. However, treatment of elders with cardiac conditions in other settings is also addressed.

Heart disease is one of the most frequent chronic conditions that occur among elders (American Heart Association, 1996; American Association of Retired Persons [AARP], 1995; O'Rourke, Chatterjee, Wei, 1987). **Cardiovascular diseases** include disorders of the heart and vascular system. These disorders can be classified as (1) diseases that primarily affect the heart such as coronary artery disease and congestive heart failure, (2) circulatory problems involving peripheral vessels such as peripheral vascular disease, and (3) circulatory problems involving the cerebral circulation.

BACKGROUND INFORMATION

During the aging process, the body experiences gradual changes. Although many of these changes are inevitable, studies show that some of the changes are less pronounced in elders who are free of cardiovascular diseases (Rodeheffer, Gersten-Blith, Becher, 1984). This is especially true for elders who have lifestyles that include regular physical activity. However, most elders experience age-related changes in their cardiovascular systems, including changes in the heart muscle and vessels, peripheral vascular disease, and an increase in systolic pressure, which makes the heart work harder (Lakatta, Yin, 1982). Valvular disease, endocarditis, and rheumatic disease may be present; however, most coronary diseases are related to lifestyle and family history. Chronic cardiac conditions include hypertension, angina pectoris, congestive heart failure, and peripheral vascular disease. Heart disease often accompanies other illnesses or conditions such as diabetes or chronic obstructive pulmonary disease (AARP, 1995).

Medical treatment varies according to the condition and other individual health factors. Thrombolytics are used to prevent muscle damage from heart attacks. Other common drugs are those used to treat hypertension, angina, heart failure, and dysrhythmias. Surgical treatments may include angioplasty or bypass for damaged arteries. In rare cases, treatment may involve a heart transplant to replace heart muscle that is irreversibly damaged. Cardiac management may include electromechanical devices such as pacemakers to achieve a normal **heart rate (HR)** and rhythm.

Circulatory heart disease may begin with a loss of elasticity in the small vessels, causing the heart to work harder to maintain blood flow to organs (Hutchins, 1980). A change in the temperature in the extremities, cyanosis, or an increase in systolic blood pressure may indicate circulatory insufficiency. Atherosclerosis is a condition in which lipid deposits accumulate on the walls of large and medium vessels (Cawson, McCracken, Marcus, 1989). This narrows the lumen of these vessels, which restricts blood flow. Atherosclerosis of coronary vessels can produce ischemia, which causes angina (chest pain) and/or a myocardial infarction (MI), which damages the heart muscle. Atherosclerosis of cerebral vessels can lead to a cerebrovascular accident, or stroke. A change in the structure of the heart valves, either from viral illness or aging, may result in heart failure, a condition in which the heart cannot deliver enough oxygen to peripheral tissues.

Valvular disease may be heard as a murmur during a routine examination. When the left side of the heart fails, fluid accumulates in the lungs, causing exertional dyspnea, orthopnea, paroxysmal nocturnal dyspnea, dyspnea at rest, pulmonary edema, weakness, and fatigue (Kloner, 1984). When the right side of the heart fails, blood backs up in the periphery, causing systemic venous congestion, dependent edema, upper right quadrant pain, anorexia, nausea, bloating, and fatigue (Kloner, 1984). Many elders with cardiovascular disease lose the ability to perform physical activities and lose independence in their daily skills.

PSYCHOSOCIAL ASPECTS OF CARDIAC DYSFUNCTIONS

Cardiac dysfunction can have profound psychosocial implications on elders and their significant others. All elders react differently to a cardiac event, but most progress through many stages of adjustments. Initially the anxiety produced by fear of death and discomfort can have a profound effect and produce overwhelming feelings. Some elders demonstrate this anxiety in behavioral changes and may act out or become agitated. This level of anxiety places a physiological demand on the cardiac system at a time when rest is important. Elders experiencing a rapid change in their care status may also have difficulty with anxiety, so antianxiety medications often are used to assist them. However, some of these medications can have unwanted side effects and lead to additional stress. Elders should be encouraged to voice their feelings and work with the health care team to alleviate their fears about the course of events. Good communication and supportive staff members are the key elements in reducing elders' anxiety levels. Fear of another cardiac event can impair functional levels, especially in the early rehabilitation phase. Education and therapeutic intervention can help to alleviate these fears. Once stable, elders should be encouraged to begin ambulation and self-care activities following the guidelines established by the therapist. This helps eliminate the helplessness elders may feel after a cardiac event. The longer these two elements are delayed, the more helpless elders may feel, which can reinforce the disability (Matthews, Foderaro, O'Leary, 1996). (Chapter 13 includes a discussion of ways to address the sexual concerns of elders with heart disease.)

As elders begin to regain some strength and control over events, denial of risk related to the disease may become evident. Denial gives some elders the mechanism necessary to cope with the cardiac event. This particular phase may be more prevalent in elders with coronary disease because the symptoms and characteristics associated with this disease are vague. COTAs must not try to break through the denial phase too soon. Facing the realities of the situation may be overwhelming and may create stress-related physical and emotional complications. COTAs can help elders by instructing them to monitor their performance carefully and thus reduce the risk of another cardiac event.

Some elders become depressed after a cardiac event. Inactivity and anxiety may trigger depression. Depression and anxiety combined can have a long-term effect on the elder's physical and emotional well-being.

COTAs can play a strong role in addressing the psychosocial aspects of cardiac disease by educating elders about the expected outcomes after a cardiac event. Relaxation training and lifestyle education are key elements in achieving emotional well-being. Informing the family of risks and precautions can assist elders in the transition to the home environment and ensure that elders have the best chance to regain their status in the home and community.

EVALUATION OF ELDERS WITH CARDIAC CONDITIONS

COTAs working with elders who have had cardiac events or who have chronic cardiac conditions should be able to monitor vital signs. It is important that COTAs accurately determine HR and take **blood pressure (BP)** during activity (Figure 25-1). Guidelines for HR and BP responses are usually written as treatment precautions. To determine the HR, COTAs should palpate the elder's pulse at the wrist, count the number of beats felt for 15 seconds, and then multiply this number by 4. This will provide a baseline HR in beats per minute (BPM) before the elder engages in activity. Although HRs vary, a normal baseline HR ranges between 60 and 100 BPM (Matthews, Foderaro, O'Leary, 1996). **Maximum HR** corresponds with performing maximal levels of exertion that involve large muscle groups in rhythmic activities such as walking and cycling. One method of predicting maximum HR is by subtracting the elder's age from 220. This figure is multiplied by 0.6 to predict the appropriate HR response for normal activity (American College of Sports Medicine, 1991). For example, a 78-year-old woman's predicted maximum HR would be 142 BPM (220 − 78 = 142). Her HR appropriate for activity would be 85 (0.6 × 142 = 85 BPM). Signs and symptoms *must* be considered when using formulas to predict activity HR values. Elders should perform activities in a symptom-free range.

Likewise, BP should be taken if a physician has so ordered or if the elder has symptoms of distress such as shortness of breath, dizziness, weakness, or cyanosis. Elders with hypertension should be monitored for excessive elevations in BP or orthostatic hypotension, which may occur as a side effect of medications. BP values greater than 140/90 indicate mild hypertension, and those greater than 160/100 indicate moderate hypertension (Joint National Committee on Detection, Evaluation and Treatment of High Blood Pressure, 1993). BP is considered hypotensive if the systolic pressure is less than 90 mm Hg. Hypotension can be associated with dizziness and light-headedness or, in severe cases, circulatory inadequacy of the extremities (Matthews, Foderaro, O'Leary, 1996). In the presence of a shunt for renal dialysis, the BP should be read on the opposite limb. Renal shunts are

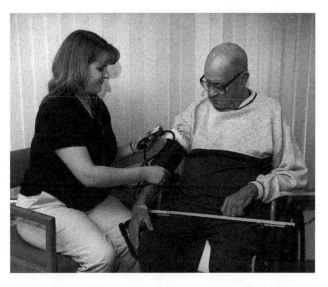

FIGURE 25-1 Elders with cardiac conditions should be monitored for HR, BP, and respiratory rate responses to activity.

fragile and cannot withstand the pressure produced by the BP cuff (sphygmomanometer) during BP monitoring. For training, COTAs should practice monitoring HR and BP with an instructor before performing care.

The COTA and OTR team should be able to perform a basic bedside activities of daily living (ADL) evaluation as part of the initial evaluation. This might include having the elder perform oral care, grooming tasks, washing of upper body, and dressing. Another area tested simultaneously is the elder's work tolerance for basic self-care activities. COTAs working with elders who have decreased endurance and low activity tolerance caused by cardiac disease may use **metabolic equivalents** (METs) as a basis for estimating the energy expended when performing an activity. The MET table provided along with HR and BP responses can help COTAs determine the cardiovascular stress and amount of work performed for specific tasks (Table 25-1). Further areas to be assessed are grip strength, muscle strength, and bed mobility.

INTERVENTIONS, GOALS, AND STRATEGIES

For interventions to be effective, COTAs must understand the functional levels that are used to classify elders with cardiac disease. There are four functional categories for cardiac disease (Box 25-1). Knowing the categories allows COTAs to make adjustments in elders' rehabilitation programs. The four phases of cardiac rehabilitation describe where the elder is in the recovery process (Box 25-2).

COTAs need to be aware of activities that can be stressful to the heart. Such activities include isometric and upper extremity activities, especially if performed at a level above the heart. The stress on the heart is reflected

TABLE 25-1

Santa Clara Valley Medical Center's Post-MI and Post–Open-Heart Surgery

Phase I Rehabilitation	
Stage	**OT**
In ICU or on ward 1.5 METs	General mobility (bed mobility, transfers to the commode, and position changes) with energy-conservation techniques (environmental setups, equipment, and pacing) Sedentary leisure tasks with arms supported (reading, writing, playing cards). OT may not treat in the ICU; OT usually starts in stage 3
In ICU or on ward 1.5 METs	Stage 1 continued with focus on sitting (5 to 30 min) Standing tasks (seconds to 2 min) Simple hygiene, semi-Fowler sitting position
On ward 1.5-2 METs	Unsupported sitting (30 to 60 min) Standing tasks (3 to 5 min) Bedside bathing (assist with feet and back) Bathroom privileges Light leisure tasks
2 METs	Standing tasks (5 to 8 min) Sustained UE activity (2 to 5 min) Total body bathing at sink
2 METs	Standing tasks (8 to 12 min) Sustained UE activity (5 to 30 min) Total hygiene, bathing, dressing at sink
2 METs	Standing tasks (10 to 30 min) with intermittent UE activity UE sustained activity (5 to 30 min) Total body mobility: bending for small objects, retrieval training Moderate leisure tasks
3-3.5 METs	Shower transfers Total showering task (hair washing, total body washing, drying, and dressing) Simple homemaking tasks Energy-conservation techniques with activity METs (or greater as indicated by ETT or GXT) Home program with ADL guidelines and recommendations for equipment as appropriate

Modified from Santa Clara Valley Medical Center: *Cardiac rehabilitation program protocol*, San Jose, Calif, 1987, The Center [unpublished].)
Education program to be performed by all team members as per *SCVMC Cardiac Education Manual.*
ICU, intensive care unit; *UE,* upper extremity; *ADL,* activities of daily living; *ETT,* Exercise tolerance test; *GXT,* Graded exercise test.

by the elder's HR and BP responses. Consequently, any activity that produces excessive increases in HR and BP may overstress the heart.

The primary goal of any cardiac rehabilitation program is to return elders to their maximum functional capacities. The COTA and OTR team must design an individualized rehabilitation program for each elder. Although the phases of rehabilitation follow certain key steps, each elder's progress will be different. Psychosocial aspects, family support, age, and medical status, as well as the desire to participate in the rehabilitation program, affect treatment progression. A rehabilitation treatment

plan for OT with MET allowances for specific activities is useful (see Table 25-1).

Phase I

Phase I consists of the period of inpatient hospitalization. Most referred elders are in the acute phase after undergoing surgery or experiencing MI. Other elders are referred for atypical chest pain. Beginning in phase I, elders are evaluated by an OTR. During the evaluation, the COTA and OTR team reviews the medical chart to obtain information on medical history and current cardiac status and interviews the elder to determine lifestyle and

BOX 25-1

The Four Functional Categories of Cardiac Disease

Class I
Elders with cardiac disease but without resulting limitations of physical activity. Ordinary physical activity does not cause undue fatigue, palpitation, dyspnea, or anginal pain.

Class II
Elders with cardiac disease resulting in slight limitation of physical activity. They are comfortable at rest. Ordinary physical activity results in fatigue, dyspnea, palpitation, or anginal pain.

Class III
Elders with cardiac disease resulting in marked limitation of physical activity. They are comfortable at rest. Less than ordinary physical activity causes fatigue, dyspnea, palpitation, or anginal pain.

Class IV
Elders with cardiac disease resulting in inability to perform any physical activity without discomfort. Symptoms of cardiac insufficiency or of anginal syndrome may be present even at rest. If any physical activity is undertaken, discomfort increases.

From New York Heart Association Inc: *Nomenclature and criteria for diagnoses of diseases of the heart and great vessels*, ed 8, Boston, 1979, Little, Brown.

BOX 25-2

The Four Phases of Cardiac Rehabilitation

Phase I
Occurs in the acute phase of hospitalization for the cardiac event. Elders qualifying for cardiac rehabilitation must be stable after event as determined by physician(s).

Phase II
Occurs during subacute period after event. Instituted once elder leaves the hospital and continues for 6 to 12 weeks. Elder is followed up by home health or outpatient service.

Phase III
Elder enters a program designed to regain former functional and performance level. Focus is on increasing duration and intensity of physical activity to achieve health benefits and to increase cardiorespiratory fitness.

Phase IV
Elder enters a maintenance phase of cardiac rehabilitation. This phase is indefinite in length and involves periodic evaluations.

Modified from Kloner R: *The guide to cardiology*, New York, 1984, Wiley & Sons.

personal goals for rehabilitation. During phase I, OT practitioners and elders work toward developing a discharge plan based on individual needs and lifestyles. Goals for meeting each of the stages in phase I are discussed (see Table 25-1). Activities and educational information are introduced as the rehabilitation process begins. Activities and exercises are initially low level. Early in phase I, COTAs educate elders regarding the need for balancing their lifestyles, which includes stress-reduction techniques (Figure 25-2). Elders are also educated to accommodate for changes in their health status. Using the occupational behavioral model of work, rest, and play, COTAs can introduce the concepts of **energy conservation** and **work simplification** while providing bedside treatment (Gibson, 1993). This gives elders the ability to regain some of their self-care and dignity while learning to work with their limitations after a cardiac event. COTAs can build rapport and support continued rehabilitation by carefully monitoring physiological responses, signs, and symptoms and structuring activities to prevent elders from feeling fatigue.

METs help establish parameters for functional activities. One MET, the oxygen consumed by the body at rest, is equal to approximately 3.5 ml O_2/kg body mass per

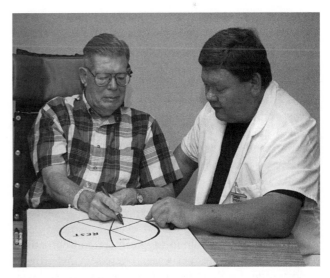

FIGURE 25-2 COTAs educate elders regarding the need for balancing their lifestyles.

minute. To translate this concept into an activity level, it takes 1.5 METs to write a letter in bed with the arms supported (Matthews, Foderaro, O'Leary, 1996). Most self-care activities range from 1.5 to 3.5 METs, and although this may seem to be light work, it can be physically demanding for elders. In some rehabilitation settings, OT does not intervene in cardiac rehabilitation until the elder is able to perform light work (1.5 to 2 METs) without symptoms of dyspnea, palpitation, or angina during or after activity. Once elders are at this level, they can attempt activities required to return home and independently perform most self-care activities. During phase I, elders are reevaluated to determine whether additional equipment or education is necessary so that they are able to return home and conduct functional activities with safe and appropriate HR, electrocardiogram (ECG), and BP responses.

Phase II

Phase II, often referred to as the *recovery*, or *healing*, *phase*, is the period immediately after hospitalization. Elders receive rehabilitation through home health or outpatient clinic services. An elder's functional performance during self-care activities is evaluated by monitoring the resting pulse and peak pulse during a task and then measuring the recovery time to a resting pulse once the activity is terminated. The elder's status is monitored during the activities by measuring HR, BP, ECG, and respiratory responses before, during, and after task completion. The course of treatment and the elder's progress are determined by the physiological responses during activities and the estimated MET level for activities. During this phase of rehabilitation, education and training continue for modifications of risk factors and monitoring of the elder's general health.

Phase III

Once elders are able to tolerate increased MET activities at greater than 3.5 METs with safe and appropriate HR, BP, and ECG responses, they are ready to move into phase III of rehabilitation. At this level of function, elders ideally have been under the care of a cardiac rehabilitation team for two to three months. Goals of phase III programs include increasing activity duration and intensity to a level sufficient to elicit cardiorespiratory training adaptations and to assist elders to make necessary lifestyle changes. Phase III of cardiac rehabilitation requires elders to be more responsible for self-monitoring and to react appropriately if signs or symptoms of a recurring cardiac event become evident. Elders in phase III programs typically attend outpatient programs 2 or 3 times per week. These sessions provide opportunities for therapists to evaluate function and performance and to facilitate progression of activity programs. Providing elders with the education and techniques necessary to maintain their new lifestyles allows them to be more successful at self-monitoring. Elders often are counseled to make dietary changes, to stop smoking, and to increase physical activity levels. COTAs are in a position to reinforce lifestyle changes. Continued

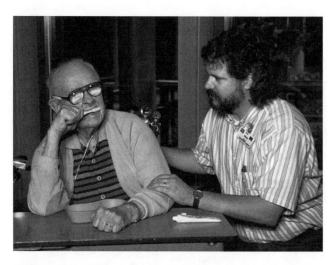

FIGURE **25-3**   Elders should perform orofacial care with arms propped on a table.

training in energy conservation and the use of assistive devices is provided to elders at functional levels III and IV. In outpatient clinics, elders can also receive training in a simulated work environment to provide guidelines for returning to a job or for avocational interests.

Energy Conservation, Work Simplification, and Other Education

During OT, elders receive education on energy conservation, work simplification, and cardiac status monitoring. Energy conservation is not only important for the elder's well-being but also is a safety monitor for routine tasks. In the acute portion of cardiac rehabilitation, this component allows elders to set the pace of their self-care routines. Energy conservation begins with basic task analysis, which includes identifying the main steps in the task, analyzing the way the task is performed, and determining the tools or skills needed to perform the task. Once analyzed, the next component of work simplification is added. Having elders perform basic orofacial care at the bedside is an example of ADL energy conservation. Using the bedside table, with arms propped for energy conservation, the elder can perform orofacial care with all the supplies and a basin of water on the table (Figure 25-3). Elders may need to be reminded to rest during the task if they experience dyspnea or an increase in HR beyond the established parameters. The task can be simplified with a complete setup of supplies, including removal of all caps from grooming supplies and provision of a light weight electric razor if appropriate. With the elder in the semi-Fowler position in bed, this task can be accomplished with no more than 1.5 METs. Other ADL functions are analyzed in the same manner, with the therapist identifying ways to reduce the energy expenditure (energy conservation) and minimize steps to perform

TABLE 25-2

Assistive Devices and Rationale for Use	
Item	**Rationale**
Long-handled reacher Long-handled shoe horn Sock aid Elastic shoe laces	These items prevent the need to bend more than 90 degrees forward flexion in trunk. This may be a precaution for bypass surgery to reduce strain over incision. Limiting trunk flexion to 90 degrees facilitates breathing by allowing full excursion of the diaphragm.
Long-handled bath sponge Bath mitt	These items reduce twisting of trunk and reaching forward in bath to wash back and lower extremities (energy conservation). Less strain is placed on heart and surgical incisions.

the task (work simplification). The addition of assistive devices may be an added benefit (Table 25-2).

Elders should be encouraged to pace themselves during activities to reduce fatigue. The work-rest-work principle is important for elders to maintain in the acute phase, especially when denial is an issue. Elders in denial about their cardiac disease may want to prove they are well by overworking or pushing themselves, placing unnecessary stress on their damaged hearts.

TREATMENT OF ELDERS WITH CARDIAC CONDITIONS IN OTHER SETTINGS

This chapter has focused primarily on cardiac rehabilitation when cardiac disease is the primary diagnosis. However, COTAs may encounter elders who have cardiac problems, perhaps as one of many chronic conditions, in settings such as nursing homes. Elders with acute cardiac conditions eventually may be transferred from the cardiac rehabilitation setting to another setting for further rehabilitation. In these settings COTAs who are not formally trained in cardiac rehabilitation need to be aware of treatment approaches and precautions. Elders with cardiac conditions in any setting need to be educated on work simplification and energy conservation. The optimal approach is to demonstrate work simplification and energy conservation during the performance of meaningful tasks.

The primary recommendation for all elders with cardiac conditions is to monitor responses to activity by measuring HR, BP, and respiratory rate at rest, during

activity, and during recovery. Activities that elicit excessive increases in HR or BP or that elicit abnormal signs and symptoms should not be performed or should be modified to ensure appropriate responses. Elders who have had coronary artery bypass graft surgery often are given lifting restrictions. Recommendations vary by physician and often include not lifting more than 10 pounds for at least 1 month after surgery. Lifting precautions also may be present for elders who have had a procedure involving catheterization of the femoral artery, such as angioplasty and stent placement. Lifting guidelines for these procedures, determined by the elder's physician, are based on the elder's lifestyle and physical status and the specific procedures performed.

Recognition of distress signals is vital in any setting when working with elders with cardiac dysfunction. Primary signs and symptoms are chest pain, shortness of breath, cyanosis, sweating, fatigue, weakness, and confusion. Elders with cardiac dysfunction often complain of burning or pressure in the chest or of upper extremity, jaw, or cervical pain. These symptoms may occur with elders who have congestive heart failure, dysrrhythmias, or a history of MI or angina. If elders demonstrate or report any of these symptoms, the COTA should monitor their BP and HR as well as ECG readings for changes in medical status. Any abnormal sign or symptom should be documented and discussed with the OTR and other health care professionals.

Another key area is the type of medication elders with cardiac or BP problems are taking. Anticoagulants are commonly used for elders who have hypertension or who have had a cerebrovascular accident or hip or knee replacement surgery. Nitroglycerin is a common medication for elders with angina pectoris. If elders have chest pain, they need to be reminded to take their medication as directed. Elders and their caregivers need to be instructed about the dosage protocol and side effects of their medications (Table 25-3). Knowledge of which medications elders are taking and their side effects is important to any therapist, but especially to those who perform therapy services through a home health agency or in a community setting.

CASE STUDY

Mrs. T. is a 65-year-old woman admitted to home health services for OT after coronary bypass surgery. She had been hospitalized for 5 days and received OT services in the acute care unit. She was educated in energy conservation and work simplification and given assistive devices to help her be more independent at home.

At the time of her referral for home health services, Mrs. T. was instructed to lift no more than 3 pounds and to maintain her work levels at no more than 2 METs. Evaluation by the COTA and OTR team determined that her HR for activity would be 94 beats per minute (BPM). To arrive at this figure, the COTA and OTR had Mrs. T. perform an activity that

TABLE 25-3

Examples of Common Medications and Potential Side Effects

Condition	Medication category (examples)	Side effects
Angina pectoris	Nitrates (nitroglycerin, isosorbide dinitrate)	Headache, orthostatic hypotension, dizziness
	β-Blockers (propranolol, atenolol)	Bradycardia, depression, fatigue
	Calcium channel blockers (verapamil, diltiazem)	Peripheral edema
Heart failure	Cardiac glycosides (digitalis, digoxin)	Cardiac dysrhythmias, GI distress, CNS disturbances
	Diuretics (furosemide)	Electrolyte disturbances, volume depletion
	ACE inhibitors (enalapril, captopril)	Skin rash
Hypertension	β-Blockers (atenolol, metoprolol)	Bradycardia, depression, fatigue
	Diuretics (hydrochlorothiazide)	Volume depletion, electrolyte imbalance
	Calcium channel blockers (diltiazem, verapamil)	Peripheral edema
	ACE inhibitors (enalapril)	Skin rash
	α-Blockers (prazosin)	Reflex tachycardia, orthostatic hypotension
	Centrally acting SNS antagonists (clonidine)	Dry mouth, dizziness, drowsiness
	Vasodilators (hydralazine)	Reflex tachyardia, dizziness, orthostatic hypotension, weakness, headaches
Dysrhythmias	Sodium channel blockers (quinidine, lidocaine)	Cardiac rhythm disturbances
	β-Blockers	Bradycardia
	Drugs that prolong repolarization (amiodarone)	Pulmonary toxicity, liver damage
	Calcium channel blockers (verapamil)	Bradycardia, dizziness, headaches
Acute MI	Narcotic analgesics (morphine)	Sedation, respiratory depression, GI distress
	Platelet-aggregation inhibitors (aspirin)	GI distress
	Thrombolytics (streptokinase, tissue plasminogen activator)	Excessive bleeding

GI, Gastrointestinal; *CNS*, central nervous system; *ACE*, angiotensin-converting enzyme; *SNS*, sympathetic nervous system.

required an approximate energy expenditure of 2 METs for 2 to 3 minutes. Her HR response to this activity was 94 BPM and was used as a guideline when she performed other activities. Mrs. T. was shown how to palpate and count her HR using the radial pulse and was encouraged to record her HR at the beginning, peak, and end of each activity in a diary. This allowed her and the COTA to monitor performance progression and helped to advance the treatment plan.

Further evaluation revealed Mrs. T. had better than fair upper body strength overall. Her endurance for tasks was approximately 5 minutes for light to moderate activity, which consisted of performing household activities including making beds, washing dishes, cooking, and dusting. Because of the incision made during her surgery, Mrs. T. was cautioned to refrain from heavier household tasks such as sweeping or mopping until she was stronger.

The treatment goals set by Mrs. T. and the COTA and OTR team were for her to complete activities at home as she had formerly done. Mrs. T. was very compliant with the therapy program and had very supportive family members who monitored her frequently to keep her on target with goal achievement. In the first week Mrs. T. increased her activity level sufficiently to allow her HR to move from a baseline of 78 BPM before beginning tasks to 110 BPM peak HR with a 10-minute recovery after task completion. Most tasks in the first phase were housekeeping chores that required no more than 10 minutes of sustained activity. In the second week Mrs. T. had a mild setback after contracting

an upper respiratory infection and had to decrease her activity levels and start taking a medication prescribed by her physician. After the respiratory infection cleared, Mrs. T. was able to resume her activity levels and increase her task levels. Her beginning MET level was 2 METs for 10 minutes of activity with a 10-minute recovery rate. During the third week of her program, Mrs. T. began to perform more complex tasks requiring 2.5 to 3.5 METs under the supervision of the COTA or a family member. Mrs. T. was able to perform tasks for 20 minutes or more and managed to keep her HR at 78 BPM before tasks and 115 to 120 BPM while performing tasks with a 5-minute recovery rate to 80 BPM. On discharge Mrs. T. was managing her routine household chores with no symptoms or discomfort. She was independent in monitoring her own HR and adjusting her work pace accordingly.

CHAPTER REVIEW QUESTIONS

1 Describe how the HR for activity was determined in Mrs. T.'s case.
2 What was her initial endurance for the task? Describe when it increased.
3 What other adaptations for tools or equipment could have been made to prevent further cardiac problems or possible injury?

4 How did the OT practitioners determine her HR?

5 What are three activities Mrs. T. should avoid? Why are these activities contraindicated?

6 Describe the effect of anxiety on elders with cardiac conditions.

7 Explain the role COTAs play in addressing the psychosocial aspects of cardiac disease.

8 Describe how maximum HRs and activity HRs are determined.

9 Describe what is involved in evaluation of elders with cardiac conditions.

10 Describe the four functional categories of cardiac disease.

11 Describe the four phases of cardiac rehabilitation.

12 What is a MET and how can the MET system be used in cardiac rehabilitation?

13 Describe how energy conservation and work simplification are used in elders with cardiac conditions.

14 What should COTAs do for elders who report symptoms of angina pectoris while washing their hair?

15 Identify a method of energy conservation for elders while dressing their lower extremities.

REFERENCES

American Association of Retired Persons: *A profile of older Americans*, Washington DC, 1995, The Association.

American College of Sports Medicine: *Guidelines for exercise testing and prescription*, ed 4, Philadelphia, 1991, Lea and Febiger.

American Heart Association: *Heart and stroke facts: 1996 statistical supplement*, Dallas, 1996, The Association.

Cawson RA, McCracken AW, Marcus PB: *Pathologic mechanisms and human disease*, ed 2, St. Louis, 1989, Mosby.

Gibson D: The evolution of occupational therapy. In Hopkins HL, Smith HD, editors: *Williard and Spackman's occupational therapy*, ed 8, Philadelphia, 1993, JB Lippincott.

Hutchins GM: Structure of the aging heart. In Welsfeldt ML, editor: *The aging heart*, New York, 1980, Raven Press.

Joint National Committee on Detection, Evaluation and Treatment of High Blood Pressure, National High Blood Pressure Education Program, Coordinating Committee: *Report of the Joint National Committee on Detection, Evaluation and Treatment of High Blood Pressure*, Bethesda, Md, 1993, National Heart, Lung and Blood Institute, National High Blood Pressure Program.

Kloner R: *The guide to cardiology*, New York, 1984, Wiley & Sons.

Lakatta EG, Yin FC: Myocardial aging: functional alterations and related cellular mechanisms, *Am J Physiol* 242(6): H927, 1982.

Mathews MM, Foderaro D, O'Leary S: Cardiac dysfunction. In Pedretti LW, editor: *Occupational therapy: practice skills for physical dysfunction*, ed 4, St. Louis, 1996, Mosby.

O'Rourke RA, Chatterjee K, Wei JY: Coronary heart disease: 18th Bethesda conference report—cardiovascular disease in the elderly, *J Am Coll Cardiol* 10:52A, 1987.

Rodeheffer RJ, Gersten-Blith G, Becher LC: Exercise cardiac output is maintained with advancing age in unhealthy human subjects: cardiac dilation and increased stroke volume compensate for diminished heart rate, *Circulation* 69:203, 1984.

Working With Elders Who Have Pulmonary Conditions

ANGELA M. PERALTA AND SHERRELL POWELL

KEY TERMS

chronic obstructive pulmonary disease (COPD), chronic pulmonary emphysema, chronic bronchitis, bronchiectasis, energy conservation, work simplification

CHAPTER OBJECTIVES

1. Define chronic obstructive pulmonary disease.
2. Identify common symptoms of chronic obstructive pulmonary disease.
3. Identify the psychosocial effect of chronic obstructive pulmonary disease on elders.
4. List conditions that affect the sexual functioning of elders with chronic obstructive pulmonary disease.
5. Describe assessment and treatment intervention for elders with chronic obstructive pulmonary disease.

Denise is a COTA who works in a large rehabilitation hospital in the South Bronx in New York City. Her clients are from lower socioeconomic backgrounds. Many of them are factory workers and manual laborers. Denise has noticed a marked increase in the number of referrals to OT of elders who have **chronic obstructive pulmonary disease (COPD)** as a secondary diagnosis. These elders are finding it difficult to carry out their activities of daily living (ADLs) because of the debilitating effects of COPD. On reviewing their social histories, Denise found that many of these elders worked with a variety of chemicals and that many of them were heavy smokers. Some of the major problems these elders must deal with include difficulty engaging in self-care activities, a decreased level of endurance, chronic fatigue, and an inability to engage in leisure activities. Many elders with COPD report a fear of not being able to breathe because of frequent episodes of shortness of breath.

COPD is also seen in elder residents of nursing homes, usually as a secondary diagnosis. No matter the setting, COTAs working with elders who have COPD must be aware of the causes, symptoms, and OT interventions for this disease.

COPD

COPD is a general disease that can include **chronic pulmonary emphysema, chronic bronchitis,** and chronic severe asthma. Chronic bronchitis and emphysema affect the upper and lower respiratory tracts and are characterized by cough, expectoration, wheezing, and dyspnea. These symptoms occur first with exercise and later when the elder is at rest. Asthma, which is characterized by an increased responsiveness of the bronchi to various stimuli, results in bronchoconstriction, inflammation of the mucosa, and an increased amount of secretions (Tamparo, Lewis, 1995). COPD is associated with airflow obstruction, which may be accompanied by airway hyperreactivity and may be partially reversible (Snyder, 1996). Clinical symptoms of COPD vary depending on the severity and duration of the diseases.

Chronic Bronchitis

Chronic bronchitis is defined as the presence of a chronic productive cough and sputum production for at least 3 months out of a year for a 2-year period. One symptom of chronic bronchitis is hypersecretion of mucus in the respiratory tract in persons for whom other causes, such as infection, have been ruled out (Snyder, 1996). The sputum of a person with chronic bronchitis is usually thick yellow to gray. A deep productive cough is the main symptom of this disease. Other symptoms include shortness of breath, wheezing, a slightly elevated temperature, and pain in the upper chest that is aggravated by cough.

A person may have a mild form of chronic bronchitis for many years. Persons with mild chronic bronchitis may have only a slight cough in the morning after being inactive at night. This cough can become aggravated after the person has an acute upper respiratory tract infection. As the condition progresses, obstructive and asthmatic symptoms appear, along with dyspnea. Chest expansion becomes diminished, and scattered rales and wheezing are frequently heard (Schell-Frazier, Drzymkowski, Doty, 1996).

Bronchiectasis, a permanent dilation of the bronchi, is the most common complication of bronchitis. Bronchiectasis is often associated with bronchiolectasis, a dilation of the bronchiole. Such dilation occurs as a result of persistent inflammation inside the airways. The dilated bronchi and bronchiole are filled with mucopurulent material that stagnates and cannot be cleared by coughing. Infection then spreads into the adjacent alveoli, and recurrent episodes of pneumonia are common. Clubbing of the fingers often develops in elders with this condition (Damjanov, 1996).

Chronic Pulmonary Emphysema

Emphysema is a chronic condition characterized by permanent enlargement of the air spaces distal to the terminal bronchioles. Emphysema is accompanied by destruction of the alveolar walls and causes the lungs to lose elasticity, resulting in decreased airflow (Tamparo, Lewis, 1995). This decreased airflow results in dyspnea. Elders with emphysema have no bronchial obstruction or irritation that would cause them to expectorate (Damjanov, 1996). The inability to exhale the carbon monoxide that is trapped in the lungs causes the chest to overexpand, a condition referred to as *barrel chest*. The elder must hunch forward while holding onto a stable object to engage the auxiliary respiratory muscles during breathing. These elders manage to oxygenate their blood by hyperventilating, which prevents cyanosis and anoxia (Damjanov, 1996).

Asthma

Asthma is defined as a reversible airway disease characterized by an increased responsiveness of the trachea and the bronchi to various stimuli. Asthma is displayed by a widespread narrowing of the airways that changes in severity either spontaneously or as a result of therapy. During an acute attack, pronounced wheezing occurs because of difficulty in inhaling and exhaling air. Dyspnea, tachypnea, and chest tightness may also occur. The elder experiencing an asthmatic attack may also perspire profusely (Tamparo, Lewis, 1995).

PSYCHOSOCIAL EFFECT OF COPD

Rehabilitation of elders with COPD should include both medical management and assistance in coping with the debilitating effects of this chronic condition. As with any chronic condition, elders adapt in different ways. Some elders accept and adapt to the changes in energy level and other accompanying symptoms of COPD. For other elders, coping with symptoms of COPD may be a frustrating and depressing experience. Furthermore, elders with COPD often have additional stressors in their lives, such as the loss of a spouses and close friends, changes in living situation, a decrease in financial status, loss of productivity, lack of family support, inability to perform ADL functions, and loss of general body function (Damjanov, 1996).

Weakness and fatigue associated with COPD may require changes in living situations including a move to a higher level of assistive living. As with any move, emotional adaptations are required. Often elders with COPD seek to live in a different environment where they believe the air is cleaner or they can breathe better; however, they may find that such a move is not the solution to their problem because it cuts them off from a social support network. A sense of isolation may cause an increase in anxiety and may lead to depression.

Additional problems related to decreases in finances may arise for elders. The primary source of income for many elders is social security payments. Funds obtained from this source may not be sufficient to pay for medications or home health services if needed. The situation can be particularly frustrating for elders with COPD who are insured by Medicare because they will not be reimbursed for rehabilitation care unless they have a change in functional status.

In addition, elders with COPD may have a sense of loss of productivity if they are unable to engage in activities that provided enjoyment in previous years. Social isolation because of concerns about a decreased energy level, shortness of breath, oxygen usage, coughing, and sputum production may contribute to depression. Elders may become afraid that engaging in any type of physical activity may cause an increase in shortness of breath. This can lead to a cycle of fear and ultimately a need for more oxygen. Some elders with COPD also experience frustration because of a decline in their abilities to perform ADL functions as a result of a decreased level of endurance. Finally, some elders with COPD may have other chronic problems such as decreased vision or perhaps a general decline in other body systems. All these stressors could contribute to anxiety and depression.

Over time some elders with COPD begin to realize that a change in emotional status, whether positive or negative, has a direct effect on the respiratory system. Fear of expressing any type of emotion becomes a reality. This situation can further perpetuate a state of isolation. These elders may rationalize, "If I cannot express my emotions, then I will stay by myself." This position may be misinterpreted by others as hostility or aloofness, thereby creating more isolation.

SEXUAL FUNCTIONING

Elders with COPD may experience some loss of sexual functioning. Factors that may affect sexual functioning are shortness of breath, a decreased level of endurance, and a lack of desire. Changes in self-concept can also affect sexuality. Some men may have difficulty maintaining or obtaining an erection, perhaps because of fears of sexual failure. However, impotence can be the result of many causes, including side effects of medication. Therefore elders who are impotent should contact their physicians. Fear of sexual failure because of shortness of breath is one of the most common causes of sexual inactivity among elders with COPD. Engaging in sexual activity involves an increase in the breathing rate. For many elders a fear of suffocation or not being able to increase the depth of breathing inhibits their abilities to engage freely in sexual activity (Kim et al, 1984). COTAs can address some of the sexual functioning concerns of these elders by being open to discussing these concerns during treatment. Providing energy conservation suggestions such as encouraging elders to have sexual relations when they are most rested may be beneficial. (A more in-depth discussion of ways to address sexual concerns with elders is provided in Chapter 13.)

OCCUPATIONAL THERAPY ASSESSMENT AND TREATMENT PLANNING

COTAs contribute to the evaluation process of elders with COPD and collaborate with OTRs in treatment planning. ADL functions and productive and leisure activities are often the primary areas of concern. Elders may experience the most disabling symptoms of COPD, such as dyspnea and fatigue, when engaging in these activities. These symptoms, along with anxiety and depression related to the chronic illness, perpetuate the vicious cycle of inactivity. The deconditioning and muscle weakness that occurs from inactivity makes it increasingly difficult for elders to perform necessary ADL functions to be independent in the home and community (Shanfield, Hammond, 1984).

The OTR and COTA assess many performance components to determine the effects of COPD on function. Performance components such as sensory awareness are assessed to determine tactile impairment. Perceptual skills are assessed to determine an elder's response during episodes of dyspnea, particularly if they become dizzy. Neuromuscular components are assessed to determine physical tolerance and endurance, shortness of breath upon exertion, muscle strength, range of motion, and posture. Cognition is assessed to determine the elder's knowledge of the disease and accompanying problems. In addition, the elder's judgment, problem-solving skills, ability to generalize learning, and awareness of safety hazards are evaluated. Psychosocial ability is assessed to determine the elder's psychological, social, and self-management skills. Elders with COPD may experience feelings of hopelessness, depression, withdrawal from social activities, and dependency on a spouse or caregiver (American Psychiatric Association, 1994). Impairment in any of these areas directly affects the elder's ability to engage in self-care, work, and leisure activities.

COTAs must be aware of certain precautions during treatment. Knowing the various symptoms associated with COPD, such as shortness of breath and asthma, as well as the environmental irritants that can affect the elder's ability to breathe, is important. These irritants c an include cigarette smoking, dust from woodworking activities, and fumes that arise from activities such as copper tooling. Other irritants include talcum powder and certain perfumes, as well as poor air quality in the clinic.

OT intervention is geared toward increasing independence in functional activities by improving strength and endurance through resistive activities. Reconditioning programs such as the Metabolic Equivalents (METs) that are used with persons who have cardiac conditions are often used with persons who have COPD (Spencer, 1993). (A more in-depth discussion of the use of METs to guide activity prescriptions is provided in Chapter 25.) Low-impact exercise places minimum stress on joints and is easier to perform than high-impact activities. Exercise programs should include functional activities that target the upper body, and they should be designed to increase the strength of respiratory muscles. Activities should be stopped if nausea, dizziness, fatigue, increased shortness of breath, or chest pain develops.

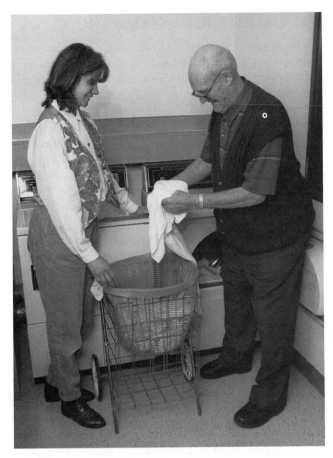

FIGURE 26-1 A COTA observes an elder practice energy conservation and work simplification techniques while he does laundry.

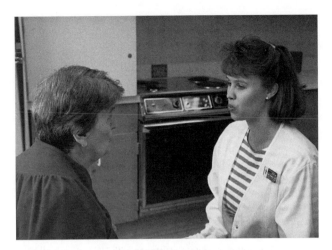

FIGURE 26-2 COTAs often must reinforce techniques such as "pursed-lip breathing" during activity.

The COTA and OTR team may also reinforce breathing techniques taught in the respiratory therapy program, such as pursed-lip breathing and diaphragmatic breathing (Figure 26-2). According to Spencer (1993), "Pursed-lip breathing creates a resistance to the flow of air out of the lungs and slows down the breathing rate. This technique is used with stressful activities to avoid shortness of breath. Diaphragmatic breathing decreases the cost of breathing and enables the elder to engage in purposeful activities." COTAs working with elders who have COPD must become efficient at administering oxygen and must be prepared to assist with controlled coughing, breathing, and other procedures.

Energy conservation and **work simplification** techniques are used with elders who are predisposed to fatigue (Figure 26-1). COTAs should try these techniques with elders rather than simply providing them with education sheets. Energy conservation and work simplification techniques should include scheduling rest periods in between activities, sitting whenever possible, reducing or eliminating steps, pushing rather than pulling, and analyzing an activity before starting it. Having all supplies for ADL functions within easy reach to avoid unnecessary trips is also beneficial. Time management is a technique that teaches elders to plan daily activities so that rest periods are "built in" to avoid some of the complications of COPD. Good time management skills may make the difference between a full, active life and a sedentary one.

Elders must develop the problem-solving skills needed to identify the fact that they are no longer able to perform a task in the customary way and when to change the process. Adaptive equipment such as a reacher, a cart to carry heavy items, and a motor scooter for outdoor activities can assist with function. In addition, COTAs can encourage elders to become involved in social activities. Teaching stress reduction techniques can help encourage elders have a sense of independence.

CONCLUSION

COPD is a common disease in the United States, especially among elders. COTA and OTR teams are becoming increasingly proactive in the treatment of this debilitating disease. They provide intervention to elders with COPD in a variety of settings. OT intervention is geared toward restoration of self-care skills, instruction in pacing of daily activities, and the restoration of physical capabilities. COTAs are instrumental in teaching compensatory techniques to be used in the performance of ADL functions and in the selection and use of assistive devices and adaptive equipment. COTAs may also become involved in teaching energy conservation and work simplification techniques. Addressing stress management may be a part of therapy; this may also help reinforce respiratory therapy breathing techniques. Ultimately the goal of OT with elders who have COPD is to maximize their level of independence as they adjust to living with a chronic condition.

CASE STUDY

M.B., a 65-year-old woman who is currently diagnosed with chronic emphysema, malnutrition, and depression, is five feet tall and weighs 80 pounds. She is a chronic smoker. M.B. is a widow and has four grown children who live nearby. M.B. has refused her children's help with ADL functions. She lives alone in a second floor apartment and does not have any assistance at home. Her children are concerned about her debilitating condition and have sought medical intervention. The physician ordered OT services at home after seeing M.B. Mark, the OTR, initiated the assessment, and Jenny, the COTA, contributed to the data collection for the assessment. OT assessment findings include the following:

1. M.B. has fair bilateral upper extremity (UE) muscle strength. Her bilateral UE range of motion is within functional limits except for 0 to 110 degrees shoulder flexion.

2. M.B. is dependent in bathing. She is unable to enter the bathtub because of low endurance and difficulty lifting her legs into the tub.

3. M.B. requires moderate assistance with UE and lower extremity (LE) dressing. She has difficulty obtaining clothes from her closet, carrying clothing items, and opening and closing drawers. UE dressing is limited by shoulder flexion of 110 degrees bilaterally.

4. M.B. is independent with simple meal preparation. However, she becomes tired after meal preparation and loses motivation to eat.

5. M.B. is unwilling to stop smoking.

6. M.B. has difficulty with ambulation within the apartment and with stairs because of a decreased level of endurance. She is unable to transport objects from one room to another or from one part of a room to another.

7. M.B. is able to drive a car. However, she fatigues easily and requires stand-by assistance to climb in and out of a car. Public bus transportation is not convenient.

8. M.B. becomes easily short of breath when washing and drying clothes. Placing clothes in the dryer is difficult for her because of the forward bending required for the task.

9. M.B. is dependent in cleaning activities.

10. M.B. does not participate in leisure activities that were of interest to her in the past, such as reading and socializing with friends. Reading is difficult because she experiences fatigue while holding a book. M.B. watches television while smoking and engages in telephone conversations with family and friends.

■ CHAPTER REVIEW QUESTIONS

1 List treatment interventions that the COTA might provide in the case of M.B.

2 Describe any community resources that might be useful to M.B.

3 Describe any psychosocial concerns for M.B. and how OT might intervene to address these concerns.

4 List the signs and symptoms of emphysema, bronchitis, asthma, and bronchiectasis.

5 Describe some psychological factors that may affect elders with COPD.

6 Describe factors relating to sexual functioning that may affect elders with COPD.

7 Describe any precautions to be aware of when working with elders who have COPD.

REFERENCES

American Psychiatric Association: Diagnostic and statistical manual of mental disorders, ed 4, Washington, DC, 1994, The Association.

Damjanov I: *Pathology for the health-related professions*, Philadelphia, 1996, WB Saunders.

Kim H et al: Psychosocial factors and pulmonary patients. In Hodgkins JE, Zorn EE, Connors JL, editors: *Pulmonary rehabilitation: guidelines to success*, Boston, 1984, Butterworth.

Schell-Frazier M, Drzymkowski JA, Doty SJ: *Essentials of human disease*, Philadelphia, 1996, WB Saunders.

Shanfield K, Hammond MA: Activities of daily living. In Hodgkins JE, Zorn EE, Connors JL, editors: *Pulmonary rehabilitation: guidelines to success*, Boston, 1984, Butterworth.

Snyder GL: Defining chronic obstructive pulmonary disease. In Calverly P, Pride N, editors: *Chronic obstructive pulmonary disease*, London, 1996, Chapman & Hall.

Spencer EA: Functional restoration: implementation of occupational therapy with adults. In Hopkins HL, Smith HD, editors: *Willard and Spackman's occupational therapy*, Philadelphia, 1993, JB Lippincott.

Tamparo CD, Lewis MA: *Diseases of the human body*, ed 2, Philadelphia, 1995, FA Davis.

CHAPTER 27

Working With Elders Who Have Oncological Conditions

LESLIE BRUNSTETER-WILLIAMS

KEY TERMS

cancer, metastasis, pathological fracture, myelosuppression, cachexia

CHAPTER OBJECTIVES

1. Identify common oncological diagnoses.
2. Discuss incidence of cancer as it relates to elders.
3. Define the role of occupational therapy in cancer care.
4. Understand the importance of the interdisciplinary team in cancer care.

The constant improvements in **cancer** treatment produced by ongoing clinical trials have resulted in better survival rates for people with cancer. Surgery, radiation, cytotoxic chemotherapy, and hormone therapy are all currently being used in cancer treatment. However, elders with cancer appear to be at a disadvantage because of their age. Clinical trials of treatment protocols are used to develop the most effective form of cancer treatments, and subjects are generally younger than 65 years of age (Ershler, Balducci, 1994). Elders are often considered rigid and untreatable, with comorbid conditions that cannot be reversed. Although comorbidity does occur with age, increasing evidence suggests that elders tolerate cancer treatments as well as their younger counterparts (Lindsey, Larson, Dodd, 1994; DiSilvestro et al, 1995). It is hoped that in the future, elders will be included in

cancer treatment trials, and improved treatment options will be made available on the basis of physiological rather than biological age.

GENERAL OVERVIEW OF COMMON CONDITIONS

This chapter discusses four types of cancer that are associated with increased risk in aging: breast, lung, prostate, and colorectal cancer (Table 27-1). With the exception of lung cancer, the 5-year survival rates for people over 65 years of age with these malignancies are significant. Therefore the need for rehabilitation of elders with cancer must be recognized. COTAs have a unique and valuable role in the interdisciplinary treatment of elders with cancer. Methods for improving overall function and quality of life are described later in this chapter.

TABLE 27-1

Five-Year Relative Survival Rates (Percent) for Common Malignancies in Persons Ages 65 Years and Over (1983-90)

Site	All races	
	65 to 74 yrs (%)	75+ yrs (%)
All sites	52.2	47.4
Lung/bronchus	12.6	8.5
Colon/rectum	60.5	56.4
Breast (females only)	82.7	81.3
Prostate (males only)	83.3	74.3

Adapted from Ries LAG et al, editors: *SEER cancer statistics review, 1973-1991: tables and graphs, national cancer institute,* [NIH Pub. No. 94-2789], Bethesda, Md, 1994, National Institutes of Health.

Breast Cancer

The incidence of breast cancer has been increasing for 40 years, with a dramatic rise occurring in the 1980s (Sondik, 1994). Earlier screening through the use of mammography may account for this increase. Earlier screening has resulted in increased early diagnoses of breast cancers (Wun, Feuer, Miller, 1995). Muss (1995) asserted that one in eight women in the United States will develop carcinoma of the breast during her lifetime and one in 28 American women will die from the disease. As with many other cancers, the incidence of breast cancer increases with age. Researchers estimate that over 43% of all new patients with breast cancer will be older than 65 years of age, with 52% of related deaths expected from this age group (Yancik, Ries, Yates, 1989). As a woman ages, her chance of developing breast cancer increases. The risk of a 40-year-old woman developing breast cancer by age 50 is 1 in 63, but by age 60, her chances increase to 1 in 26, and by age 70 the risk becomes a startling 1 in 14 (Garfinkel, Boring, Heath, 1994). In a report published by the American Association of Retired Persons (AARP) (1995), the population over age 65 has grown more than eightfold since the beginning of this century. The report also noted that in 1994 the ratio of females to males in this age group was 146 to 100. As the average length of life and the number of older women increase, researchers predict a corresponding increase in the number of elders with breast cancer being treated in health care settings.

Because breast cancer is increasingly being diagnosed at an early stage, the person is often asymptomatic at the time of diagnosis. The diagnosis is made when a breast mass is found to be malignant. Whether the surgical approach involves a lumpectomy with lymph node dissection or a modified radical mastectomy with removal of the entire breast and axillary lymph nodes, the elder must deal with important decisions. These decisions concern the future course of treatment and the psychological ramifications of dealing with a life-threatening illness.

Lung Cancer

Cancer of the lung is the most prevalent cancer in the Western world, and its incidence among women has increased significantly in recent years. This increase probably corresponds to the increase in the number of women who smoke. Lung cancer is now the leading cause of cancer-related death among women in the United States (Bruderman, 1994). The frequency of lung cancer increases up to the age of 70 years, with more than 40% of deaths attributable to lung cancer in people over 65 years of age (Byrne, Carney, 1993). Between 1973 and 1991, a 16.2% increase occurred in deaths caused by lung cancer in people under the age of 65 in the United States. The mortality rate increased sharply (67%) in those 65 years of age and older with the same disease (Ries, 1994). From 1987 to 1991 the incidence rate in people 65 years of age or older was estimated to be at an average of 317 per 100,000 cases (Ries, 1994).

The majority of lung malignancies have an infiltrative pattern of growth, which means that the tumor spreads within the mucosa of the lung and then through the lymphatic system (Bruderman, 1994). Because of the aggressive nature of this disease, it metastasizes early, frequently by the time of diagnosis (Bruderman, 1994). Because many people who develop lung cancer are or were smokers, the presence of cough or dyspnea (shortness of breath) may be nonspecific and usually is not the presenting symptom. Hemoptysis, or the presence of blood in the sputum, may be the symptom that brings the elder to the doctor for evaluation. If metastasis has occurred, chest pain in the midline of the chest or on the side of the tumor may be experienced as severe and debilitating.

Prostate Cancer

A report entitled "Trends in Prostate Cancer: United States, 1980 to 1988" (*Oncology,* 1993) identifies carcinoma of the prostate as the second most common cancer. This cancer most often affects men over the age of 70 years (Byrne, Carney, 1993). As with breast cancer the recent trends in prostate cancer may reflect improved screening practices. Diagnosis is made through blood tests, specifically the prostate-specific antigen (PSA) test (Brawer et al, 1992). This test is widely available and appears to be responsible for increased early detection and treatment.

If prostate cancer is diagnosed early and the tumor has a well-differentiated cytology, the disease can be slow and progressive. However, the cancer can be aggressive if poorly differentiated. Treatment involves surgical removal of the prostate gland and hormonal therapy. In cases of advanced metastatic disease, radiation therapy may be used as a palliative measure (Byrne, Carney, 1993).

Colorectal Cancer

Colorectal cancer is the second most common cause of fatal malignancies in the United States (DeCosse, Tsioulias, Jacobson, 1994). Individuals have a 1 in 20 risk of developing colorectal cancer, and this risk increases with age (Seidman et al, 1985). From 1987 to 1991 the incidence was 18.1 per 100,000 for persons under 65 years of age, increasing to 323.1 per 100,000 for those 65 years of age and older (Ries, 1994). Researchers have estimated that in 1996 a total of 133,500 new cases of colorectal cancers will be diagnosed (Parker, et al, 1996). As these statistics show, colorectal cancer will be increasingly treated in elders.

Initial presenting symptoms of colorectal cancer may include changes in bowel habits, the presence of blood in stools, and progressive weight loss. The primary tumor may be localized in the rectum, distal colon, or proximal colon areas. Surgery may be used as a curative treatment. If surgery is indicated, colostomy may be necessary. The elder's adjustment to this situation will need attention. Local invasion of colorectal cancer is evaluated at the time of diagnosis, and the course of treatment is outlined. Depending on the extent of tumor spread, treatment to control distant metastases may include surgery, radiation, and chemotherapy.

Metastases

Metastases occur when malignant or cancerous cells spread from the primary site of origin to other organs or systems of the body. This spread may be local, occurring in tissues surrounding the primary tumor site, or distant, traveling to another site in the body. This migration occurs via the blood vessels or the lymphatic system. Common sites of **metastasis** include breast cancer to bone, lungs, or brain; lung cancer to brain, liver, or bone; prostate cancer to bone; and colorectal cancer to liver or lungs.

Lung metastasis is commonly seen secondary to breast cancer but may also be found in progressed colorectal cancer. When lung metastasis occurs or lung cancer is the primary disease, pulmonary functions may change. This alteration may limit functional capacity and respiratory potential. Rehabilitation efforts can be beneficial in these situations. Rehabilitation works to maximize functional abilities through adaptation, pacing, and correct body mechanics.

Skeletal, or bone, metastasis may be seen secondary to breast, prostate, and colorectal cancers. When weight-bearing or long bones are affected by metastases, they become weakened in structure and susceptible to easy breaking or **pathological fractures.** A pathological fracture may occur with the placement of very little weight or pressure on the bone. For example, if an elder's humerus has a metastatic lesion, an activity such as taking out the trash or picking up a carton of soda could actually precipitate a fracture at that site. When upper extremities are affected by a fracture, immobilization, surgical reduction, and radiation therapy may be used alone or in combination. During this period the elder can use only one-hand and may require training in self-care tasks. Should the hip or femur be affected, partial or total hip replacement surgery may be performed to restore integrity and return weight-bearing potential to the hip joint. (Refer to Chapter 24 for details on this type of surgery.) After surgery, rehabilitation efforts should include instruction in total hip precautions during ADL functions, including adaptive equipment to allow for limited hip flexion and adduction. If healing does not occur after surgery and the joint remains unstable, use of a walker during ADL functions and avoidance of weight-bearing on the affected hip joint may be necessary. If metastasis involves the spinal column, pain can be a major problem. Medical treatment includes epidural nerve blocks to the spinal area, radiation treatments, and surgical stabilization of the spine. During rehabilitation, emphasis should be placed on use of correct body mechanics in functional tasks to protect the spine and prevent further damage.

PSYCHOSOCIAL ASPECTS OF ONCOLOGICAL CONDITIONS

When dealing with cancer, elders have varying emotional needs depending on the stage of the illness. Stages include initial diagnosis, treatment, disease recurrence, and the terminal stage of the illness. The elder's reaction(s) to the diagnosis might include anxiety, denial, worry, anger, and depression (Mor, Allen, Malin, 1994). Helplessness, uncertainty, and fear are also common. Fear may be related to a loss of control. It may also originate in a fear of pain, which has been associated with cancer. For example, in the case of early-stage lung cancer, pain may be caused by the chest tumor or metastatic areas in the bone. Lack of sufficient pain control may exacerbate fears of dying (Bernhard, Ganz, 1994). COTAs can help by actively listening to elders, allowing them to express feelings and fears and providing emotional support. The diagnosis of cancer suggests images of death and dying to most people, but in fact, with improved screening and more effective treatments, many elders can continue to lead productive, satisfying lives.

During the early phase of diagnosis and treatment the establishment of trust between the elder and health professional is essential in helping the elder adjust to treatment and maintain compliance (Bernhard, Ganz, 1994). When elders and families are given information regarding treatment and potential toxicities, fear of the unknown may decrease.

The successful treatment of cancer, whether it includes chemotherapy, radiation, surgery, or a combination of any of these, often brings adverse side effects with which the elder must deal. Elders often have one or more chronic conditions already present, such as arthritis, heart disease, orthopedic impairments, diabetes, and visual impairments (AARP, 1995). These comorbid conditions may compound the problematic side effects of cancer treatment. Alopecia, or hair loss, may occur as a side effect of certain chemotherapeutic drugs. Total-brain irradiation for brain cancer may also cause alopecia. This change in body image can negatively affect elders' self-esteem, sometimes causing them to avoid social activities that were once important to them. Social support is important for elders with cancer. If elders neglect previously important activities, they also lose opportunities for emotional assistance. Women may have difficulty adjusting to the loss of a breast after a mastectomy and experience changes in their feelings about femininity and sexuality. In both cases, losses have occurred that will precipitate the grieving process (Bloch, Kissane, 1995).

Cytotoxic drugs can affect the bone marrow by impairing its ability to produce needed white blood cells, red blood cells, and platelets. This phenomenon is called **myelosuppression.** Myelosuppression renders elders susceptible to infection, anemia, and easy bruising. Elders may need to limit their contacts with others during this period to prevent infection. This may decrease the emotional support available, adding to feelings of isolation. COTAs can encourage solitary activities such as putting photos in albums, which promotes reminiscence; rewriting recipe cards; and communicating with friends through letter writing.

During the course of cancer treatment, fatigue is common. Performing everyday tasks such as bathing and dressing may be difficult and may require assistance. Adjustment to this loss of independence may be difficult for elders, and a profound feeling of loss of control may surface. Social support and referral to community resources that provide assistance with daily living activities can be beneficial during this period.

During cancer treatment the chronic nature of the disease may become evident. Routines include regular medical appointments for treatment and blood work. Periodic radiographic scans are also necessary to assess response to treatment. Transportation to and from clinics may present a problem for many elders. This stress, compounded with anxiety about the possible recurrence of cancer, may result in emotional difficulties.

If the cancer recurs, initial feelings of denial and anger may resurface. At this point, uncertainty about the future becomes a real concern (Mor, Allen, Malin, 1994). If recurrence results in loss of function or strength, family

roles may change, and family education and support by the health care team are essential. Cancer has been called a "family affair," and its effect on the family is evident throughout all stages of the illness (Mor, Allen, Malin, 1994). According to a report published by the AARP (1995), 68% of elders lived in a family setting in 1994. An example of the effects of cancer on the family follows. An active man with lung cancer is no longer able to meet the physical demands of meal preparation and homemaking, duties that he previously performed. Although his wife might need to assume these duties, he can still participate in menu planning and grocery shopping, thereby contributing to the family needs.

Many community cancer support and self-help groups exist. Both elders with cancer and their caregivers may find these groups beneficial. Meeting others who are dealing with similar changes and problems can help alleviate fear and anxiety. The health care team should facilitate referrals to these community groups when the need is identified. Examples of available support organizations are Reach to Recovery (for people who have undergone breast surgery), the American Cancer Society, the local YMCA (for indoor exercise or swim programs), and hospital-based support groups.

Quality of life is an elusive term, one that continues to be studied by many professionals with diverse perspectives. The four areas generally included in defining quality of life are physical, functional, emotional, and social status (Balducci, 1994). The ultimate goal in the rehabilitation of elders with cancer is to maintain quality of life. Because these different areas overlap, each area must be thoroughly explored. However, functional status is likely to influence all other domains (Balducci, 1994). The way elders perceive their functional status influences emotional adjustment and ultimately affects their abilities or desires to seek out needed social support. Therefore maintaining functional status becomes the primary goal in treatment.

When elders reach the terminal stage of the cancer process, family support and education are critical. The identification of needed home care services, such as a homemaker, hospice intervention, and occasional respite care, becomes the primary focus of the health care team. Measures provided should alleviate suffering while maintaining dignity. All home care services should be coordinated, promoting the emotional adjustment and support of the entire family. (Chapter 28 contains further information regarding the hospice philosophy and approach.)

OT TREATMENT
Evaluation and Treatment Plan

Elders who have cancer require a holistic approach to treatment. Intervention should be tailored to all stages of the disease: diagnosis, treatment, recurrence, and in the terminal stage for palliation of symptoms. The first step in the OT evaluation of elders with cancer is a thorough review of the client's medical record. Particular attention should be paid to radiographic studies in the event of known skeletal metastasis and laboratory blood studies, which may reveal myelosuppression.

After reviewing the medical record, the OTR and COTA collaborate in the evaluation of the elder. The elder's functional status should remain the focus of assessment, with both deficits and functional capabilities identified. Sensorimotor performance should be assessed, particularly the elder's functional endurance and strength. During the evaluation process, communication with the family is especially important. The family can describe the elder's functional status before admission. COTAs should ask about adaptive equipment at home and whether the elder has received previous instruction in adaptation so that this information can be incorporated into the treatment plan.

COTAs then develop a treatment plan, which includes problem areas that can be improved through adaptation, strengthening, and education. The goals of treatment must be objective and measurable and should reflect the elder's personal values and goals. At this point, communication with other team members is important to provide the most beneficial and comprehensive plan. During the treatment process, the COTA and OTR should meet regularly to discuss complications and the elder's tolerance of treatment and improvements. The medical record must be periodically checked to monitor the elder's response to medical treatment, progression of the disease, and changes in blood counts. Treatment is adapted to meet the changing needs of the elder. During the treatment process, the family or primary caretaker should be included in treatment and education. This participation enables them to understand the capabilities of the elder, as well as the type and amount of assistance that will be necessary after discharge. If changes in family roles or duties are necessary, COTAs can provide support and assistance in renegotiation of role functioning (Lloyd, Coggles, 1990). As discharge nears, important topics for discussion include home care needs, equipment needs, and assistance required in the client's care. (Further discussion follows in the section titled "Discharge Planning.")

Treatment Goals and Strategies

The primary purpose and ultimate goal of OT intervention is to maximize the elder's functional independence within the limits of the disease. The desired outcome is that elders gain an increased sense of control over the environment, feel improved self-esteem, and take more responsibility for their lives (Lloyd, Coggles, 1990). To meet this goal, COTAs work to improve the elder's abilities in independent living skills through training in dressing, bathing, feeding, homemaking, functional am-

bulation, transfers, and leisure activities. If needed, adaptive equipment can provide a means to complete activities. COTAs should instruct clients in the use of this equipment and encourage them to practice using it. The family should also be included in the education process. If weakness or deconditioning limits elders' functional independence, COTAs may suggest some general strengthening exercises to increase functional capacity.

As noted, fatigue is a common problem among elders with cancer. Conservation of energy becomes an important aspect of preventive OT. COTAs can provide instruction in energy conservation and work simplification in ADL functions (Figure 27-1). These techniques may include learning to prioritize daily tasks, use improved body mechanics, organize work centers, and rest frequently. To understand elders' feelings and help address them, families must also understand the effects of fatigue and the purpose of energy conservation techniques (Lloyd, Coggles, 1990). In the case of an elder man with prostate cancer that had metastasized to his spine and pelvis, adapting his position during bathing by use of a shower bench allowed him to be independent. This change kept him from bending, thus limiting stress on his spine while conserving energy and helping prevent a fall. COTAs may provide written materials on body mechanics and energy conservation to elders and family (Boxes 27-1 and 27-2).

OT treatment may include various orthotic devices designed to protect and support joints, maintain functional position, relieve pain, promote healing, support fractures, reduce deformities, and improve functioning (Lloyd, Neven, 1989). Examples of devices frequently seen are lumbosacral supports, arm elevators, slings, and braces. COTAs may need to fabricate an upper or lower extremity splint to provide needed joint support and

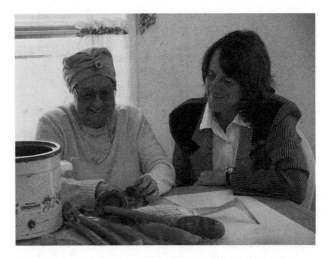

FIGURE 27-1 COTAs provide instructions in energy conservation and work simplification during meal preparation tasks.

BOX 27-1

Body Mechanics to Decrease Stress on Bones and Skeletal System

1. Pain may arise from sitting in one position for prolonged periods of time; therefore change positions frequently.
2. While working at a desk or table, make sure the work surface is the correct height so that your shoulders are not raised or lowered and your neck is not bent forward.
3. While sitting for activities, place a small pillow or rolled towel at your lower back for added support. Also, keep your knees higher than your hips by using a low stool to slightly raise your feet.
4. Stooping and bending are not advised, but if you must perform an activity in a bent position, interrupt the position at regular intervals **before** the pain starts. This may be done by standing upright or sitting down briefly.
5. Avoid bending your neck backwards; you may need to rearrange your kitchen to prevent reaching and looking up for items on high shelves.
6. While driving, move the seat forward enough to keep your knees bent and back straight. Using a small pillow or supportive roll behind your lower back may be helpful while sitting in the car.
7. When moving from a lying position to a sitting position, first roll on your side and bring your legs up toward your chest; then, as you swing your legs off the bed, push up with your arms.
8. Usually a good firm bed with support is desirable. If your bed is sagging, slats or plywood supports between the mattress and base will help add firmness.
9. Whenever lifting, follow these rules:
   - Stand close to the object
   - Concentrate on using the small curve, or lordosis, in your lower back
   - Bend at your knees and keep your back straight.
   - Get a secure grip and hold the load as close to you as possible
   - Lean back slightly to stay in balance and lift the load by straightening your knees
   - Take a steady lift, and do not jerk
   - When upright, shift your feet to turn and avoid twisting the lower back

BOX 27-2

Work Simplification Techniques to Decrease Stress on Bones and Skeletal System

1. Avoid stairs whenever possible. Use ramps or elevators. When you must use stairs, take them one at a time to decrease stress on your joints.
2. Whenever possible, sit rather than stand while working. Any activity that lasts longer than 10 minutes should be done from a seated position.
3. Avoid sitting or lying on low surfaces such as beds or chairs. Use foam or pillows to raise the seat.
4. Avoid kneeling or squatting. If you absolutely must squat, use heavy objects nearby to help pull yourself up.
5. Slide objects rather than lifting or carrying, and push rather than pull objects whenever possible.
6. Do not reach up high for an object; instead, use a stool or long-handled reachers.
7. Never start an activity that cannot be stopped immediately if it proves too strenuous.
8. When performing a daily activity with equipment or tools, use lightweight tools. Stand near the work rather than reaching.

maintain the joint in a functional position. Once the orthotic device is in place, treatment should include instruction of elders and their families regarding purpose, proper positioning, methods of donning and doffing, wearing schedule, and care of the device or support.

Cancer affects the entire family, and as physical and functional changes occur, alterations in family roles may become necessary. The loss of a contributory role may be difficult for elders to accept, and COTAs can help in this adjustment by suggesting alternative roles that may be more practical. Rather than being involved in the physical jobs of homemaking or yardwork, for example, elders may now become involved in checkbook balancing and decision making. Inclusion of the family in discussion and planning is important to determine the amount of assistance needed and fully understand the elder's abilities (Lloyd, Coggles, 1990).

OT practitioners should address both the emotional and physical needs of elders. Ideally, treatment goals for elders who have cancer should combine these needs with recognition of the psychological effects of cancer. COTAs need to maintain and communicate respect for the client, as well as demonstrate empathy. Maintaining eye contact and listening carefully convey the message that the elder with cancer continues to be valued as a human being (Lloyd, Coggles, 1990). If elders are extremely anxious, COTAs may suggest relaxation exercises such as visual imagery and deep breathing. Music has been shown to decrease anxiety, depression, and feelings of isolation (Cook, 1986). The appropriate use of therapeutic touch is also helpful in treatment and reminds elders that they will not be rejected because of their illness (Lloyd, Neven, 1989). As mentioned earlier, alopecia may cause decreased self-esteem. In the case of an elder woman with lung cancer who loses her hair after chemotherapy, the COTA may provide or suggest a turban, scarf, or wig. The COTA may also coordinate a facial or makeover, which could help restore the elder's self-esteem.

Special Considerations in Treatment Planning and Implementation

The treatment of elders with cancer requires awareness of certain considerations unique to this population. Because of the abnormal resting energy expenditures found in hospitalized cancer patients, attention must be given to the effect of fatigue on rehabilitation (Lloyd, Neven, 1989). **Cachexia,** or general ill health and malnutrition, is manifested in overall weakness, generalized muscle atrophy, and loss of body mass. Cachexia occurs when energy intake decreases because of biochemical abnormalities or loss of appetite. Progressive activity is difficult to promote in elders with cachexia. The elder's physical tolerance to the treatment provided and current nutritional intake should be considered when working toward functional achievement.

Elders with cancer who are experiencing depression and fatigue may show a lack of interest in participating in treatment. The combination of depression and fatigue makes ongoing emotional support by all team members essential. Involving elders in identifying meaningful goals of treatment may help increase their motivation. If additional supportive care is needed, formal psychosocial interventions may be necessary.

One of the greatest challenges in working with elders who have cancer occurs when physical changes take place or when functional abilities are lost because of disease progression. At this point, COTAs should reassess clients' capabilities and develop new, realistic, goals with them. They should also provide frequent encouragement and reassurance during this process.

Complications Related to Cancer and its Treatment

Complications of inactivity may occur as a result of fatigue. Metabolic and physiological changes occur secondary to prolonged bed rest (Mellette, Blunk, 1994). Reports also indicate changes in cardiovascular functions, muscle wasting, joint stiffness, and ligament weakness when inactivity is continuous (Rose, Rothstand, 1982; Greenleaf, 1984; Akeson et al, 1987). These problems can complicate the rehabilitation process and require a carefully monitored progressive treatment program. Complications from cytotoxic (cell-damaging) chemotherapeutic drugs require on-going monitoring. If myelosuppression occurs, changes in the daily treatment plan may become necessary. For example, with decreased normal white blood cells, or granulocytopenia, resistance to infection decreases. Therefore keeping elders away from potential sources of infection (for example, other elders) is important. Good hand-washing techniques and frequent cleaning of equipment are also essential. If the normal production of platelets is decreased (thrombocytopenia), sharp objects should be avoided during treatment. Decreasing the amount of physical resistance used in exercise may be necessary. These strategies lessen the risk of unnecessary bleeding, which further compromises the elder's status. Other complications may occur secondary to cancer treatment or the disease process itself (Table 27-2). The COTA must be aware of potential complications and modify treatment accordingly if these occur.

Lymphedema, or swelling that results from an abnormal collection of protein-rich fluid, is sometimes seen after lymph-node removal or radiation treatment for breast cancer (Passik et al, 1993). If the lymph nodes are absent after dissection or rendered ineffective after radiation, the normal pathway for fluid removal in the affected upper extremity is interrupted. The fluid accumulates, and the upper extremity swells (Figure 27-2). Lymphedema can also occur in the lower extremities if the inguinal lymph nodes are involved. This condition may also be accompanied by chronic inflammation, pain, and fibrosis (Passik et al, 1993). Lymphedema can be a major problem, interfering with the ability to wear certain types of clothing, negatively affecting body image and hindering the performance of daily activities. Rehabilitation approaches include applying pressure to the extremity with compression garments or bandages, exercise, massage therapy (known as *manual lymph drainage*), and sequential pumps. Treatment can improve skin texture and overall appearance, decrease limb girth, and increase functionality.

Discharge Planning

Because of the short duration of hospital stays and the push for the earliest possible discharge, discharge planning must begin early and continue throughout treatment. This preparation and discussion occurs as an ongoing process between the team members, elders, and their families. A weekly team meeting is a good way to bring all the team members together to share concerns, identify the needs of elders, and develop a comprehensive plan for their discharge.

Necessary home equipment that will improve safety and independence in the home should be discussed. The family should be present to help identify potential problems in daily activities. When equipment needs have been identified, COTAs can assist in the selection of this equipment and provide instruction in its proper use, set-up, and care. If a caregiver must assist the elder in using the equipment, the caregiver should also be trained in its use. If assistance is required in any daily activity, COTAs can instruct caregivers and family members in proper methods of care, including proper transfers and bathing assistance.

TABLE 27-2

Complications in Elders With Cancer

Complication	Clinical symptoms	OT treatment implications
Granulocytopenia (decreased white blood cells)	Increased susceptibility to infection	Good hand-washing technique, frequent cleaning of equipment, wearing of mask if in reverse isolation; treatment in client's room
Thrombocytopenia (decreased platelets)	Easy bruising, potential for bleeding, CNS bleeding	Avoidance of sharp objects, resistive exercises, participation in less strenuous activities
Anemia (decreased red blood cells)	Easy fatiguing, shortness of breath	Frequent rest periods, client monitored for fatigue, treatment modified according to client's tolerance
Hypercalcemia (excessive calcium in blood; normal level: 8-10.5 mg Ca^{++})	Confusion, giddiness, mental status changes, drowsiness, polyuria, polydypsia	Consultation with physician before beginning activity, reality orientation
Hyperkalemia (abnormally high level of potassium)	Weakness, paralysis, ECG changes, renal disease if severe	Decrease in physical demands of treatment
Airway obstruction (emergent situation caused by tumor impingement on trachea)	Coughing, SOB, acute difficulty breathing	Immediate notification of medical staff
Increased intracranial pressure (caused by primary tumor or metastatic lesion in the brain)	Headaches, blurred vision, nausea or vomiting, seizure	Avoidance of physically active tasks, avoidance of tasks requiring fine vision, quiet environment for treatment
Spinal cord compression (caused by tumor impingement on spinal cord)	Back pain, leg pain or weakness, sensory loss, bowel or bladder retention	Consultation with physician before treatment, avoidance of resistive exercise, extreme care in client transfers, immediate notification of any changes in sensation or strength
Skin desquamation (breakdown of outer layer of skin)	Open ulcers on skin, fragile epidermis	Protection of skin surfaces during treatment, avoidance of abrasive contact
Cardiac toxicity (decreased cardiac output or function)	Limited cardiovascular tolerance, SOB, dizziness	Selection of activities that do not exceed client's tolerance, monitoring of client's pulse and blood pressure during treatment
Peripheral neuropathy (impaired sensory pathways in upper or lower extremities)	Impaired sensation; loss of coordination; unsteady gait, foot-drop	Adaptive equipment, splints, compensation techniques

CNS, Central nervous system; *ECG*, electrocardiogram; *SOB*, shortness of breath.

In some cases, OT treatment at home may be beneficial. An assessment within the home by an OTR and COTA team ensures proper set-up of equipment and use of the best space available for ADL functions. The team can also give the caretaker and family needed support in bringing their loved one home.

CASE STUDY

Mrs. D. is a 70-year-old woman who underwent a right modified radical mastectomy, secondary to a diagnosis of infiltrating ductal carcinoma that was detected through an abnormal mammogram and confirmed through biopsy. A postsurgical metastatic workup revealed that metastatic lesions were present in her thoracic spine and pelvis. The ax-

illary lymph node dissection revealed that 12 of the 18 nodes removed were malignant, indicating lymph node metastasis. Postsurgical systemic chemotherapy was recommended, followed by irradiation treatments to her thoracic spine and pelvis. Mrs. D.'s past medical history includes hypertension and degenerative arthritis of the spine. Before this admission, Mrs. D. lived with her husband of 35 years and performed all homemaking duties, was active in a bridge club and in church activities, and volunteered at a nursing home. Her hobbies included gardening and needlework. Mrs. D. has two grown children, both living in other states.

In the OT assessment, the OTR and COTA found that Mrs. D. was right-hand dominant and had limitations in active range of motion at her right shoulder since her sur-

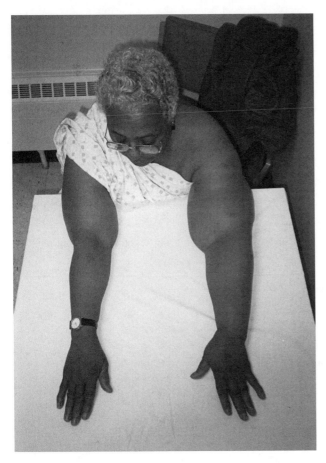

FIGURE 27-2 Lymphedema is swelling that results from the abnormal accumulation of protein-rich fluid. This condition is sometimes seen after lymph node removal or radiation treatment for breast cancer.

gery. Active shoulder flexion and abduction were limited to 90 degrees 4 days after surgery, with mild numbness or paresthesia in her axilla. Because of her limited range of motion, Mrs. D. was unable to perform grooming and bathing independently and was fearful of moving her arm. She had previously experienced back pain intermittently as a result of arthritis in her spine; now she has questions regarding ways to move without injuring herself. Mrs. D. was found to have good endurance. She is anxious to return home and resume her previous activities.

■ CHAPTER REVIEW QUESTIONS

1 Considering the case study above, identify independent living skills that could be used to help Mrs. D. in the gradation of shoulder range of motion to facilitate full return of movement.

2 The upper extremity precautions after breast surgery include avoidance of cuts, pinpricks, or infections in the affected arm to prevent the occurrence of lymphedema. During what activities will Mrs. D. need to take particular precautions for this? What might she do to protect her arm?

3 What principles of body mechanics should the COTA teach Mrs. D. to protect her spine and pelvis? What principles should be covered to prevent falls?

4 What are some examples of adaptive equipment that could help Mrs. D. maintain her independence while protecting her from pathological fracture?

5 When should the COTA include Mr. D's. husband in the OT treatment?

6 What needs should the COTA communicate to the other team members during discharge planning to ease the transition from hospital to home?

7 What other special considerations in treatment apply to Mrs. D?

8 Research has shown an increased incidence of breast cancer and lung cancer among elder women. To what are these increases attributed?

9 If a pathological fracture occurred in the hip, what would the rehabilitation approaches include?

10 Discuss the psychological symptoms that may occur with elders who have cancer at various stages.

11 Why is involvement and education of the client's family important in the treatment process?

12 Describe the role of the COTA in discharge planning.

REFERENCES

Akeson WH et al: Effects of immobilization on joints, *Clin Orthop* 219:28, 1987.

American Association of Retired Persons: *Profile of older Americans*, Washington, DC, 1995, The Association (brochure).

Balducci L: Perspectives on quality of life of older patients with cancer, *Drugs Aging* 4(4):313, 1994.

Bernhard J, Ganz P: Psychosocial issues in lung cancer patients. In Hansen H, Hansen, editors: *Cancer treatment and research*, Zurich, 1994, Kluwer Academic Publisher.

Bloch S, Kissane D: Psychosocial care and breast cancer, *Lancet* 346 (8983):1114, 1995.

Brawer MK et al: Screening for prostatic carcinoma with prostate specific antigen, *J Urol* 147:841, 1992.

Bruderman I: Bronchogenic carcinoma. In Baum GL, Wolinski E, editors: *Textbook of pulmonary diseases*, Boston, 1994, Little, Brown.

Byrne A, Carney D: Cancer in the elderly, *Curr Probl Cancer* 17(3): 145, 1993.

Commentary, *Oncology* 7(4):18, 1993.

Cook JD: Music as an intervention in the oncology setting, *Cancer Nurs* 9(1):23, 1986.

DeCosse JJ, Tsioulias GJ, Jacobson JS: Colorectal cancer: detection, treatment, and rehabilitation, *Cancer J Clinicians* 44(1):27, 1994.

DiSilvestro PA et al: You may think I'm too old, but can't you treat my cancer? *R I Med* 78(5):143, 1995.

Ershler WB, Balducci L: Treatment considerations for older patients with cancer, *In Vivo* 8(5):737, 1994.

Garfinkel L, Boring CC, Heath CW: Changing trends: an overview of breast cancer incidence and mortality, *Cancer* 74 (suppl 1):222, 1994.

Greenleaf JE: Physiologic responses to prolonged bed rest and fluid immersion in humans, *J Appl Physiol* 57(3):619, 1984.

Lindsey AM, Larson PJ, Dodd MJ: Comorbidity, nutritional intake, social support, weight, and functional status over time in older cancer patients receiving radiotherapy, *Cancer Nurs* 17(2):113, 1994.

Lloyd C, Coggles L: Psychosocial issues for people with cancer and their families, *Can J Occup Ther* 57(4):211, 1990.

Lloyd C, Neven J: Occupational therapy and the elderly cancer patient, *Phys Occup Ther Geriatr* 6(3-4):87, 1988.

Mellette SJ, Blunk KL: Cancer rehabilitation, *Semin Oncol* 21(6):779, 1994.

Mor V, Allen S, Malin M: The psychosocial impact of cancer on older versus younger patients and their families, *Cancer Suppl* 74(7):2118, 1994.

Muss H: Chemotherapy of breast cancer in the older patient, *Semin Oncol* 22(suppl 1):14, 1995.

Parker SL et al: Cancer statistics, 1996, *Cancer J Clinicians* 46(1):5, 1996.

Passik S et al: Psychiatric consultation for women undergoing rehabilitation for upper extremity lymphedema following breast cancer treatment, *J Pain Symptom Manage* 8(4):226, 1993.

Ries LAG et al, editors: *SEER cancer statistics review, 1973-1991: tables and graphs* (NIH Pub. No. 94-2789), Bethesda, Md, 1994, National Cancer Institute.

Rose SJ, Rothstein JM: Muscle mutability, part I. General concepts and adaptations to altered patterns of use, *Phys Ther* 62(12):1773, 1982.

Seidman H et al: Probabilities of eventually developing or dying of cancer: United States, 1985, *Cancer J Clinicians* 35(1):36, 1985.

Sondik EJ Breast cancer trends, incidence, mortality, and survival, (suppl 3): *Cancer* 74(suppl 3):995, 1994.

Wun LN, Feuer EJ, Miller BA: Are increases in mammographic screening still a valid explanation for trends in breast cancer incidence in the United States? *Cancer Causes Control* 6(2):135, 1995.

Yancik R, Ries LG, Yates JW: Breast cancer in aging women, *Cancer* 63:976, 1989.

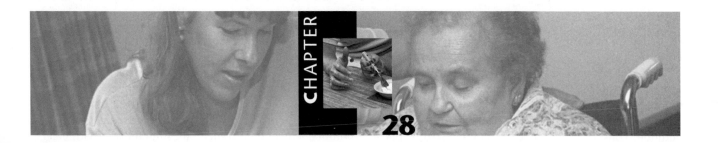

CHAPTER 28

Working With Elders in Hospice

SUE BYERS-CONNON AND JEAN VANN

KEY TERMS

hospice, palliative, terminal illness, communication, caregivers, cultural differences

CHAPTER OBJECTIVES

1. Define and discuss the hospice concept.
2. Define the role of the COTA in hospice care.
3. Discuss the role of the hospice team.
4. Explain the fears of the dying person.
5. Relate ways of communicating with the dying person.
6. Discuss ways to teach and communicate with caregivers.

"You Matter Because You Are You . . .
You Matter To The Last Moment Of Your Life . . .
And We Will Do All We Can . . .
Not Only To Help You Die Peacefully . . .
But Also To Live Until You Die."
Dame Cicely Saunders, St. Christopher's Hospice, London

Hospices originated in medieval times as way stations where weary travelers rested. They were usually located in monasteries, and monks set the precedent of nurturing and caring that established the philosophy of **hospice** today.

With a holistic background as a nurse, social worker, and physician, Dame Cicely Saunders began the modern hospice movement in 1969. She established St. Christopher's Hospice in London according to a model of **palliative** care for the dying that provides symptom control and emphasizes quality of life.

The first U.S. hospice opened in 1971 in New Haven, Connecticut. The National Hospice Organization was organized in the 1970s and incorporated in 1978. Medicare hospice guidelines were established in 1982. Soon after, most hospice organizations sought Medicare hospice accreditation (Hamilton, Reid, 1980).

In a Medicare-certified hospice the primary physician must document that the elder has an estimated life span of 6 months or less and is not seeking active treatment. Care should be provided by a Medicare-participating hospice program, using only palliative, or pain-relieving, treatment (Health Care Financing Association, 1993). Occupational therapy services are available to elders, at least on a contract basis, in Medicare-certified hospice programs (Thiers, 1993).

Hospice no longer refers to a specific place; it suggests instead a concept of care. Most of this care is provided in the individual's home but may also occur in hospitals, free-standing hospices, group homes, foster care homes, nursing homes, and adult day-care centers. Regardless of the setting, the primary mission is to help dying people and their families handle the burdens and trauma of dying. Maintaining the client's dignity is a major concern.

This chapter provides COTAs with examples of OT interventions in the hospice setting. The importance of working effectively with family members, caregivers, and members of the hospice team is also discussed. In addition, considerations for COTAs interested in practicing in a hospice setting are covered.

THE HOSPICE PHILOSOPHY

The American Occupational Therapy Association (AOTA) position paper on hospice states the following:

> "The hospice philosophy states that dying is a normal process of life whether or not resulting from disease. Hospice exists neither to hasten nor to postpone death. Rather, hospice exists to affirm life by providing support and care for those in the last phases of an incurable disease, so that the person live as fully and comfortably as possible. Hospice promotes the formation of caring communities that are sensitive to the needs of patients and their families at this time in their lives so that they may be free to obtain that degree of mental and spiritual preparation for death that is satisfactory to them" (AOTA, 1981).

THE ROLE OF THE HOSPICE TEAM

The hospice team can include a physician, nurse, social worker, home health aide, OT practitioner, RPT, pastoral counselor, volunteer coordinator, well-trained volunteers, bereavement counselor, speech-language pathologist, and dietitian. The roles of the hospice team members are defined as follows. A physician serves as the medical director of the team. An elder may also have a personal physician. The medical director is present at staff meetings and available to the team at all times. One of the medical director's primary roles is to collaborate with the elder's primary physician on medical matters. The elder's primary physician should have the major responsibility for care. The medical director also advises members of the hospice team. Nurses generally direct the hospice team and also serve as the primary team managers. Nurses provide pain management, monitor physical symptoms, dispense medications; and meet the elder's overall medical needs. Nursing services are available on an intermittent basis 24 hours a day through home visits and telephone consultations. Social workers provide information pertaining to resources, counseling, financial assistance, and emotional support for the elder, family members, and caregivers. Home health aides assist with personal care and bathing and can perform light household tasks. RPTs are concerned with safe mobility, equipment needs, and sometimes physical agent modalities for pain relief. Speech-language pathologists (SLP) may be called on to provide assistance to clients who are having difficulties in communicating and swallowing. Pastoral counselors provide spiritual support or contact a counselor from the elder's own church if requested to do so. All members of the hospice team provide emotional support for family members and caregivers. The volunteer coordinator recruits and trains volunteers and assigns them to clients. The volunteers provide respite care for families, allowing caregivers to leave home for a few hours. They can also spend meaningful time with elders. The bereavement counselor follows each family for 1 year after the death of the elder and may also suggest support programs in the community. Dietitians advise about nutrition.

The role of OT is discussed throughout this chapter. The common thread that links hospice and OT is quality of life. Both hospice and OT use a holistic approach and foster self-actualization (Brown, 1984). Interventions include providing adaptations, teaching energy conservation and relaxation techniques, providing meaningful activities, training caregivers, and helping elders maintain autonomy in their life roles. All team members should communicate regularly and work together for the benefit of the individual. "A degree of role blurring inevitably occurs among the disciplines, and this needs to be permitted" (Hospice Task Force, 1987). According to Flanigan (1982), "to serve the best interests of the patients who are striving for a meaning in a limited life, we must be able to sidestep the defined limits of our traditional roles and cooperate in providing hospice care."

HOW HOSPICE DIFFERS FROM TRADITIONAL SETTINGS

Hospice differs from traditional settings in several ways, and COTAs who have worked in conventional rehabilitation settings must understand the hospice philosophy. The role of COTAs in rehabilitation settings focuses on helping clients become independent. In hospice care, COTAs work with people who have declining abilities (Table 28-1).

Reimbursement is another area in which hospice differs from traditional settings. Elders over 65 years of age almost always receive Medicare benefits. In traditional Medicare settings, elders pay a portion of each bill and all medication costs. In a Medicare-certified program the participating hospice is reimbursed on a per-patient capitated basis. From this amount, all team visits and prescriptions related only to the terminal disease are paid. Necessary and approved equipment is also covered. Sometimes, no copayment is required from patients for these services. The family is relieved of all Medicare paperwork and billing.

OCCUPATIONAL THERAPY EVALUATION

Most Medicare and insurance regulations, as well as state licensure laws, require that OTRs be responsible for the evaluation. COTAs contribute to the assessment process under the supervision of OTRs (AOTA, 1993).

TABLE 28-1

Differences in Treatment Between a Rehabilitation and a Hospice Approach

	Rehabilitation	Hospice
Treatment philosophy	Focuses on adapting to disability and maximizing independent functioning	Focuses on a caring environment, enhancing quality of life and dealing with spiritual, physical, and emotional aspects
Approach to death and dying	Deals with issues related to living and coping with a disability	Deals with issues of life and death, particularly the elder's need to come to terms with dying
Treatment goals	Are specific and measurable with functional outcomes	Are short term, usually changing from session to session, and focused on enhancing quality of life and finding meaning in dying
Treatment approach	Fast paced, with a push for discharge within a reasonable time period	Treatment is slow, and unhurried, with an emphasis on quality time
Application of activities (occupations)	Used to increase endurance, strength, ROM, coordination, and ADL functions.	Used to increase meaning of life
Role of ADL functions	Used to enhance functional abilities	Used to maintain function, if meaningful
Role of exercise	Used to enhance functional abilities	Used only if important to the elder and if it will increase safety and comfort and maintain functional abilities
Role of energy conservation	Some education with certain diagnoses	Strongly emphasized
Role of relaxation training	Varies by practitioner	Used to increase energy and decrease pain and stress
Role of environmental adaptations and adaptive equipment	Used to increase safety and function	Used to increase safety, compensate for functional abilities, maintain function, and improve comfort
Role of caregiver training	Done for safety reasons and follow-through with the treatment	Done to improve body mechanics, energy conservation, bed mobility, communication systems, safety, and decrease burnout
Treatment discontinuation	Focus on discharge to another setting or home within a timely period	Focus on maintaining quality of life during the dying process; often includes planning for death

ROM, Range of motion.

Ultimately, COTAs, OTRs, and elders collaborate on the evaluation. When seeing the elder for the first time, the OTR should initiate a general functional assessment. Because almost all persons in hospice have limited endurance, the assessment should be done in a timely manner. Included in the assessment are the physical abilities, activities, interests and roles of the elder; the roles and abilities of the caregiver(s); and the environment in which the elder and caregiver reside.

The role of COTAs in the assessment process is to contribute to the data collection, which involves interviewing elders on past and present interests and activities to determine what is meaningful. Therefore COTAs should ask elders what they would like to do and document this information. COTAs must also determine

whether activities are possible with or without adaptation. The role of the elder within the family and community is noted, and the family is treated as a unit of care. The environment is assessed for safety, function, and comfort. The caregiver's role, skills, and abilities are assessed. Most important is the caregiver's ability to safely transfer the elder while using good body mechanics.

After the assessment is complete, OTRs and COTAs should collaborate on formulating a treatment plan. The goals should be individual driven, with input from members of the hospice team to ensure that a holistic approach is used. Hospice care is based on the dying person's perspective, not a medical diagnosis (Pizzi, 1983).

COTAs must be flexible to adjust to the changing needs of elders and modify treatment accordingly.

COTAs and OTRs regularly discuss treatment and changes in each client's condition. The treatment plan should reflect these changes. New short-term goals are usually made for each session.

ADDRESSING FEARS AND LOSSES OF THE DYING PERSON THROUGH OT INTERVENTION

Fear is a common reaction to impending death, and is apparent in people who are dying and all others around them. Losses contribute to fears.

Loss of Abilities

Grief usually accompanies each loss. The loss of physical, cognitive, and psychosocial abilities in daily life affects clients' self-esteem and sense of identity. Relying on others to hold a glass of water, place a bedpan, and perform other routine activities serves as a grim reminder of the loss of self-determination and can lead to sadness, depression, and anger (Tigges, Marcil, 1988). COTAs possess skills to help elders make the most of their remaining physical abilities. They help elders develop compensatory methods, including use of adaptive equipment. COTAs also teach elders nondominant handwriting, suggest ways to conserve energy, and recommend equipment placement.

Cognitive loss can impair clients' abilities to perform daily living skills. For example, a woman with cognitive deficits may frequently dial the wrong number when attempting to phone her daughter. The COTA could suggest interventions such as using speed dialing or saying the number while dialing it.

The loss of the ability to participate with others in meaningful activities affects psychosocial needs. COTAs can work with elders on activities they find meaningful. This may involve almost any activity, such as cooking simple meals, doing art projects, and writing in a journal. Arranging photos in an album could result in a parting gift for a loved one, while providing the elder with an opportunity for reminiscing. OT practitioners believe that participation in meaningful activities promotes a sense of competence and mastery, leading to a sense of personal worth (Cusick, Lawler, Swain, 1987). Kubler-Ross stated that OT practitioners have used arts and crafts projects to show clients that they can still function at some level (Dawson, 1982).

Many elders in hospice programs would benefit from the use of energy conservation techniques to help them gain control of their environments. The example of Katie illustrates this point. She is a 76-year-old elder in hospice who refused to try energy conservation and exerted herself in the morning hours. As a consequence, she quickly became fatigued and was in bed the rest of the day. After learning energy conservation principles, she paced herself better and was able to attend activities such as an evening birthday party for her grandchild. An afternoon nap and cutting back on her activities allowed her to participate in activities that were meaningful to her.

Loss of Relationships and Roles

Dealing with psychosocial loss can be devastating to dying people. Their roles in life and relationships with family members may be totally altered or relinquished. COTAs can facilitate adjustments to new roles. For instance, a terminally ill man had become bed bound. He had a car that would not run and was teaching his teenage granddaughters to repair it. After working on the car the granddaughters would return to him for feedback and further instructions. They were successful in getting the car on the road, and he was able to continue his involvement in their lives. The COTA's expertise in analyzing the role of this grandfather led to this successful outcome. OT is invaluable in a hospice setting because it promotes feelings of self-worth and competence and helps elders be productive (Tigges, Sherman, Sherwin, 1984).

Many elders have a strong work ethic. Their self-concept is directly related to their abilities to be productive. Men in particular have traditionally been the providers for their families. As their abilities to be productive decrease, so may their self-concept. To improve productivity and self-concept, the COTA may identify an activity that matches the elder's interests and abilities. For example, Sam, who was a carpenter for 40 years, made and sold custom tables. As his disease progressed, he was no longer able to be productive in this manner. The COTA helped Sam use his woodworking skills to make bird houses for the Audubon Society. In addition, they completed a life review to help Sam realize his self-worth apart from his past work role.

Loss of Control

Loss of control is a major concern for most people in hospice programs, possibly because it entails a loss of mastery over themselves and their environment. Encouraging elders to make decisions, if they can be made safely, promotes this sense of control. COTAs can also help dying people regain control of the environment through adaptations and positioning. Touch-on lamps, speaker phones, and ramps are examples of adaptations. This control may include planning a funeral and writing an obituary.

Loss of the Future

"The presence of a terminal illness not only threatens one's immediate life, but also abruptly confronts the future goals one has set in life" (Parad, Caplan, 1960). A **terminal illness** may force a person to reevaluate goals and set more realistic ones. For example, a terminally ill photographer wanted to say good-bye to all the meaningful people in her life. This would mean extensive traveling to several cities, which she was unable to do. The COTA suggested that she take a photograph representing each particular relationship as a way to say good-bye. This example illustrates a way COTAs can offer suggestions to help clients realize their dreams. Some future goals, such as seeing a grandchild grow up and graduate, may be impossible, and elders need the opportunity to grieve.

Fear of Pain

One of the primary goals in palliative care is the control of pain and relief of other discomforting symptoms (Park, 1991). One of the most significant reasons people choose hospice care is to control the severe and unrelenting pain that often accompanies terminal illness (Marcil, Tigges, 1988; Park, 1991). Many terminally ill people fear pain. Physical pain can be decreased and controlled with medication in almost all cases, allowing clients to remain alert and functional. The individual's perception of pain is important. Pain sensation may be localized or appear to occupy the entire body. One man described his intense pain as feeling as though he were being cut in two. This perception should be reported to the hospice team for medication adjustment. COTAs can also help alleviate pain by using relaxation techniques.

Emotional and Spiritual Pain

Emotional and spiritual pain can be overwhelming and is therefore as important as physical pain (Brown, 1984). Elders may confuse deep emotional and spiritual pain with physical pain. The fears they experience, as well as the anticipated loss of everyone and everything, is very painful. Dame Cicely Saunders distinguished emotional and spiritual pain from physical pain, claiming that the former is often more severe and long lasting. Emotional and spiritual pain encompasses the loss of one's own life and separation from not only loved ones but all humanity. This pain exists regardless of the presence or absence of religious values (Carr, 1995). One woman often wept and said, "You will cry over the loss of me, but I am crying over the loss of everyone I know." Some elders and families have difficulty discussing feelings and may unknowingly project their own emotional pain to others. COTAs can help by being available as nonjudgmental listeners, fostering creative expression of feelings, and encouraging dying people to leave a gift of themselves to loved ones. COTAs can also help by acknowledging this pain and saying some words of encouragement in a caring manner. A referral to the pastoral counselor is often appropriate.

Fear of Dying

Some elders may be fearful of dying, such as the person who said, "I don't know how to die because I've never died before." COTAs can assure elders that they have

some control over the dying process. Facing the unknown is much more frightening than knowing the possibilities ahead. The assurance that they have some control helps. This control can be expressed through writing one's own obituary or requesting the company of family members or a spiritual counselor at the time of death. Some elders even seem to control the time of death to coincide with a significant anniversary, arrival of a loved one, or resolution of an issue. By the time dying people enter a hospice program, they have often, but not always, dealt with the fear of death. Almost all deaths that occur in hospice are peaceful.

Although elders in hospice rarely die when the COTA is present, their condition can change rapidly. The COTA must be able to recognize the signs of impending death and share these with family members, who may be frightened by it (Table 28-2).

COMMUNICATING WITH THE DYING PERSON

In working with dying people, COTAs must have effective **communication** skills. Kubler-Ross (1974) suggests that dying people communicate in three languages: plain English, nonverbal language, and symbolic verbal language. Plain English is clearly stated verbally and conveys a literal meaning. Nonverbal language is communicated through obvious behaviors such as gestures, actions, and drawings. Symbolic verbal language conveys a message that transcends its literal meaning (Rando, 1984).

Attending behaviors signify that COTAs are listening to clients. These behaviors include eye contact, attentive body language, and verbal following (Rando, 1984). Minimizing the physical distance between speaker and listener is important. COTAs should maintain a relaxed position, lean forward, or kneel to be at the speaker's eye level. Verbal following is another way for COTAs to communicate attentiveness. This may be accomplished by summarizing or reflecting on elders' comments.

GUIDELINES FOR EFFECTIVE COMMUNICATION

The following guidelines can provide COTAs with tools to communicate with dying people and families.

1. Keep speech simple and concise. Avoid wordiness.
2. Avoid medical jargon—it may alienate some people.
3. Use open-ended questions to provide opportunities for stating opinions.
4. Do not be judgmental. Keep an open mind.
5. Allow time for elders to speak. This may take longer for those who are in poor health.

TABLE 28-2

Signs of Impending Death	
Signs	**Comfort measures**
Circulation Arms and legs feel cool to touch Skin of hands, arms, feet, and legs deepen in color and develop a mottled appearance Other areas of body become dusky or pale	Keep client warm with blankets or hot water bottle Avoid using electric blankets
Metabolism Periods of sleep increase during day Waking the client from sleep in increasingly difficult Elder seems confused about time, place, and people Increased restlessness occurs Anxiety, fear, and loneliness increase at night Need for food and drink decreases	Plan to be with client during alert periods or at night, when the presence of a familiar person might be comforting Mention your name, the date, and time when talking with the elder Use a calm and confident tone of voice when speaking Cool, moist wash cloths applied to head, face, and body may relieve effects of dehydration
Secretions Oral mucus increases and collects in the back of throat ("death rattle") Increased secretions result from decreased fluid intake and inability to cough up saliva	Use a cool mist humidifier to increase room humidity Provide ice chips and sips of fluid through straw
Respirations Breathing pattern is irregular 10- to 30-second periods of no breathing (apnea) occur	Elevate head of bed or prop head and chest at an angle with pillows

Elimination
Elder loses control (incontinence) of bladder and bowel
Urine darkens and decreases in amount
	Put layers of disposable pads between the elder and mattress
	Consult nurse regarding the following:
	    Hygiene techniques for cleanliness
	    Catheter (urinary bladder tubing) care

Senses Vision decreases in clarity and becomes dim or blurred Hearing is usually the last sense to decrease	Leave indirect lights on Never assume elder cannot hear Continue to touch and speak to elder as reassurance of your presence

Modified from Visiting Nurse Association: *Signs of impending death*, Portland Ore., 1992, The Association.

6. Do not interrupt or finish sentences.
7. Do not give too much information in one visit, or none will be retained. Give demonstrations during teaching and provide both verbal and written instructions. Adapt them for visual difficulties as needed.
8. Allow comfortable periods of silence.
9. Do not argue with elders about the way they perceive their condition. Unrealistic views may represent a defense mechanism necessary until the elder is able to face reality.
10. Talk to clients and include them in all conversations at which they are present. Do not talk exclusively to caregivers, even when the client is in a coma.
11. Be aware of decreased energy levels, and leave before clients become too tired.
12. Provide appropriate touch, such as holding a hand, if the elder permits it.
13. Respect **cultural differences** in communication.
14. Help elders write if they are unable to speak. Use alphabet boards, prewritten messages, computers, and even eye blinks as methods of communication.
15. Encourage elders to express important thoughts.
16. Encourage caregivers to let the dying person know that they will survive.

TABLE 28-3

Strategies for Training COTAs to Work With Caregivers	
Caregiver needs	**COTA intervention**
Help with physical aspects of care	Teach good body mechanics, safe transfer, and energy conservation techniques
Help in assisting with personal care	Teach provision of personal care by simple methods that involve energy conservation and maintain the client's dignity.
	Obtain needed adaptive equipment and teach safe use.
	Arrange for removal of adaptive equipment.
Help with caregiver's psychosocial needs	Allow the caregiver to express emotion
	Encourage input in treatment planning
	Facilitate a realistic view of everyone's abilities
	Encourage a balance of life roles
	Offer therapeutic touch if the caregiver permits this.
	Suggest additional counseling support
Help with resources	Explore availability of support from family, friends, church, and social groups
	Access resources in the community
Help with spiritual needs	Allow expression of spiritual beliefs and accept differences
	Suggest spiritual support from members of caregiver's religious community
Help with preparing for the person's death	Discuss and educate caregivers about signs and symptoms of impending death
	Help caregivers obtain closure
	Suggest ways to make the environment meaningful
	Review procedures to follow at the time of death
Support after death	Listen and be supportive
	Attend funeral or memorial service

17. Consider safety factors if a nonverbal person is left alone. A prerecorded message near the telephone could alert others to an emergency.

OCCUPATIONAL THERAPY INTERVENTION AND CAREGIVER TRAINING

Caregiver training is an important safety factor. **Caregivers** should be educated to follow through with the OT interventions. The challenges and responsibilities of caring for dying people can be emotionally and physically draining.

During the progression of a terminal illness, major demands are placed on significant others. The transition from living to dying is rarely smooth. Sometimes, dying people lead normal lives with minimal changes. At other times, symptoms may severely curtail any semblance of a normal life. In either case, dying people wish to be treated as they were before their illness, despite the increasing assistance needed from caregivers (Park, 1991).

Sometimes, caregivers do too much for dying people out of concern or guilt, leaving them weaker, with decreased self-esteem. Other caregivers deny the decreasing abilities of dying people and expect them to do more than they are capable of doing. Most caregivers, however, are realistic. COTAs can help caregivers understand the need for dying people to participate in meaningful activity and remain active within physical limits.

Some resources are available to help caregivers live a more balanced life. COTAs can refer them to the volunteer coordinator for help. Elders in certified Medicare hospice programs are eligible for 5 days per year respite care in an approved facility.

COTAs should not impose their values on dying people and their families. Their support and willingness to learn from dying people and their caregivers can improve the quality of care they deliver. Some caregivers find touch comforting; hospice workers often hug caregivers when this is acceptable. COTAs can also help caregivers understand that laughing and having a sense of humor are acceptable. The therapeutic use of self is essential when working in hospice care. COTAs should receive thorough training in working with caregivers (Table 28-3).

PROVIDING SUPPORT FOR THE CAREGIVER RELATING TO DEATH

COTAs can help families and caregivers understand the importance of their roles as death nears. COTAs can convey to caregivers the importance of telling elders who are dying that they are appreciated and loved. Rando (1984) emphasizes the need for the family to be present at the time of death if possible. Individuals who have been keeping vigil but are not present at the actual moment of death often feel guilty afterward.

CONSIDERATIONS FOR WORKING IN HOSPICE

COTAs may consider the following questions:

1. Have you ever been around someone who is terminally ill? By being around someone who is terminally ill, you can better understand the feelings of clients and family members.
2. Have you ever experienced the death of a loved one, including pets? Experiencing the death of someone held dear helps you understand the depth of caregivers' grief.
3. How did you handle this death? If handling a personal loss was extremely difficult and time consuming, dealing with the many losses that occur in hospice can be overwhelming.
4. What helps you relieve stress in your life? OT stresses the importance of maintaining balance in life. Exercising, engaging in creative activities, and networking with other team members can help relieve stress associated with this type of work.
5. What are your own spiritual views about death? Are you familiar with and willing to accept other religious and cultural views? As a health care provider, the COTA must accept people exactly as they are—physically, emotionally, culturally, and spiritually. This acceptance increases the comfort of clients and decreases their anxiety.

CONCLUSION

COTAs interested in working in hospice settings should have a holistic background so that they can address both physical and psychosocial needs. An understanding of terminal illness and the progression of disease is essential for COTAs to understand the elder's condition, make appropriate changes in treatment, and recognize the point at which the elder is actively dying. COTAs must be able to accept people and their beliefs about dying without being judgmental. Effective interpersonal communication skills are vital when interacting with families, elders, and hospice team members.

CASE STUDY

Vivian was a lively woman with a great sense of humor and a quick wit. She enjoyed being with others, especially family members. Vivian was living independently when she was diagnosed with ovarian cancer. She continued living alone until she was physically unable. At that time, she moved to her daughter's home in another state. This new home was warm, accepting, and busy. Vivian's presence made this a

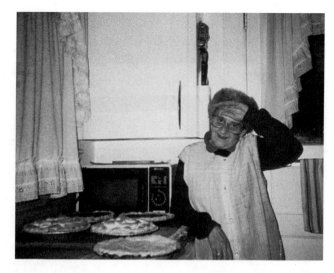

FIGURE 28-1 Baking pies was one of Vivian's favorite activities. (Courtesy Sue Byers-Connon.)

delightful four-generation home. Another daughter and her family, including a great-granddaughter, lived nearby.

Throughout her life, Vivian was very active. She worked in a neighborhood tavern for 30 years. Her many interests included playing billiards, reading, listening to music, going to movies, playing cards, and working crossword puzzles. Baking was her specialty, and she delighted her family with lemon meringue pies (Figure 28-1).

When her condition worsened, Vivian was referred to hospice by her oncologist. The hospice team, including the COTA, worked with Vivian. The role of the COTA was to provide necessary equipment for safety and comfort. A tub transfer bench was installed, and Vivian and her family were taught safe transfers. Other adaptations included a safety frame on the toilet and later a bedside commode. A trapeze was placed over the bed. A portable device that allowed moving Vivian in bed was designed and fabricated. A baby monitor was used as a communication system. After meeting these initial needs, the COTA concentrated on enhancing Vivian's life.

Scheduling rest periods between activities conserved Vivian's declining energy. The most necessary or desired activities were chosen in order of importance. Relaxation tapes helped alleviate her pain. Listening to these tapes led Vivian to express an interest in music. She particularly enjoyed tapes of popular music from the 1940s. Her family often heard her over the communication system, singing as she listened to the music.

A special bond existed between Vivian and her 3-year-old great-grandson, who lived in the home. He would eat breakfast with her and then climb on her hospital bed and cuddle with her (Figure 28-2). This special relationship was mutually rewarding and engendered in the child a respect for elders regardless of their physical or mental status.

Vivian was an active participant in family activities. She helped with cooking and preparing meals. The entire family read aloud together and played cards and board games. Vivian rewrote and organized recipe cards, including humorous notes to be found later by her daughter. She ate meals

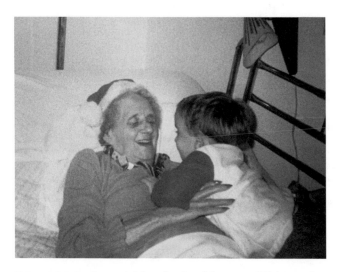

FIGURE **28-2** A special bond existed between Vivian and her 3-year-old great-grandson. (Courtesy Sue Byers-Connon.)

with the family, and when getting out of bed became difficult for her, the family ate meals in her room. Keeping in touch with family and friends in other states was important to her, and she frequently wrote letters and made phone calls.

The family shared caregiving responsibilities, including shopping, helping with personal care, running errands, arranging respite care, preparing meals, and helping with household chores. Vivian's room was cheery, with family photos on the walls. A bird feeder was placed outside the window. Frequently used items such as her tape recorder were close at hand on a bedside table. The family brought in fresh flowers from the yard. She operated the television by remote control to watch her favorite programs. As time passed and her condition declined, she was unable to participate in activities. She requested that her door remain open so she could hear the laughter and conversation of family members. She died with her family at her side.

CHAPTER REVIEW QUESTIONS

1 Considering Vivian's case, what was the role of the COTA in working with Vivian?
2 How can COTAs make life as normal as possible for elders in hospice, as illustrated by the case study?
3 What are some specific examples of ways to encourage participation in these activities, as illustrated by the case study?
4 What are some suggestions that COTAs can make to the family to enhance the environment, and how is this done in the case study?
5 In reference to the whole chapter, how could an elder benefit from a hospice program?
6 What previous experience should COTAs have before considering hospice work?

7 Define the roles of the following members of the hospice team: physical therapist, nurse, physician, dietitian, bereavement counselor.
8 Discuss two losses a dying person may experience.
9 Describe physical pain and emotional and spiritual pain.
10 List 10 effective ways to communicate with dying persons and their families.
11 What are five differences between a rehabilitation and a hospice approach to treatment?

EXERCISE

The purpose of this exercise is to enhance sensitivity. Find a partner and ask him or her to lie on the floor looking up. Stand nearby and start a conversation, continuing for 5 minutes. Observe body language, and ask about your partner's feelings. How can you use this exercise with clients in hospice? Reverse positions with your partner, and repeat the exercise.

REFERENCES

American Occupational Therapy Association: Occupational therapy and hospice position paper, *Am J Occup Ther* 40:839, 1981.
American Occupational Therapy Association: Occupational therapy roles, *Am J Occup Ther* 47(12):1087, 1993.
Brown P: The growth of the hospice movement: a role for occupational therapy, *OT in Health Care* 1:119, 1984.
Carr WF: Spiritual pain and healing in the hospice, *America* 173(4): 26, 1995.
Cusick A, Lawler R, Swain M: Chemotherapy, cancer, and the quality of life: an occupational therapy approach, *Austr Occup Ther J* 34:105, 1987.
Dawson S: The role of occupational therapy in palliative care, *Austr Occup Ther J* 28(3):119, 1982.
Flanigan K: The art of the possible: occupational therapy in terminal care, *Br J Occup Ther* 45:274, 1982.
Hamilton M, Reid H, editors: *A hospice handbook: a new way to care for the dying*, Grand Rapids, Mich, 1980, William B. Eerdmans.
Health Care Financing Administration: *Medicare administration handbook* (GPO Publication No. HCFA-10050), Baltimore, Md, 1996, Government Printing Office.
Hospice Task Force: *Guidelines for occupational therapy services in hospice*, Rockville, Md, 1987, The American Occupational Therapy Association.
Kubler-Ross E: The language of dying, *J Clin Child Psychol* 3:22, 1974.
Health Care Financing Administration: *Medicare administration handbook* (GPO Publication No. HCFA-10050), Baltimore, Md, 1996, Government Printing Office.
Parad HJ, Caplin G: A framework for studying families in crisis, *Social Work* 5:3, 1960.
Park S: *The role of the occupational therapist on a hospice care team*, 1991, Unpublished manuscript.
Pizzi M: Occupational therapy in hospice care, *Am J Occup Ther* 36: 597, 1983.
Rando TA: *Grief, dying and death: clinical intervention for caregivers*, Champaign, Ill, 1984, Research Press.

Saunders DC, editor: *St. Christopher's in celebration: twenty-one years at Britain's first modern hospice*, London, 1988, Hodder & Stoughton.

Thiers N: Hospice care helping bring life full circle, *OT Week* 7(36): 14, Sept 9, 1993.

Thompson B: *Occupational ther with the terminally ill.* In JM Kiernat, editor: *Occupational therapy and the older adult*, Gaithersburg, Md, 1991, Aspen.

Tigges KN, Marcil WM: Maximizing quality of life for the housebound patient: specialized ramp allows accessibility to outdoors, *Am J Hospice Care* 3:21, 1988.

Tigges KN, Sherman LM, Sherwin FS: Perspectives on the pain of the hospice patient: the roles of the occupational therapist and physician, *Occup Ther Health Care* 3:55, 1984.

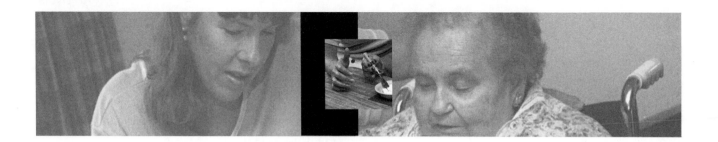

Appendix

HOW TO OBTAIN GUIDELINES FOR THE MDS

Information about the MDS is contained in The OBRA Resident Assessment Instrument Regulations and User's Manual, effective January 1, 1996. All therapists working in nursing facilities are strongly advised to become familiar with this HCFA (Health Care Financing Administration) manual—MDS 2.0 Part I: The Regulations HCFA State Operations Manual Transmittal 275: Appendix R and Part II: The User's Manual HCFA's Instruction Guidelines. Nursing facilities should have copies of this manual, or it can be obtained by writing the Center on Long Term Care, Health Standards and Quality Bureau, Health Standards and Quality Bureau, Health Care Financing Administration, 7500 Security Boulevard, Baltimore, MD 21244-1850.

RESTRAINT REDUCTION RESOURCES

Chairs

Adirondack chairs (estate chairs) manufactured by Rubbermaid. Available from outdoor furniture stores.

Alerting Systems

Sentry II Wireless Attendant Station
MRW World, Inc.
15 Central Way, Suite 313
Kirkland, WA 98033
(206)826-6299, FAX (208)889-9779

Developed to meet specific needs of foster care and assisted living settings, the call/alerting system requires no wiring to install and is simply plugged in. Basic attendant console ($96) handles up to eight residents. Cost of transmitters varies with type ($45-$68 ea). The system is flexible: in addition to call/alerting exit from each room, and a bedside beam sensor and a perimeter alert bracelet unit which alarms exit for only the individual wearing the bracelet, are also available. The exit door alarm costs approximately $465 per exit.

Baby nursery monitors
Available from Fisher-Price and other companies, nursery monitors allow caregivers to hear whether someone is moving about or calling for assistance.

Personal Alarms

Ambularm
Alert Care Inc.
Shelter Point Business Center, Suite 2125
591 Redwood Hwy.
Mill Valley, CA 94941
(800)828-7444

This lightweight, position-sensitive alarm worn on the thigh costs approximately $170. New Ambularm Plus can be converted to position-change, pressure-change, and tether or exit alarm system by adding different components.

Bed-Check
Bed-Check
4408 S. Harvard #A
Tulsa, OK 74135
(800)523-7956

Chair Sentinel
Powderhorn Industries
931 N Park Ave.
P.O. Box 1443
Monrose, CO 81402

This releasable wheelchair seatbelt emits an alarm when it is unfastened and costs $150.

Code Alert
RF Technologies, Inc.
3720 N. 124th St.
Milwaukee, WI 53221
(800)669-9946 FAX (414)466-1506

Mugger Stopper
Safety Technology International, Inc.
2306 Airport Road
Waterford, MI 48327
(313)873-9898 or (800)888-4784
This device must be adapted to use as position-change alarm but costs only $15.

Personal Alarm
Radio Shack (check phone directory for nearest outlet).
This device must be adapted but costs only between $10 and $15.

Posey Sitter
Posey Co.
5635 Peck Rd.
Arcadia, CA 91006-0020
(800)44-POSEY or (818)443-3143

TABS Mobility Monitor
WanderGuard, Inc.
941 "O" Street, Suite 205
Lincoln, NE 88501
(800)824-2996, FAX (402)475A281
Cost $195.

Signs

Stopper Kit
Clock Medical
P.O. Box 620, Winfield, KS 67156
(800)527-0049
This kit includes "stop" and "do not enter" signs, as well as mesh strips to put across doors, and costs $24.95.

Other Adaptations

Dycem
AliMed
297 High Street
Dedham, MA 02026
(617)329-2900, FAX (617)329-8392
This nonslip, rubberlike plastic material (16 in. × 2 yds) is placed in chair seats to prevent sliding. It costs $34.95 and is available in many sizes and configurations. It can also be obtained from many health equipment companies.

Posey Grip
See phone and address under Posey Sitter above.

Scoot Gard
Designed for use in boats and recreational vehicles, this material is washable, with anti-microbial properties to inhibit bacteria and mildew. It is available in many stores and costs $.79/ft or $8.99 for 1 × 12 ft roll.

Foam/Cushions

Armrest (padded flipaway)
Therafin Corp.
1974 Wolf Rd.
Mokena, IL 60448
(708)479-7300, FAX (708)479-1515, order line (800)843-7234. Cost $144.95.

Cheese Leaner Cushion
Clock Medical Supply
118-124 E. 9th
Winfieki, KS 67156
(800)527-0049
This cushion prevents lateral slumping in wheelchairs, recliners, and gerichairs. It costs $25 with cotton cover, $32 with naugahyde.

Foam elevating inserts
Fred Sammons
P.O. Box 32
Brookfield, IL 60513
(800)323-5547, FAX (800)547-4333. Cost $30. (For use with trough BK-6462-01.)

Inflatable seat cushions
Roho
P.O. Box 658
Belleview, IL 62222
(800)851-3449, FAX (618)277-6518
Cost $385.

LiteNest
Orthopedic Products Corp.
10381 W. Jefferson Boulevard
Culver City, CA
(800)235-4661
This ultralight portable system weighs less than 4 lb. It also incorporates an integrated seat and back design with a multidensity foam pad. It costs $199 (an incontinence cover is also available).

PASS (Patient Autonomy Safety Systems)
Skill-Care
167 Saw Mill River Rd.
Yonkers, NY 10701
(800)431-2972
These safety systems include self-release devices and positioning cushions. A video is available at no cost on a 30-day loaner basis.

Super Constructa Foam
AliMed
297 High Street
Dedham, MA 02026
(617)329-2900, FAX (617)329-8392

This dense, closed cell foam is easily cut to form custom-made positioning wedges and supports. Its cost varies with size—call for information.

Ultra-Form Wedge Cushion
American Health Systems, Inc.
P.O. Box 26688
Greenville, SC 29616-1588
(800)234-6655

This wedge-shaped cushion prevents sliding in addition to preventing pressure relief. The cost is $91.60 for a case of 4 without covers. Prices for covers are as follows: protective—$30 ea., durable—$35 ea. Call local representative for estimate.

Varilite Chair Cushion
Cascade Designs, Inc.
4000 1 St Ave. S.
Seattle, WA 98134
(800)527-1527, FAX (206)467-9421

This lightweight cushion/seating system comes with firm or soft base with two to four self-inflating modular cushions that compensate precisely for posture deviation. The cost ranges between $250 and $350, depending on the number of cushions required.

Firm Wheelchair Seats

Drop seats (hardware)
Adaptive Engineering Lab, Inc.
4403 Russell Rd. 2S-3
Mukilteo, WA 97275-5018
(800)327-6080

Seat cushions and backs
Jay Medical, Ltd.
P.O. Box 18656, Boulder, CO 83038-8656
(800)648-8282

Solid seat inserts
AliMed
297 High Street
Dedham, MA 02026
(617)329-2900, FAX (617)329-8392

Wheelchair inserts eliminate discomfort caused by sling seats and create a flat, stable seating surface. They also come in wedge shapes. Two sizes are available: 16 × 18 (product #1192) and 16 × 16 (#1193). The cost is $25 ($35 if covered).

Walkers

Able Walker
Brandt Enterprise
P.O. Box 491
Donald, OR 97020
(800)426-6857

This four-wheeled walker comes with brakes and a shopping basket that converts to a seat. It costs $349.

Chariot Ambulator
First Choice International
12 Westerville Square #335
Westerville, OH 43081
(800)235-0370

This adult walking frame is designed for elders with good trunk balance who stand or walk unsteadily. The cost is $495 in the continental United States, plus $38.50 for shipping and handling.

Next Step & Rover
Noble Motion, Inc.
P.O. Box 5366
58T1 Center Ave.
Pittsburgh, PA 15206
(800)234-9255

This four-wheeled, 8-inch solid tire walker is equipped with hand brakes. Additional accessories are available. The cost ranges from $375 to $450, with free delivery.

Ultimate Walker, (formerly Merry Walker)
Direct Supply
6761 N. Industrial Rd.
Milwaukee, WI 53223
(800)634-7328

This adjustable-wheeled walking frame made of PVC pipe allows wheeling in standing or sitting position. It is useful for elders who stand unsteadily or are unsafely mobile on their own. The cost is approximately $300, plus shipping and handling.

Printed Material

Christenson M: *Aging in the designed environment,* Bingham, NY, 1990, Hawthorne Press.

This book provides detailed information on ways to adapt the physical environment to compensate for sensory changes associated with aging, enhance independence in the home, and redesign long-term care facilities. This is an excellent resource for modifying the environment ($19.95).

Rader J: *Individualized dementia care: creative, compassionate approaches,* New York, NY, 1990, Springer Publishing Co. [(212)431-4370. $37.95, plus $3.50 shipping.]

Robinson A, Spencer B, White L: *Understanding difficult behaviors: some practical suggestions for coping with Alzheimer's disease and related illnesses,* Ann Arbor, Mich, 1989, The Alzheimer's Program, P.O. Box 981337, Ann Arbor, MI 45198, phone (313)487-2335. Written for professional and family caregivers, this book explains the causes of behaviors such as wandering, resistance, incontinence, and agitation. Problem-solving strategies for managing behaviors are also suggested ($14, including shipping).

Untie the elderly, The Kendal Corp., P.O. Box 100, Kennett Square, PA 19348. This newsletter on restraint reduction is available by request.

Fell N: *Validation: the Fell method*, Cleveland, Ohio, 1989, Edward Fell Productions (4614 Prospect Ave, Cleveland, OH 44103.)

This book provides information regarding interaction with disoriented elders ($10, plus $2.50 shipping).

RESOURCES TO ASSIST THE OLDER DRIVER
General
The Handicapped Driver's Mobility Guide
American Automobile Association
Traffic Safety Department
1000 AAA Drive
Heathrow, FL 32746

(Provides state-by-state listing of driver evaluation programs and vehicle modification vendors.)

Drivers 55 Plus: Test Your Own Performance
Self-rating form of questions, facts, and suggestions for safe driving.
Available from the American Automobile Association
Foundation for Traffic Safety
1730 M Street, N.W., Suite 401
Washington, D.C. 20036

(Also offers other publications and videos related to the older driver, as well as general information related to driving)

Older Driver Skill Assessment and Resource Guide
American Association of Retired Persons
601 E. Street, N.W.
Washington, D.C. 20049

Association of Driver Educators for the Disabled (ADED)
P.O. Box 49
Edgerton, WI 53534
(608)884-8833

(Provides information related to drivers with disabilities, such as information on Driving Rehabilitation Specialists and others in the fields of driver education and transportation equipment modification and educational conferences)

Architectural and Transportation Barriers Compliance Board
1331 F Street NW, Suite 1000
Washington, DC 20004-1111
(202)272-5434

(Issues accessibility guidelines for the ADA; ensures compliance with standards issued under the Architectural Barriers Act of 1968)

Equipment for Hearing Impaired Drivers
HARC Mercantile, Ltd.
1111 W. Centre
P.O. Box 3055
Kalamazoo, MI 49002
1-800-445-9968

Source For Key Holders and Door Openers
Sammons Preston
P.O. Box 5071
Bolingbrook, IL 60440-5071
(800)323-5547

North Coast Medical
187 Stauffer Boulevard
San Jose, CA 95125-1042
(800)821-9319

HEARING DEFICITS
Information on hearing aids that may assist COTAs and elders is available through the AARP (American Association of Retired Persons), *Product Report: Hearing Aids* (D13766), AARP (EE0458), PO Box 22796, Long Beach, CA 90801-5796.

LOW VISION
American Foundation for the Blind
15 West 16th Street
New York, NY 10011

National Library Service for the Blind and Physically Handicapped
Library of Congress
Washington, DC 20542

New York Times/Large Type Weekly
New York Times Company
Large Print Edition
P.O. Box 2570
Boulder, CO 80302

Reader's Digest Large Type Edition
P.O. Box 241
Mt. Morris, IL 61054

Guideposts
Guideposts Associates, Inc.
Carmel, NY 10512

FAMILY AND CAREGIVERS
Publications
Many practical, hands-on guidebooks and personal accounts for family and professional caregivers are available. Many books are written in an easy-to-read style

that is user-friendly and nontechnical, presenting key information on caregiver concerns. Of particular interest are books that assist the caregiver in learning ways to keep clients engaged through meaningful activities, preventing caregiver burnout, and coping with wandering and other difficult behaviors. Books that offer personal accounts written by patients experiencing dementia assist us in gaining empathy for our patients and family members.

Carroll D: *When your loved one has Alzheimer's disease*, New York, 1989, Harper & Row.

Carter R, Golant S: *Helping yourself help others*, New York, 1994, Times Books.

Cohen D, Eisdorfer C: *Loss of self: A family resource for the care of Alzheimer's disease and related disorders*, New York, 1986, WW Norton Co.

Dolan MJ: *How to care for aging parents and still have a life of your own*, New York, NY, 1992, Mulholland Press.

Greenberg VE: *Your best is good enough: aging parents and your emotions*, Philadelphia, 1989, Lexington Books.

Greenberg VE: *Children of a certain age: adults and their aging parents*, Philadelphia, 1994, Lexington Books.

Faloon I, Boyd J, McGill C: *Family care of schizophrenia*, New York, 1984, Guilford Press.

Friel D: *Living in the labyrinth: a personal journey through the maze of Alzheimer's disease*, New York, NY, 1993, Bantam, Doubleday Dell.

Mace NL, Rabins PV: *The 36-hour day*, Baltimore, 1981, John Hopkins.

Morris A, Hunt G: *A part of daily life*, Bethesda, Md, 1994, The American Occupational Therapy Association (Includes a video and resource booklet).

New York City Alzheimer's Resource Center: *Caring: a guide to managing the Alzheimer's patient at home*, New York, 1985, The Center.

Oakley F: *Understanding the ABCs of Alzheimer's disease: a guide for caregivers*, Rockville, Md, 1993, American Occupational Therapy Association.

Reisburg B: *A guide to Alzheimer's disease for families, spouses and friends*, New York, 1983, Free Press.

Sheridan C: *Failure-free activities for the Alzheimer's patient: a guidebook for caregivers*, San Francisco, 1987, Cottage Books (Available in Spanish, Japanese and Dutch translations).

Susik DH: *Hiring home caregivers: the family guide to in-home elder care*, New York, 1995, Impact Books.

Torrey EF: *Surviving schizophrenia: a family manual* (revised edition), New York, 1988, Harper & Row.

Support Groups and Referrals

Alzheimer's Association

The Alzheimer's Association has an impressive network of more than 200 chapters and 1500 support groups nationwide. Most major cities have local chapters of the Alzheimer's Association. It was founded in 1980 by family caregivers and provides programs and services to assist families in their communities. Information on Alzheimer's disease, current research, patient care, and assistance for caregivers is available. Support groups allow families to share their experiences in an emotionally supportive environment. This association has practical suggestions, educational handouts, pamphlets, videos, and publications to assist families and caregivers. The Alzheimer's Association has a web server with information on the association, its local chapters, caregiving (which includes some online publications), public policy, and upcoming conferences and events devoted to Alzheimer's disease and related disorders. To locate a Chapter near you, contact the national office.

By e-mail: WWW server feedback and suggestions: webmaster@alz.org

24-hour information and chapter referral: (800) 272-3900, TDD: (312) 335-8882, By mail: Alzheimer's Association, 919 North Michigan Avenue Suite 1000, Chicago, IL 60611-1676

American Academy of Ophthalmology

This organization offers information about the National Eye Care Project and referrals to free or low-cost eye care to financially disadvantaged older adults.

P.O. Box 7424, San Francisco, CA, 94120-7424; 800/222-EYES

American Association of Homes and Services for the Aged

This organization offers a brochure on the selection of a nursing home or assisted living facility that can be obtained free of charge by calling (202)783-2242 or by writing the Association at Suite 500, 901 E Street, NW, Washington, DC, 20004-2837

American Association of Retired Persons (AARP)

This organization provides caregivers with a resource kit when they write for Item #D15267, AARP 601 E Street, N.W., Washington, DC 20049.

American Dietetic Association

This organization offers free information and publications by mail: Suite 800, 216 W. Jackson Blvd., Chicago, IL, 60606 (312/899-0040)

Area Agencies on Aging (AAA)

These are local offices that can direct family or professional caregivers to sources of help for elders with limited incomes. Resources include subsidized housing, food stamps, Supplemental Security Income, Medicaid, and the Qualified Medicare Beneficiary program. Family members may be eligible for services provided through the AAA, including home health aide services, transportation, home-delivered meals, assistance with chores, home repair, and legal aid. It also provides a registry of home care workers for hire and information on home care agencies and volunteer groups that provide various services. This agency may also provide an assessment of the elder's needs. AAA can also provide information on senior center and adult day care programs and assist in arranging respite care. The national office can provide the numbers of local Agencies on Aging. (112 16th Street, NW, Suite 100, Washington, DC 20036; (202) 296-8130; e-mail: http://howard.hbg.psu.edu/psdc/AGING.html)

Children of Aging Parents (CAPS)

This organization serves as a national clearinghouse for caregivers, matching existing support groups to individuals looking for groups on a national level. CAPS has developed a national directory of caregiver support groups and private geriatric care managers. It also offers community education programs and assists caregivers in gaining access to community resources. Peer counseling, manuals, and materials are available through this organization. Programs sponsored by CAPS include workshops and seminars for caregivers and professionals, inservice training programs for health care agencies; educational presentations and consultations for programs and services to elders; and an annual conference for caregivers and professionals. For more information, contact this organization at 1609 Woodbourne Road, Suite 302A, Levittown, PA 19057-1511 [(215)945-6900 (Voice); (215)945-8720 (Fax)]

Concerned Relatives of Nursing Home Patients
PO Box 18820, Cleveland Heights, OH, 44118 [216/321-0403]

Courage Stroke Network
This network links stroke survivors, family members, and professionals. It promotes the development of support groups and provides information and educational materials about stroke. [7272 Greenville Ave., Dallas, TX 75231-4596; (800)553-6321]

National Academy of Elder Law Attorneys
This organization offers a free brochure on selecting an elder law attorney. [Suite 108, Alvernon Place, 655 N. Alvernon Way, Tucson, AZ, 85711; (602)881-4005; Web site at: http://www.primenet.com/~rbf/lawyer.html]

National Alliance for the Mentally Ill (NAMI)
This organization provides grassroots self-help, support, and advocacy. [2101 Wilson Blvd., Suite 302, Arlington, VA 22201 (703)524-7600]

National Association of Meal Programs
204 E. Street, NE, Washington, DC, 20002 [(202)547-6157]

National Association of Private Geriatric Care Managers
Suite 108, 655 N. Alvernon Way, Tucson, AZ 85711 [(602)881-8008]

National Citizens' Coalition for Nursing Home Reform
Suite 301, 1224 M Street NW, Washington, DC 20005 [(202)393-2018]

National Consumers' League
Information about medigap insurance and long-term care services. 815 Fifteenth St., NW, Washington, DC 20005 [(202)639-8140]

National Mental Health Consumers' Association
311 Juniper St., Philadelphia, PA 19107

National Institute of Mental Health (NIMH)
NIMH provides free publications for professionals and the general public on various topics related to mental illness. Information can be gained through Public Inquiries, Room 15C-05, 5600 Fishers Lane, Rockville, MD 20857 [(301)443-4513]

National Institute of Neurological Disorders and Stroke
Fact sheets, current reports; and brochures on neurological disorders are available by writing the Office of Scientific and Health Reports, Building 31, Room 8A16, 9000 Rockville Pike, Bethesda, MD 20892 [(301)496-5751]

Nursing Home Information Service
National Council of Senior Citizens, 1331 F Street NW, Washington, DC 20004 [(202) 347-8800]

Stroke Connection of the American Heart Association
This organization maintains a listing of over 1000 stroke support groups across the nation for referral to stroke survivors, their families, caregivers and interested professionals and will provide information and referral. *Stroke Connection* magazine offers a forum for stroke survivors and their families to share information about coping with stroke. This association offers additional publications of stroke-related books, videos, and literature for purchase. [7272 Greenville Avenue, Dallas, TX 75231; (800)553-6321 (Voice); (214)696-5211 (Fax)]

United Seniors Health Cooperative
A list of publications are available from this organization on topics of importance to older consumers, including insurance and Medicare, nursing home selection, finances, caregiving, and health. [1313 H Street NW, 5th Floor, Washington, DC 20005; (202)393-6222.]

WORLD WIDE WEB

An additional great source of information is accessible through your computer on the World Wide Web and the internet. Although all the groups, associations, and agencies using this method of information exchange are too numerous to mention here, the following URLs are recommended:

http://www.aoa.dhhs.gov/aoa/webres/craig.htm

This home page produced by the U.S. Administration on Aging is the best source of URLs and direct links to community services and agencies. This site provides over 175 direct links to other Web sites on aging.

http://www.ice/net/~kstevens/ELDERWEB.HTM

This site pulls together from numerous sources hundreds of documents dealing with many concerns of elder consumers, including health care; living arrangements; aging, death and dying; social, mental, and spiritual care; financial concerns; law and legislation; demographics; state-specific information; and provider locations.

http://www.nbn.com/people/elder/alzheimer/html

This is the web page of Elder Books, a publisher of practical books for family and professional caregivers of persons with Alzheimer's Disease.

http://www.aoa.dhhs.gov/aoa/pages/postlst.html
http://www.crm.mb.ca/scip/other/postlist.html
gopher://una.hh.lib.umich.edu/77/inetdirsstacks/
.waisindex/index?aging
http://moondog.usask.ca/pinnacles
http://www.wimsey.com/~bgraham/gerontology.html

These are all Web addresses for pages that provide a variety of information related to the concerns of elders. All sites offer the option of topical searches that permit explorations of information and resources all around the world.

Government Agencies Online
Social Security Administration: http://www.ssa.gov/
U.S. Department of Health and Human Services: http://www.os.dhhs.gov/
GSA's Catalog of Federal Domestic Assistance Programs: http://www.sura.net/gsa.

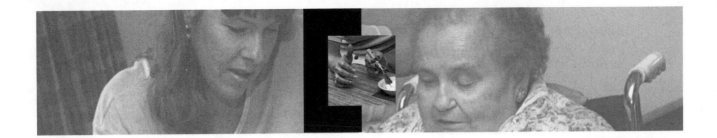

Glossary

A

arrhythmias Variations from the normal rhythm, especially of the heartbeat.

acalculia A form of aphasia characterized by the inability to solve simple mathematic calculations.

acetylcholine A neurotransmitter substance widely distributed in body tissues with the primary function of mediating synaptic activity of the nervous system and skeletal muscles.

acute Beginning abruptly with marked intensity or sharpness, then subsiding after a relatively short period of time.

amyloid Combining forms: starch of polysaccharide nature or origin.

angina Spasmodic choking or suffocative pain; now used almost exclusively to denote angina pectoris.

angioplasty The reconstruction of blood vessels damaged by disease or injury.

ankylosing spondylitis A chronic inflammatory disease of unknown origin that first affects the spine and adjacent structures and commonly progresses to cause eventual fusion of the involved joints.

anosognosia An abnormal condition characterized by a real or feigned inability to perceive a defect, especially paralysis, on one side of the body; possibly attributable to a lesion in the right parietal lobe of the brain.

anoxia An abnormal condition characterized by a lack of oxygen.

Definitions from Anderson KN, Anderson LE, Glanze WD, *Mosby's medical, nursing, and allied health dictionary*, ed 4, St Louis, 1994, Mosby; Miller BF, Keane C, editors: *Encyclopedia and dictionary of medicine, nursing, and allied health*, ed 5, Philadelphia, WB Saunders; *Taber's cyclopedic medical dictionary*, ed 17, Philadelphia, 1993, F.A. Davis; Miller BF, Keane C, editors: *Saunder's encyclopedia and dictionary of medicine, nursing, and allied health*, ed 4, Philadelphia, 1987, WB Saunders; McDonough JT, editor: *Stedman's concise medical dictionary*, ed 2, Baltimore, 1994, Williams & Wilkins; The American Psychiatric Association: *Diagnostic and statistical manual of mental disorders*, ed 4, Washington DC, The Association.

antecedent Something that comes before something else; a precursor.

antioxidant A chemical or other agent that inhibits or retards oxidation of a substance to which it is added.

atrophy A wasting or diminution of size or physiological activity in a part of the body because of disease or other influences.

axis I Psychiatric disorder usually diagnosed in infancy, childhood, or adolescence, excluding mental retardation.

axis II Psychiatric personality disorder and mental retardation.

B

bradycardia A circulatory condition in which the myocardium contracts steadily but at a rate of less than 60 contractions a minute.

bronchiole A small airway of the respiratory system extending from the bronchi into the lobes of the lung.

C

calcification The accumulation of calcium salts in tissues.

catastrophic Sudden downturn; a pattern of medical and nursing care that involves intensive, highly technical life-support care of an acutely ill or severely traumatized patient.

chronic Developing slowly and persisting for a long time, often for the remainder of the individual's lifetime.

cochlea A conic, bony structure of the inner ear, perforated by numerous apertures for passage of the cochlear division of the acoustic nerve.

cohort A collection or sampling of individuals who share common characteristics such as persons of the same age or same sex.

collagen A protein consisting of bundles of tiny reticular fibrils that combine to form the white, glistening, inelastic fibers of the tendons, the ligaments, and the fascia.

contralateral Affecting or originating in the opposite side of a point of reference, such as a point on the body.

cyanosis Bluish discoloration of the skin and mucous membranes caused by an excess of deoxygenated hemoglobin in the blood or a structural defect in the hemoglobin molecule.

cytology The study of cells, including their formation, origin, structure, function, biochemical activities, and pathology.

cytoxic chemotherapy Any pharmacological compound that inhibits the proliferation of cells within the body.

D

decubitis ulcer stage III Stage characterized by broken skin, loss of skin, full thickness of skin, possible damage to subcutaneous tissues, and possible serous or bloody drainage.

decubitus ulcer stage IV Stage characterized by formation of a deep, craterlike ulcer, loss of the full thickness of skin, and destruction of subcutaneous tissues; exposure of fascia connective tissue, bone, or muscle underlying the ulcer, causing possible damage; an inflammation, sore, or ulcer over a bony prominence.

deleterious Harmful or dangerous.

detrusor urinae muscle A complex of longitudinal fibers that form the external layer of the muscular coat of the bladder.

diaphragmatic breathing A type of breathing exercise that patients are taught to promote more effective aeration of the lungs; movement of the diaphragm downward during inhalation and upward with exhalation.

DNA Deoxyribonucleic acid: a large nucleic acid molecule found principally in the chromosomes of the nucleus of a cell that carries genetic information.

dopamine A compound, hydroxytramine, produced by the decarboxylation of dopa; an intermediate product in the synthesis of norepinephrine.

DRG Diagnosis-related group; a group of patients classified for measuring delivery of care in a medical facility; used to determine Medicare payments for inpatient care.

durable power of attorney for health A document that designates an agent or proxy to make health care decisions for a patient who is unable to do so.

dyspnea A shortness of breath or a difficulty in breathing that may be caused by certain heart conditions, strenuous exercise, and anxiety.

E

edema The abnormal accumulation of fluid in interstitial spaces of tissues, such as in the pericardial sac, intrapleural space, peritoneal cavity, and joint capsules.

elastin A protein that forms the principal substance of yellow elastic fibers of tissue.

embolus A foreign object, a quantity of air or gas, a bit of tissue or tumor, or a piece of thrombus that circulates in the bloodstream until it becomes lodged in a vessel.

endocorditis An abnormal condition that affects the endocardium and the heart valves and is characterized by lesions caused by a variety of diseases.

erosion The wearing away or gradual destruction of a mucosal or epidermal surface as a result of inflammation, injury, or other effects; usually marked by the appearance of an ulcer.

expectoration The ejection of mucus, sputum, or fluids from the trachea and lungs by coughing or spitting.

extertional dyspnea Shortness of breath during exertion or exercise.

G

gastrostomy Surgical creation of an artificial opening into the stomach through the abdominal wall; performed to feed a patient who has cancer of the esophagus or tracheosophageal fistula or one who is expected to be unconscious for a long period.

glomerular filtration The renal process whereby fluid in the blood is filtered across the capillaries of the glomerulus and into the urinary space of the Bowman's capsule.

glycogen A polysaccharide that is the major carbohydrate stored in animal cells.

gracilis The most superficial of the five medial femoral muscles.

H

health care proxy A person designated to make health care decisions for a patient who has become incapacitated.

hemiparesis (hemiplegia) Paralysis of only one side of the body.

hemorrhage An escape of blood from the blood vessels.

I

IADL Instrumental activities of daily living, including health management community living skills, safety management, and home management.

intermediary A Blue Cross plan, private insurance company, or public or private agency selected by health care providers to pay claims under Medicare.

intrinsic Originating from or situated within an organ or tissue.

ipsilateral Pertaining to the same side of the body.

irradiation Exposure to any form of radiant energy such as heat, light, and x-ray.

J

jejunostomy A surgical procedure to create an artificial opening to the jejunum through the abdominal wall.

L

lumen A cavity or channel within any organ or structure of the body.

M

motor planning The ability to plan and execute coordinated movement.

mucosa Mucous membrane.

mucopurulent Characteristic of a combination of mucus and pus.

myelosuppression The inhibition of the production of blood cells and platelets in the bone marrow.

N

nasogastric tube Any tube passed into the stomach through the nose.

neurons Functional cells of the nervous system.

O

ombudsman A person who investigates and mediates patients' problems and complaints regarding hospital services.

opacification Making something opaque.

orthopnea An abnormal condition in which a person must sit or stand to breathe deeply or comfortably; usually accompanies cardiac and respiratory conditions.

orthostatic hypotension Abnormally low blood pressure occurring when an individual assumes the standing posture.

ossification The development of bone.

osteoarthritis A form of arthritis in which one or many joints undergo degenerative changes, including subchondral bony sclerosis, loss of articular cartilage, and proliferation of bone and cartilage in the joint, forming osteophytes.

osteomalacia An abnormal condition of the lamellar bone characterized by a loss of calcification of the matrix, resulting in softening of the bone, accompanied by weakness, fracture, pain, anorexia, and weight loss.

P

palliative Affording relief (for example, a drug that relieves pain).

parenteral nutrition The administration of nutrients by a route other than through the alimentary canal, such as subcutaneously, intravenously, intramuscularly, and intradermally.

Parkinson's disease A slowly progressive, degenerative, neurological disorder.

paroxysmal nocturnal dyspnea A sudden onset of shortness of breath while sleeping.

pharynx A tubular structure in the throat about 13 cm long that extends from the base of the skull to the esophagus and is situated just in front of the cervical vertebrae.

Pick's disease A form of presenile dementia occurring in middle age that produces neurotic behavior and the slow disintegration of intellect, personality, and emotions.

polyuria The excretion of an abnormally large quantity of urine.

presbycusis A loss of hearing sensitivity and speech intelligibility associated with aging.

psychodynamics The study of the forces that motivate behavior.

R

RNA Ribonucleic acid; a nucleic acid found in both the nucleus and the cytoplasm of cells that transmits genetic instructions from the nucleus to the cytoplasm.

S

Semifowler's position Placement of the patient in an inclined position, with the upper half of the body raised by elevating the head of the bed approximately 30 degrees.

senile Pertaining to or characteristic of old age or the process of aging, especially the physical or mental deterioration accompanying aging.

stent A compound used in making dental impressions and medical molds.

subacute Somewhat acute; between acute and chronic.

subluxation A partial abnormal separation of the articular services of a joint.

supraglottic swallow Coordinated muscular contractions of swallowing in the region of the mouth and pharynx.

syncope A brief lapse in consciousness caused by transient cerebral hypoxia.

synovium Synovial membrane; the inner layer of an articular capsule surrounding a freely movable joint.

T

thrombophlebitis Inflammation of a vein, often accompanied by formation of a clot.

thrombus An aggregation of platelets, fibrin, clotting factors, and the cellular elements of the blood attached to the interior wall of a vein or artery.

thrombotic stroke Obstruction by the thrombus of the blood supply to the brain, causing a cerebral vascular accident.

trachea A nearly cylindrical tube in the neck composed of cartilage and membrane that extends from the larynx at the level of the sixth cervical vertebra to the fifth thoracic vertebra, where it divides into two bronchi.

tracheobronchial tree An anatomical complex including the trachea, bronchi, and bronchial tubes that conveys air to and from the lungs and is a primary structure in respiration.

U

urodynamic The study of the hydrology and mechanics of urinary bladder filling and emptying.

utilitarianism A doctrine stating that the purpose of all action should be to bring about the greatest happiness for the greatest number of people and that value is determined by utility; often applied in the distribution of health care resources, such as in decisions regarding the expenditure of public funds for health services.

V

Valsalva's maneuver Any forced expiratory effort against a closed airway, such as when an individual holds the breath and tightens the muscles in a concerted, strenuous effort to move a heavy object or change position in bed.

valvular heart disease An acquired or congenital disorder of a cardiac valve characterized by stenosis and obstructed by valvular degeneration and regurgitation of blood.

vital capacity A measurement of the amount of air that can be expelled at the normal rate of exhalation after a maximum inspiration; represents the greatest possible breathing capacity.

Index

Dexterity, manual, 149
Diabeta; *see* Oral hypoglycemics
Diabetes, common medications for, 147
Diabetic retinopathy, 176, 177
Diabinese; *see* Oral hypoglycemics
Diagnostic and Statistical Manual of Mental Disorders, 236
Diagnostic-related groups, 58, 82, 299
Diarrhea, 196
Diary, medication, 151
Diet; *see also* Nutrition
  cancer prevention, 47
  dysphagia, 209
  incontinence, 197
Digitalis, 264
Digoxin, 147, 264
Diltiazem, 264
Dinitrate, 264
Direct Supply, 293
Disability, community transportation, 167-168
Disabled parking placard, 167
Discharge planning
  cancer, 277-278
  documentation, 94
Discrimination, 103
Discussion group, 141, 142
Disease prevention, 38-45
Disengagement theory of aging, 16
Displaced fracture, 246
Distal radius fracture, 248
Distraction technique in Alzheimer's disease rehabilitation, 230
Distributive justice, 115
Disuse syndrome, 41
Diuretics
  incontinence, 195
  side effects, 147, 264
Diversity, cultural; *see* Cultural diversity
Dizziness
  falls, 163, 164
  as medication side effect, 148
DNA; *see* Deoxyribonucleic acid
Documentation, 89-99
  content and quality of, 95
  creative, 114
  evaluation, 91-92
  informed consent, 90-91
  reimbursement, 95
  restraint reduction, 158
  screening, 90
  treatment plans and goals, 92-95
Door opener, 294
Doorbell, 190
Dopamine, 299
Drawing, 240
Dressing
  stroke, 199
  total hip replacement, 251
  urinary and fecal incontinence, 199
DRGs; *see* Diagnostic-related groups
Driver rehabilitation specialist, 167
Drivers 55 Plus: Test Your Own Performance, 294
Driving
  accident as cause of fracture, 246
  hearing-impairment, 294
  resources, 294
  safety, 165, 169-171
Drop seats, 293

Drug abuse, 242
Drugs, 145-154
  adverse reactions, 146-147
  cardiac, 264
  common terminology, 146
  drug interactions, 147-148
  inappropriate use, 146
  medication diary, 151
  nutritional concerns, 209-210
  polypharmacy, 146
  for restraint, 156
  self-medication
    assistive aids, 150-153
    programs for, 152, 153
    skill required, 148-150
Dual diagnosis, 242
Dura mater, 26
Durable power of attorney for health, 299
DVT; *see* Deep venous thrombosis
Dycem, 292
Dycem mat, 208
Dying; *see* Hospice care
Dysarthria, 214
Dysfunction
  defined, 22, 64
  Model of Human Occupation, 76
Dyskinesia, tardive, 241
Dysphagia, 204-210
  adaptive devices, 207-208
  case study, 211-212
  dietary concerns, 209
  direct intervention, 208-209
  environmental concerns, 205-206
  etiology, 204
  following stroke, 214
  nursing/caregiver instruction, 210
  positioning techniques, 206-207
  precautions, 209-210
Dyspnea, 299
  paroxysmal nocturnal, 300
Dysrhythmia; *see* Arrhythmia
Dysthymic disorder, 236, 237

E

Ear; *see* Hearing
Eastern Orthodox, 106
Eccentric viewing, 182
Economic factors, 9, 40
Edema, 299
Editorial intent in documentation, 95
Education
  disease prevention and health promotion, 46
  family and caregiver, 122
    Alzheimer's disease and dementia, 233
    dysphagia, 210
    hospice care, 287-288
    incontinence, 198
    medication administration, 152, 153
  old old age group, 8
  restraint reduction, 157
  sexuality, 132, 133-134
Ego-adaptive skills, 68
Elastin, 299
Elavil; *see* Antidepressants
Elbow
  cerebrovascular accident assessment and rehabilitation, 219